THREE DIMENSIONAL FACIAL SCULPTING

THREE DIMENSIONAL FACIAL SCULPTING

EDITED BY

EDWARD O. TERINO

Plastic Surgery Institute of Southern California
Thousand Oaks, California, U.S.A.

informa
healthcare

New York London

Informa Healthcare USA, Inc.
270 Madison Avenue
New York, NY 10016

Printed in the United States of America on acid-free paper
10 9 8 7 6 5 4 3 2 1

International Standard Book Number-10: 1-57444-816-1 (Hardcover)
International Standard Book Number-13: 978-1-57444-816-0 (Hardcover)

Visit the Informa Web site at
www.informa.com

and the Informa Healthcare Web site at
www.informahealthcare.com

Foreword

Over the last quarter century or so, face-lifts have evolved from a skin-pulling procedure into the current form which we now refer to as "facial rejuvenation." The evolution has taken us from skin lifts, where the skin was pulled and stretched not only to remove excess skin but also to shift and reposition deeper tissues, to deep procedures involving the superficial muscular aponeurotic system and periosteum for directly repositioning the deeper tissues, thereby limiting the skin portion to removal of the excess skin. Even with deep tissue repositioning and excess skin removal, a piece was still missing. Over the last decade the final piece fell into place with the realization that aging leads to loss of facial volume and that true rejuvenation was not complete, indeed not possible, without volume replacement.

Edward Terino was ahead of the curve. He recognized the role of volume in facial rejuvenation and facial reshaping long before it became a trend and a routine part of facial rejuvenation. I believe that Dr. Terino's pioneering work with facial implants was a precurser to current volumetric facelifts. It is a tribute to him and his work that he has been able to gather a truly international group of experts to discuss the role of volume in facial rejuvenation. These authors, from six countries on three continents, bring their expertise and an international perspective on facial volume correction.

Three-dimensional facial sculpting is now not only state of the art, but perhaps the standard in facial rejuvenation. I commend Dr. Terino on his vision. I admire his dedication and perseverance and congratulate him on putting together this timely international text.

Foad Nahai, MD
Atlanta, Georgia, U.S.A.

Preface

Aesthetic surgery of the face has undergone a dramatic evolution since the early 1970s and 1980s. A transitional paradigm shift has occurred whereby aesthetic facial techniques have become more oriented towards sophisticated three-dimensional, restorative, and rejuvenative operations rather than the previous standard two-dimensional planar "elevate and tighten" procedures.

In the 1970s and coming from my early life's interest and background in art, I became interested in exploring the limits and boundaries for using the alloplastic material silicone rubber to contour faces in three dimensions. Other surgeons soon adopted the three dimensional model also, so that today there are many different techniques for "sculpturing" a face, which include an array of alloplastic materials as well as autologous tissues such as fat.

The alloplastic techniques are permanent due to the volume and mass dimensions in implants. Autologous techniques are not as predictably permanent. The degree of their persistence is still somewhat controversial and certainly variable from surgeon to surgeon and from one area of facial anatomy to another.

In order to change any face favorably by three-dimensional means, a philosophy of aesthetic facial balance and beauty must be embraced by the surgeon. My personal perception involves an evaluation and alteration of interrelating volume-mass units in the face, which results in "ideal facial form." The major aesthetic facial units are the forehead, nasal prominence, cheek-midface and chin-jaw line or mandible segments. There are a myriad of additional subunits, all of which, when increased or decreased by surgical manipulation, produce significant, although perhaps more subtle, effects.

The onset of subperiosteal upper and midfacial suspension techniques in the 1980s has also contributed significantly to the creation of faces with three-dimensional sculptural improvements and has encouraged the interest of plastic surgeons worldwide to explore this new emerging technology, which may well be the "final chapter" in facial aesthetic surgery. Because there are now many unique and creative surgeons on various parts of the planet who are diligently working on the challenge of three-dimensional facial sculpting surgery, I thought it would be exciting to gather a select group of them who are experienced investigators in this field to be contributors to this book.

The book, therefore, is unique. Its purpose is to comprehensively cover the subject of sculpting faces in three-dimensions from an international perspective. It includes original works from pioneers in this field that can provide useful guidelines for all interested practitioners who wish to acquire the skills necessary to use these new tools for enhancing their own three-dimensional sculpturing of facial architecture.

I wish to dedicate this book to the numerous plastic surgery colleagues worldwide who over many years have asked for my advice and assistance regarding patient facial contour surgeries and the complications thereof, and who have consistently urged me to continue providing them with the latest information about innovative and new techniques to assist them on their own personal journey into this most intriguing subspecialty in plastic surgery.

It is my fondest desire that this book will prove invaluable to them.

Edward O. Terino, MD

Contents

Contributors

Carlos Raul Barcelo International Craniofacial Institute, Dallas, Texas, U.S.A.

Thierry Besins Plastic Surgeon, Paris, France

Abel Chajchir Department of Plastic Surgery, Barrancas Medical Center, Buenos Aires, Argentina

O. Onur Erol Department of Plastic and Reconstructive Surgery, ONEP Plastic Surgery Science Institute, Istanbul Bilim University, Istanbul, Turkey

David G. Genecov International Craniofacial Institute, Dallas, Texas, U.S.A.

Silvia Gonzalez Jalisco Plastic Surgery Institute and Mexico Graduate School, University Center of Health Sciences, and University of Guadalajara, Jalisco, Mexico

Fernando Guerrerosantos Jalisco Plastic Surgery Institute and Mexico Graduate School, University Center of Health Sciences, and University of Guadalajara, Jalisco, Mexico

José Guerrerosantos Jalisco Plastic Surgery Institute and Mexico Graduate School, University Center of Health Sciences, and University of Guadalajara, Jalisco, Mexico

M. Keith Hanna Paces Plastic Surgery, Atlanta, Georgia, U.S.A.

Fernando Molina Department of Plastic, Aesthetic, and Reconstructive Surgery, Hospital General "Dr. Manuel Gea Gonzalez," Mexico City, Mexico

Foad Nahai Paces Plastic Surgery, Atlanta, Georgia, U.S.A.

Fernando Ortiz-Monasterio School of Medicine, Universidad Nacional Autónoma de México, Mexico City, Mexico

Malcolm D. Paul Department of Surgery, Aesthetic and Plastic Surgery Institute, University of California, Irvine, California, U.S.A.

Ivo Pitanguy Department of Plastic Surgery, Pontifical Catholic University of Rio de Janeiro and The Carlos Chagas Institute of Post-Graduate Medical Studies, Rio de Janeiro, Brazil

Yong-Chen Por International Craniofacial Institute, Dallas, Texas, U.S.A.

Oscar M. Ramirez Johns Hopkins University School of Medicine, Baltimore, and Esthétique Internationale, Timonium, Maryland, U.S.A.

Kenneth E. Salyer International Craniofacial Institute, Dallas, Texas, U.S.A.

Edward O. Terino Plastic Surgery Institute of Southern California, Thousand Oaks, California, U.S.A.

Frank Trepsat Clinique de Genolier, Geneva, Switzerland

Charles R. Volpe Esthétique Internationale, Timonium, Maryland, U.S.A.

Michael J. Yaremchuk Massachusetts General Hospital and Harvard Medical School, Boston, Massachusetts, U.S.A.

1 The Third Dimension in Aesthetic Surgical Contouring of the Face: Combining Alloplastic and Suspension Technology

Edward O. Terino
Plastic Surgery Institute of Southern California, Thousand Oaks, California, U.S.A.

THE SIGNIFICANCE OF A FACE

We are all unique and individual. We recognize others by their facial features. When we address our fellow humans, we focus our attention on their face. We perceive their eyes, nose, lips, eyebrows, and hair. These are only adornments on the basic facial framework. A person's attractiveness is really determined by the shape and form of their face. Shape and form are three-dimensional representations of volume and mass. In the context of a human face, these consist of both skeletal and soft-tissue contours. These contours are judged attractive according to both their underlying bony characteristics and their overlying subcutaneous soft-tissue substance.

The facial skeleton represents the underlying foundation. The overlying subcutaneum is the upholstery padding that creates a fashionable or unfashionable appearance. Finally, the overlying skin becomes the "canvas" over the face. In youth it is distributed over the bony and soft-tissue entities in a smooth manner that presents a youthful appearance. With the passing of years, this canvas becomes worn, coarse, wrinkled, and stretched. Moreover, the subcutaneum and its fatty elements shrink and atrophy, reducing the volume and soft contours to display the harshness of the underlying bony architecture, especially around the orbital eye sockets. These phenomena alter the face into an "image of age." In youth, lips are well defined, full, and sensuous, and possess a prominent cupid's bow. Eyes are considered attractive or even beautiful when there is a medial-to-lateral tilt of the palpebral fissures, producing a "doe-eyed" or "almond-shaped" configuration. Eyebrows contribute a desirable accent to the eyes when they are well demarcated and arched at the junction of the medial two-thirds with the lateral one-third.

Finally, the facial features form a pattern enveloped in the canvas of the skin and integrated with an aesthetic balance of the volume–mass relationships of the face. These laws are straightforward, universal, and unchangeable.

THE POWER OF BEAUTY

Mankind through the ages has universally acknowledged that perceived beauty bestows admiration and power on its possessor. Although standards of beauty change from century to century, decade to decade, and generation to generation, the profound effects that beauty bestows upon both those who perceive it and those who possess it are without question. Facial beauty represents an even more desirable goal because all communication with others is directed at the eyes and facial region. The rest of the body is camouflaged with clothing most of the time.

Facial aesthetics, therefore, is important in today's world where anatomic surgical alterations to improve attractiveness have become a reality rather than a sci-fi fantasy. The "sculptural" shape of faces has been known by artists from time immemorial. By a face being sculptural, we are referring to its three-dimensional form, including its many integral parts whose volumes and masses interrelate through juxtaposition. The location of these elements and their relative size and shape constitute what plastic surgeons now call facial contours. Therefore, facial contouring surgery means the art of manipulating specific anatomic features in specific locations to alter facial topography in a manner that either creates or enhances facial attractiveness. This involves working with both the skeletal foundation and the soft tissues.

The skeletal foundation lends definition and structure to faces. Our present culture considers facial structure and definition to be attractive or beautiful, both in youth and, even more so, during the aging process. The shape of the facial skeleton determines the contours of the overlying soft tissues even when aging fat atrophy occurs.

Therefore, skeletal augmentation with alloplastic materials provides plastic surgeons with the ability to aesthetically sculpture faces in the third dimension.

Autologous soft-tissue manipulations add versatility to the armamentarium of the aesthetic plastic surgeon. In the opinion of this author, these are less predictable and less precise than skeletal and soft-tissue additions provided by alloplastic methods.

GOALS OF AESTHETIC SURGERY

The primary goal of facial aesthetic surgery is to enhance natural beauty by maintaining or restoring youthful qualities whenever possible. Youth is the common historical and cultural denominator of beauty. Facial changes of aging, such as sagging, drooping, bulging, puffiness, tissue laxity, and coarsening of surface texture are regarded as highly undesirable in our society, which is heavily oriented toward youth, fitness, and beauty.

The three goals of aesthetic facial surgery are to restore, to rejuvenate, and to enhance. Restoration is a form of reconstructing early aging changes to return a person to his or her younger appearance. Rejuvenation is an attempt to alter aging changes in the face to make it more youthful in appearance and therefore more attractive. This doesn't necessarily restore a person to his or her previous and natural appearance. Enhancement improves or augments the attractiveness of a face at any age. Therefore, coronal brow surgery and alteration of basic facial structure through rhinoplasty, malar-midface, and jawline contouring produce the most significant improvements in the aesthetic appearance of the face (Fig. 1).

The term "profileplasty" traditionally was applied to nose–chin relationships. However, because traditional chin implants were small, centrally placed, and poorly designed, excessive reduction in the nasal bridge frequently occurred during attempts to improve profile relationships. This not only resulted in misshapen, artificial nasal contours, but also a protuberant, button-like, and abnormally bulging central chin mound (Fig. 2). Newer implants permit extended premandible augmentation across the entire lower third facial segment, thereby facilitating a natural-looking jawline contour. They eliminate the need for overreduction in nasal surgery.

FACIAL CONTOURING

The term "contour" may be applied to augmentation of the facial skeleton through the use of Silastic onlay implants. These implants are placed on the deepest or fourth plane, the

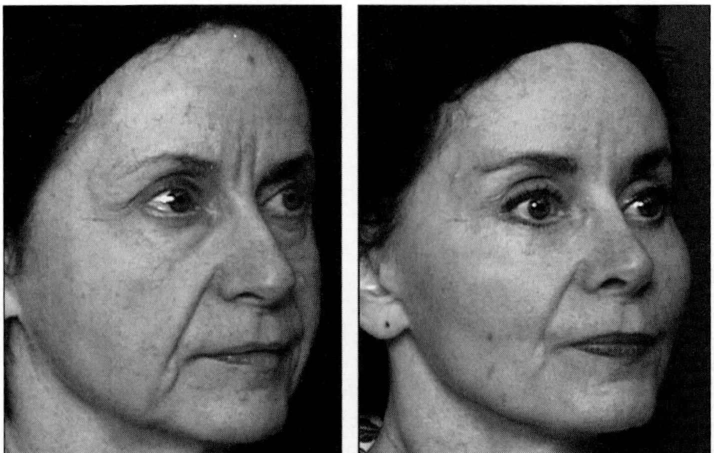

Figure 1 Example of dramatic results produced by facial contouring consisting of upper midfacial suspension, lateral brow and temple contouring, palpebral eye shaping, malar augmentation, rhinoplasty, and rhytidectomy of the lower face and neck.

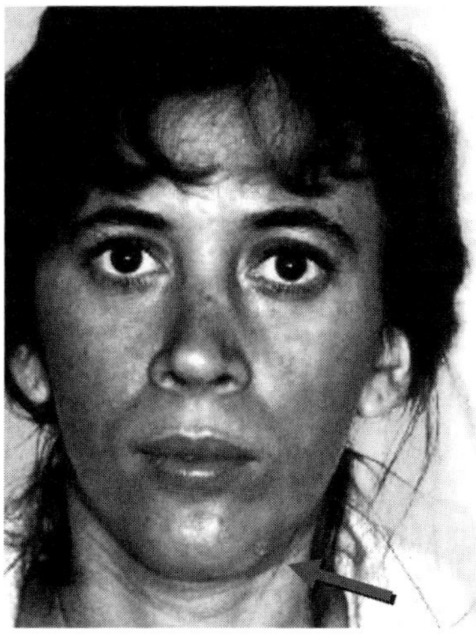

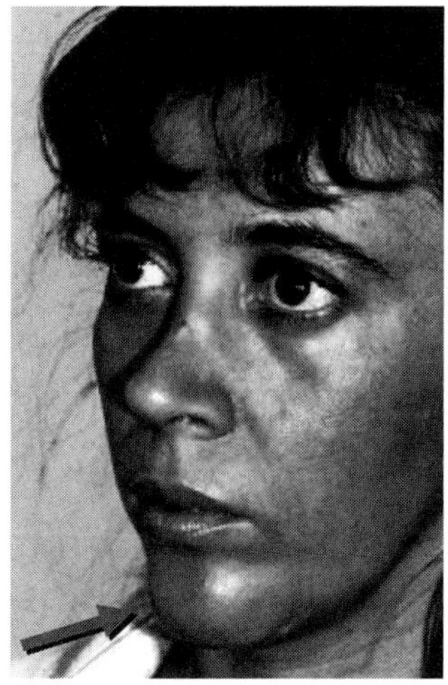

Figure 2 Example of small, poorly designed traditional chin implant that produced a protuberant, button-like, abnormal and bulging central chin mound contour associated with an overly reduced nasal dorsum.

facial skeleton. The other three planes defined in facial surgery are the skin, the subcutaneous fat, and the submuscular aponeurotic system (SMAS). Despite the most radical, extensive, BI-Planar, and SMAS techniques, facial contour does not significantly change. Only judicious alterations of mass and volume carefully placed in different anatomic regions produce contour changes.

It is a balance of three major regions of volume and mass on the face that creates classic beauty. These three fundamental facial promontories, in order of importance, are the nose, malar-midface, and jawline regions (Fig. 3). Alloplastic implants can alter and modify, in either a subtle or dramatic way, the facial promontories with ease and predictability. The diminution or enhancement of any one of these three promontories directly or inversely affects the aesthetic significance of the others. In other words, reduction of the nose gives the illusion of a stronger chin, jawline, and midface region.

The surgical creation of facial aesthetics is the art and science of perceiving and creating a correct balance in these three major promontories of facial skeletal anatomy (Figs. 4 and 5). Technically, this is accomplished through selecting implants of the proper size, shape, and design and by controlling their position on the facial skeleton. In the near future, computer-engineered technology will be able to determine and manufacture individualized implants according to precise design, dimensions, and positioning. Present limitations of surgical technique and implant selections do not always permit unerring accuracy in creating a patient's ideal appearance. However, the superb advantage that Silastic implants have over other facial skeletal augmentation biomaterials is that the implants are readily exchangeable should the

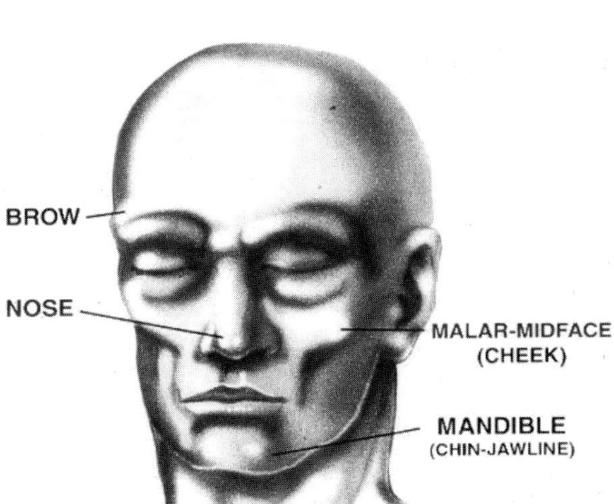

Figure 3 Artist's rendering of facial architecture illustrating major promontories of mass and volume: the nose, malar-midface, and mandible jawline.

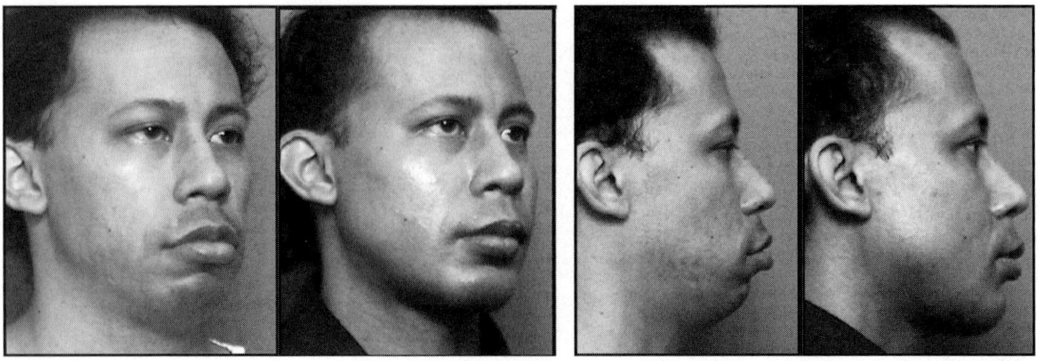

Figure 4 Example of a 36-year-old male with disproportion and imbalance of malar-midface and mandibular jawline aesthetic segment, showing an improvement in facial harmony by augmenting the central mentum, mandibular angles, and malar region.

need arise. The simple elevation of the soft-tissue envelope of the face to create space for alloplastic implants results in infinitely less morbidity and fewer complications than the intricate dissection of the SMAS in and around the neuromusculature of facial animation.

STANDARDS OF FACIAL BEAUTY

Throughout history, standards of facial beauty have always been associated with anatomic contours of facial form. These contours exist as a result of the location, volume, and size of the facial soft tissues and their relationship to the three-dimensional architecture of the underlying facial skeleton. During some centuries roundness and fullness of facial soft tissues were the cultural standard of artists; while in other time periods more defined and dramatic skeletal contours in the malar and jawline region were considered ideal. During the Renaissance, many artists depicted the ideal female face as heart-shaped, exhibiting weak lower face, chin, and mandible contours.

Contemporary standards of female beauty embody stronger structural contours. The jawlines that contemporary females request, have more anterior projection, a wider midlateral (ML) region, and stronger posterolateral (PL) angle definition. Malar-midface cheek contours are also strong and defined.

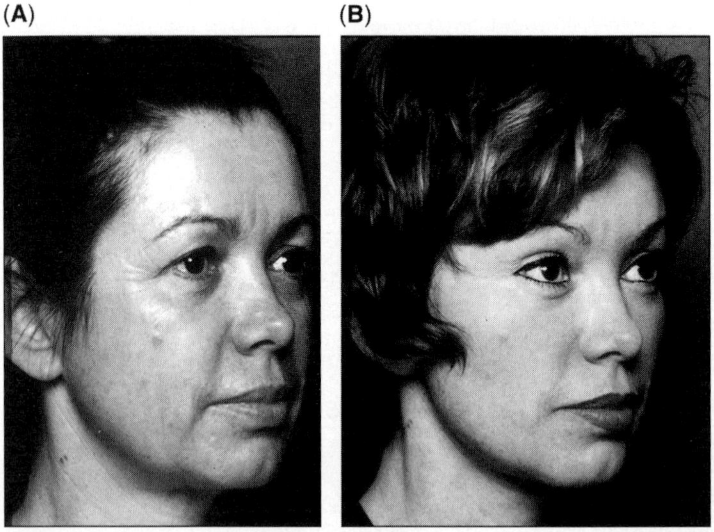

Figure 5 A 52-year-old female with midface submalar triangle soft-tissue deficiency. Her youthful appearance was restored by malar Zone 1 and submalar Zone 5 augmentation using a 4-mm shell. A midface suspension procedure was also performed. (**A**) Preoperative and (**B**) postoperative views.

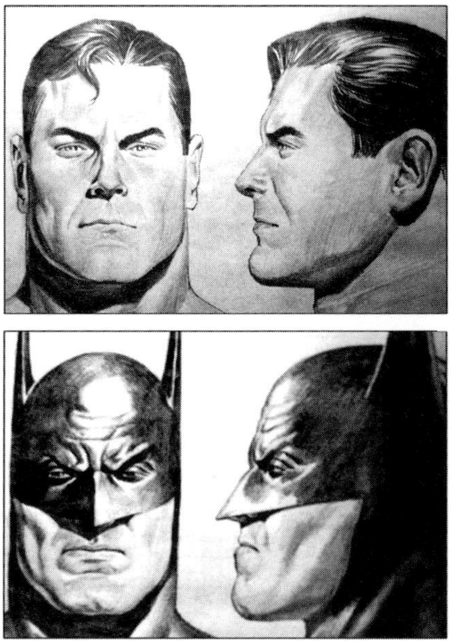

Figure 6 Example of contemporary desires of male images.

CONTEMPORARY CULTURAL IDEALS

Venus de Milo and the cherubic women painted by the artist Rubens are symbols of ideal feminine faces and figures of past cultures. Today, the standards have changed dramatically. In the new millennium, male images have superhero characteristics. Jawlines such as those of Captain Marvel, Superman, the Lone Ranger, Batman (Fig. 6), and others, are easily seen in fashion magazines, on television, on soap operas, and in the cinema. The images of Kirk Douglas, Errol Flynn, and Gregory Peck have been replaced by the jutting jaws of Mel Gibson, Brad Pitt, Johnny Depp, and a new generation of other strong muscular faces. The Amazonian exotic facial contours of Wonder Woman (Fig. 7) are typified today by Michelle Pfeiffer, Cameron Diaz, Rebecca Romijn, and others.

Cosmetic surgery has achieved respectability. A growing population of upwardly mobile, affluent patients aged 20 to 50 years are demanding surgical alternatives to their inherited facial characteristics. This desired change especially pertains to midface and jawline contours. Nasal surgery and chin implants have been well accepted by plastic surgeons and the public for 20 to 30 years. More extensive alterations of the face are recently becoming a sought-after commodity. The most commonly requested changes are stronger, squarer, angular jawlines, and more accented midface and malar bone structures (Fig. 8).

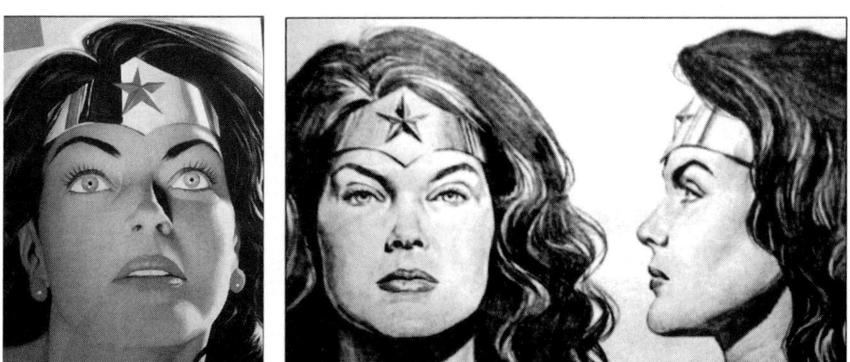

Figure 7 Example of contemporary desires of female images.

(A)

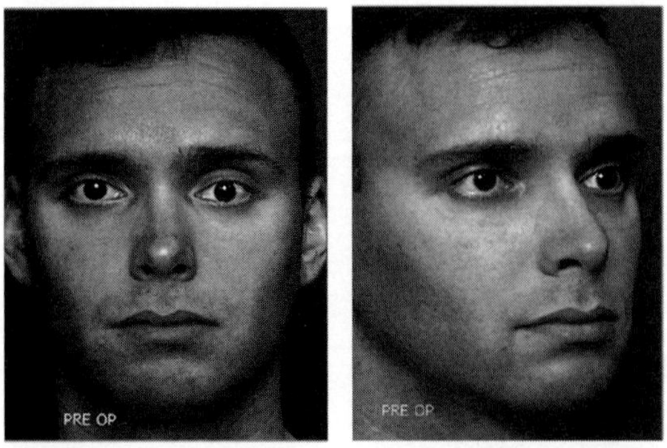

(B)

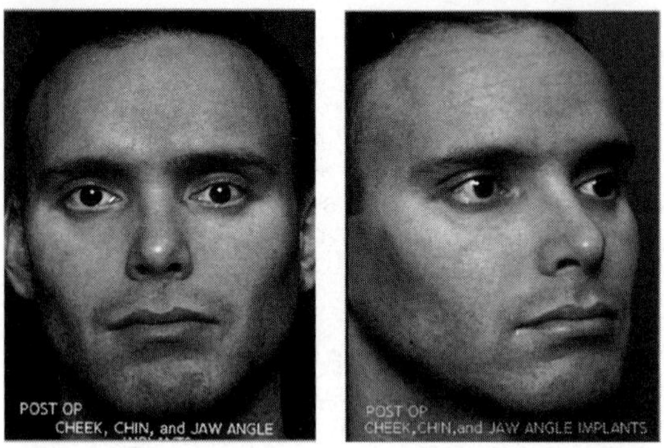

Figure 8 The most commonly requested facial contours are stronger, more severe, 34-year-old male angular jawlines, and a more accented malar cheek form. (**A**) Preoperative view. (**B**) One year postoperative view after placement of central (central mentum) and angle (posterolateral) implants and 4-mm shells.

HISTORICAL PERSPECTIVE

The evolution of the author's personal technique for alloplastic augmentations of the face originated from his experiences as a resident in training in plastic and reconstructive surgery at the Universities of North Carolina and Florida under the teachings of Drs. Erle Peacock and Maurice Jurkiewicz. The medical centers associated with these training programs treated a large volume of head and neck trauma and cancers. As residents, we became experienced in handling these problems. Unfortunately, present-day power tools and techniques for stabilizing craniofacial skeletal anatomy with bone plates and screws were not available. Instead, the "norm" consisted of dental fixation with wires, which was "state of the art" at that time in oromaxillofacial surgery.

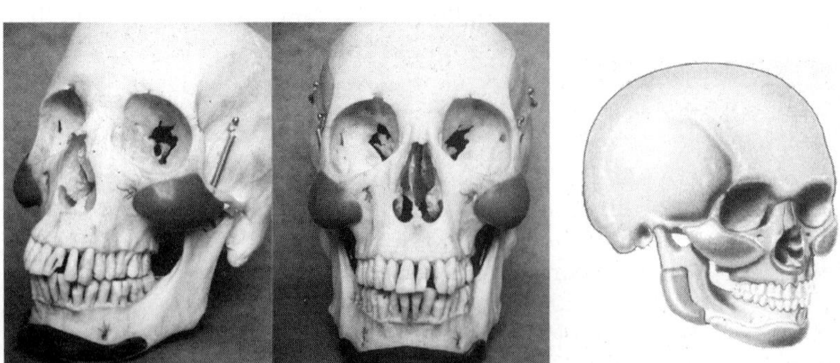

Figure 9 Anatomic-style implants designed in the 1980s by the author to imitate natural bony and soft tissue contours in malar-midface and premandible regions.

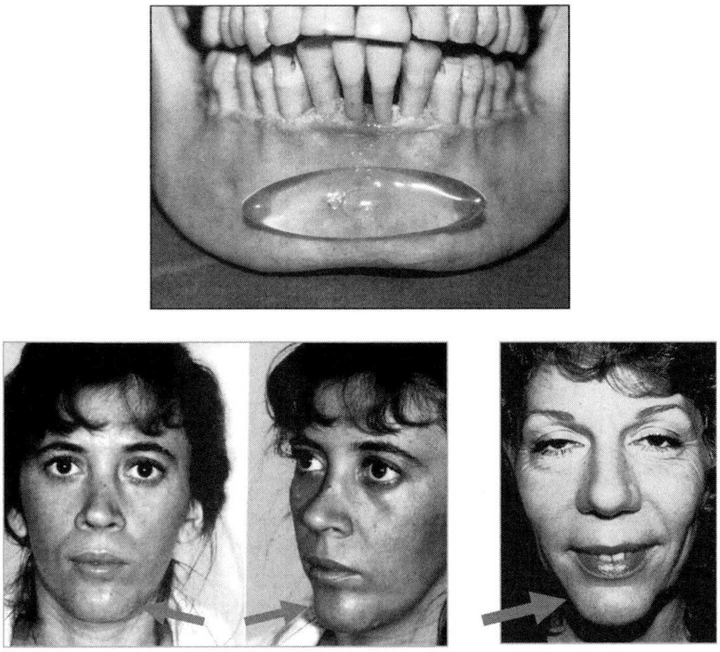

Figure 10 Example of archaic 1960s and 1970s traditional silicone gel implants for the chin and cheek regions. They produce protuberant and unnatural anatomic contours.

Poorly reduced facial fractures in both the maxillary and mandibular areas, and defects secondary to trauma or surgical extirpation of tumors were common. We were able to perform satisfactory reconstructions in many cases through the use of individually fashioned, customized alloplastic implants. The material most frequently used at that time was Silastic sponge. Although the results were less than perfect, the aesthetic benefit to these unfortunate patients was substantial. Both surgeons and patients were pleased by these alloplastic, reconstructive, yet aesthetic accomplishments.

Such cases provided the impetus for the author in the early 1970s to feel confident that the mere manipulation of implant designs into anatomic shapes would provide the key for opening the door to more sophisticated and successful cosmetic alterations, useful for both reconstructive and aesthetic facial surgery (Fig. 9).

Previously implants for the "chin" and "cheek" regions had been used but their crude and bulky geometric rather than anatomic shapes did not provide natural nonartificial aesthetic results (Fig. 10).

MIDFACE IMPLANTS: EVOLUTION

I began designing and augmenting faces with anatomic-style implants in 1973. An evolutionary phase of 10 to 12 years was necessary to conceptually develop and design implants that produced optimum and natural contours. These "final-phase" implants were not available until 1983.

In early procedures, a small trapezoidal implant was designed to augment only the malar bone. Postoperative evaluations revealed that the final malar/zygomatic contour was not fully evident until one year following surgery. Subsequent augmentation procedures confirmed the fact that one-year results are essential for final definition of midfacial form. Even then, further improvement over time occurs. Therefore, it became necessary to modify the author's early designs each and every year for 10 to 12 years to determine those that would produce an optimum natural malar/submalar contour. The current anatomic "malar shell"–style implants and the combined "malar/submalar shell" implants are the end result of this evolution. Although minor modifications may still be possible to create the perfect and universal implant, the commercially available "shells" suffice for the vast majority of cases. The results from using them are far superior to the earlier models, dating back to the 1970s (Fig. 11).

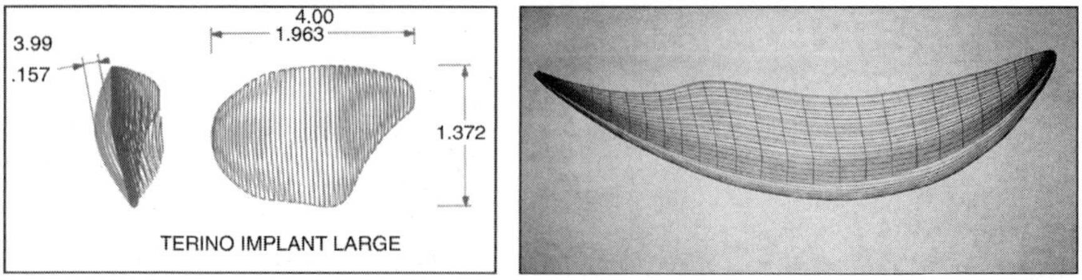

Figure 11 Original technical design drawings for Terino Malar Shell (1982), a new anatomic design-concept.

Anatomic implants of the 1970s were designed by the author in two styles, one to give a high cheekbone appearance and another to provide a rounder, lower cheekbone appearance. It became apparent after the first series of operations that to give a rounder, "apple-cheek" appearance, implant dimensions had to be vertically greater to extend beneath the malar bone and placed onto the masseter tendon into what has been named the Zone 5 submalar space. Therefore, correction of a submalar atrophic aesthetic contour deficiency is accomplished with a malar/submalar augmentation using a midface shell with an expanded surface area and greater vertical dimensions. Placement should be to bridge the malar bone and extend down into the submalar space or to reside entirely within the submalar zone to fill that region only.

The initial implants designed by this author had zygomatic extensions into the middle of the zygomatic arch and even more posterior. These proved to be unnecessary and, in fact, more dangerous to insert. They also included extensions up the lateral orbital rim, the idea being that this would also contribute to creating a more natural appearance. These extensions could produce an abnormal appearance if slight shifting of the implant occurred after placement. Without these extensions, the current modified malar shells have been designed so that a certain amount of displacement or rotation can occur without significantly disturbing an optimum contour, either visibly or palpably.

ALLOPLASTIC AUGMENTATIONS OF THE FACIAL SKELETON

The Six Basic "P" Principles

Six basic "P" principles apply to alloplastic-volume alterations of any aspect of facial anatomy:

1. Purpose—The purpose of the alterations aligns completely with the optimum goal of aesthetic facial surgery, which is the three-dimensional restructuring of facial form and balance.
2. Practice—Practice is absolutely necessary to understand fully the remarkable aesthetic changes that can be realized from alloplastic augmentation. The technical expertise to use facial implants with predictability and precision can only be gained from experience.
3. Precision—Because alloplastic implants are volume devices with a noncompressible shape and form, their size and location are extremely critical. Small changes in the measurements, shape, and anatomic location of a facial implant create a much greater difference than does the two-dimensional tightening of autogenous elastic facial tissues. This fact becomes more valid as aging and attenuation of the elastic subcutaneum occurs (Fig. 12).
4. Principles of aesthetics—Alloplastic-volume alterations follow the basic principles of aesthetics described previously. They are highly effective in establishing the facial balance that results from the symbiotic interrelationship of volume differentials and deficiencies within the zones of anatomy and the aesthetic regional segments of the face. The correction of deficiencies and the improvement of size (volume and mass) in specific regions and zones constitute aesthetic balance (Fig. 13).
5. Predictability—Alloplastic implants do not change over time. The materials from which they are made remain stable; moreover, implants are fixed in location by the encapsulating fibrosis that constitutes a normal physiologic response.
6. Permanence—The shape, size, and configuration of facial contours produced by alloplastic implants remain permanent. When smooth Silastic rubber implants are used, regional contours can be altered readily by an easy implant exchange. If the changes are considered

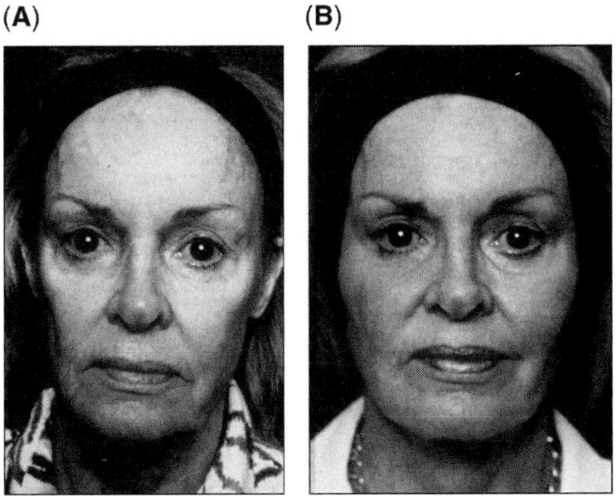

Figure 12 During the aging process, attenuation of the elastic subcutaneous tissues occurs so that implant augmentation of the midface becomes even more significant than traditional two-dimensional facelift tightening techniques. (**A**) Preoperative and (**B**) postoperative submuscular aponeurotic system rhytidectomy using submalar shell implants.

undesirable, removal of the implants in most instances produces complete reversibility to the previous natural state without deformity or disfiguration.

The advantages of alloplastic augmentation of the facial skeleton with Silastic rubber are many: (*i*) It provides volume, mass, and shape to the various natural promontories of the face. The most important of these promontories are the malar/midface and jawline/premandible regions. The nose is a third major promontory. Great aesthetic advantage is derived from augmenting or diminishing its volume. However, alloplastic augmentation of the nose is still very controversial. (*ii*) Alloplastic materials do not need harvesting operations on other areas of the body. (*iii*) The operations take a relatively short time. (*iv*) Placement under the periosteum and directly on bone produces rapid immobilization from surrounding fibrotic capsular formation. (*v*) Depending upon the material used, the biologic compatibility of the host to resist "rejection" and infection is very high.

The author favors silicone rubber because resolution of surrounding infections can be accomplished in nearly all cases without the necessity of implant removal. Antibiotics and drainage procedures will abolish infection around such implants as long as they are nonporous. Porous materials such as Gore-Tex®, hydroxyapatite, and Medpor™, when infected, may have to be removed because infectious processes can lodge within the interstices of these nonsmooth materials and challenge body defenses.

Another major advantage of alloplastic facial augmentation especially when using a smooth material that is flexible (silicone rubber), is easy removability, reversibility, and

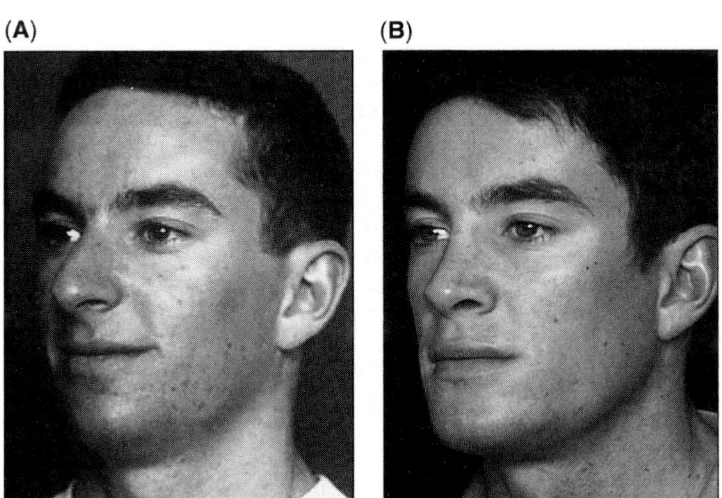

Figure 13 Dramatic improvement in facial aesthetics of a 24-year-old patient produced by rhinoplasty and alloplastic augmentation of the entire mandible including the angles. (**A**) Preoperative and (**B**) postoperative two years.

changeability. Silicone rubber implants are very flexible and can be introduced and removed through small incisions. Other materials such as Medpor, which integrate with surrounding soft tissues, have to be "carved out" with considerable difficulty, excessive bleeding, and trauma to tissues and nerves that may produce permanent dire consequences.

While it is true that removal of large implants from the central chin region may produce soft-tissue ptosis of the central chin mound, this problem is much less likely to happen when introduction of the implant does not transect the mentalis muscle in a horizontal fashion and the dissection is performed vertically through the midline pillars of the muscle. In a rare case, a patient may request removal of a mandibular angle or malar-midface implant. In this author's series, no cosmetic or functional problem has ever resulted from removal.

The major disadvantages of the use of alloplastic materials are several: (*i*) Possibilities of severe infection, especially with porous materials that stimulate fibrous ingrowth. Such soft-tissue integration makes for a risky and dangerous undertaking. (*ii*) Contour abnormalities of an unattractive or possibly disfiguring nature when implants used do not have the proper shape, size, and positioning. (*iii*) Possibilities of facial nerve and musculature damage due to excessive and inappropriate trauma during dissections to introduce or remove implant materials.

Good indications for alloplastic facial augmentation are determined by relative or absolute deficiencies of contour volumes in various anatomic regions due to either heredity, aging, and trauma from accidents, surgeries, or ablation. Contraindications exist when there is (*i*) a severe deficiency of overlying soft-tissue coverage (e.g., severe HIV subcutaneous atrophy) and (*ii*) volume deficiency in the facial areas which do not have a stable skeletal base such as the orbital and oral apertures.

OPTIMUM QUALITIES OF FACIAL IMPLANTS

Alloplastic implants for facial augmentation should have several ideal features (Table 1).

Such implants should have: (*i*) an anatomic configuration, which has a posterior surface contouring to the external surface of the facial skeleton, and an external implant shape that imitates a desired natural anatomic configuration. (*ii*) They should be readily implantable and nonpalpable. Implant margins must be tapered to blend onto the bony surface so that they will not be felt through the soft-tissue covering. (*iii*) Facial implants should be readily exchangeable. They should have no fixation, fenestration, or fabrics to immobilize them within the tissue. The natural encapsulation process ensures their immobility. (*iv*) They should be malleable and comfortable. This largely depends on the consistency of the silicone. (*v*) There should be host acceptability with high resistance to infection so that the need for removal should be rare. (*vi*) Implants should be easily modifiable by the surgeon before and during the procedure. (*vii*) Silastic implants fully meet the above-listed qualifications. When placed directly on bone they become fixed and immobilized by encapsulating fibrosis. They can, however, easily be removed and exchanged by open capsulotomy when desirable.

Porous implants such as Medpor, which permit ingrowth, fenestrated implants, and implants with Dacron backing are inconsistent, unpredictable, and have a greater incidence of infection that necessitates removal. More important is the fact that they are infinitely more difficult to exchange and modify. Silastic implants seem to survive the presence of inflammation and gross purulence. Irrigation with copious volumes of antibiotic solutions

Table 1 Ideal Qualities for Facial Implants

Ideal qualities	Silicone rubber	Gore-Tex® soft form	Porex Medpor®	Hydroxyapatite
Biocompatible	4	3	4	4
Modifiable	4	2	3	3
Exchangeable	4	2	1	1
Resistant to infection	3	1	3	2
Anatomic contours	4	1	2	2
Visible, palpable	3.5	1	2	2

Note: 4, most optimum; 1, least optimum.

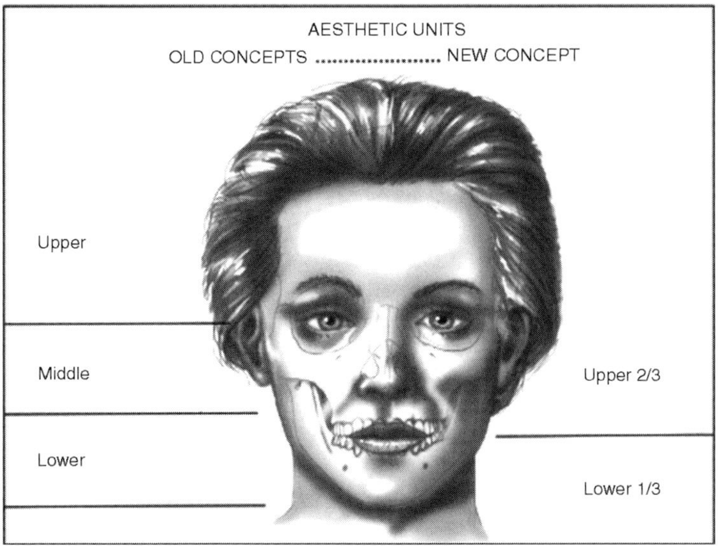

Figure 14 Traditional vs. contemporary perceptions of facial balance. The volume elements of the upper two-thirds of the face are of greater aesthetic significance than the lower third neck jawline segment.

and prophylactic use of antibiotics throughout the original augmentation procedure are important in preventing infection.

It is important to realize that any anatomic region on the surface of a bone covered by muscle and soft-tissue attachments can be augmented on the subperiosteal bone level. The natural biologic encapsulation process immobilizes Silastic implants so that they are unmovable either during muscle activity or by external palpation. The augmented bone segment will have a completely natural contour as long as the implant is designed properly with subtle geometric contour and finely tapered margins. Any segment of the premandible region can, therefore, be augmented to create a chin and jawline contour of the patient's preference. This equally applies within any area on the facial principle skeleton. When desired by the surgeon or indicated in a specific patient situation, customized implants can be manufactured rapidly by extracting data from CT scans and skeletal X rays[a].

FACIAL AESTHETICS

Indications for alloplastic facial contouring arise from considerations of facial aesthetics. Facial aesthetics is the study of facial attractiveness. Facial beauty relates fundamentally to a harmony and balance of various parts of facial anatomy. Facial balance and aesthetic beauty consist of the specific interrelationship of adjacent elements of three-dimensional volume and mass which create an appearance that is universally pleasing to the eye.

The major elements of facial volume and mass are four promontories: (*i*) the nose, (*ii*) the malar/zygomatic cheek prominence, (*iii*) the chin and jawline, and (*iv*) the forehead and supraorbital volumes. Secondary considerations are the temple contours, the premaxilla, and the suborbital region. These areas contribute more subtle and yet important nuances to overall aesthetic facial balance.

Tertiary contour considerations involve small increases or decreases in soft-tissue volumes of the face. These exist: (*i*) along the jawline as "jowls," (*ii*) within the perioral and nasolabial region as creases and folds, (*iii*) in the suborbital tear trough valley as hollowness, and (*iv*) around the central perinasal premaxilla as a retrusion or protrusion (Fig. 14).

Contours in these areas also have major relevance to facial form and balance.

It is the interplay between the topographic soft-tissue collections and the underlying skeletal promontories that architecturally determine the contours that are perceived as facial harmony, balance, and beauty.

The three major architectural aesthetic facial segments are: (*i*) upper, (*ii*) midface, and (*iii*) lower. The fundamental and basic principle of facial balance dictates that a diminution or

[a] Accuscan®, Implantech Corporation, Ventura, California, U.S.A.

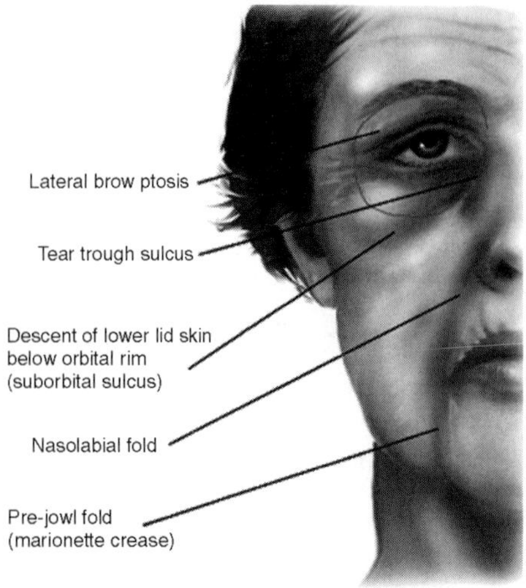

Figure 15 Universal aging changes of the face.

enhancement of volume (size) in one facial segment directly and inversely affects the aesthetic impact on the others. This principle applies equally to all of the primary, secondary, and tertiary volume/mass contour subunits described above. A more recent perception of the author subscribes to the greater significance of the upper two-thirds of the face and its volume mass elements as they relate to the lower third mandibular jawline aesthetic segment (Fig. 15).

Whereas, the larger volume/mass changes are the most significant in matters of facial balance, even minor alterations of facial subunits are equally important to observe and understand because they too have a major visual impact on facial aesthetic balance and attractiveness. Such examples exist when augmenting the nasolabial sulcus, the suborbital "hollow" region, the glabella, and other more minor subcutaneous contours.

Significant aesthetic improvement is only possible when all three facial segments are evaluated precisely and comprehensively for possible simultaneous alteration. Alloplastic augmentation permits the surgeon to adjust both the major and minor promontories with equal ease and predictability and in a subtle or dramatic fashion. Modifying facial contours involves three-dimensional change, whereas traditional face-lifting procedures are severely limited because of their two-dimensional nature.

Recent suspension techniques of the upper facial segment (brow and forehead) as well as the malar/midface segment significantly complement the three-dimensional changes that provide alloplastic regional volume enhancement when performed alone (Fig. 16). Nonetheless, it is only through the use of alloplastic techniques that permanent, precise, and extremely valuable changes to facial contours can be produced.

Patients with round, full, fleshy facial contours and abundant subcutaneous fat, and substantial muscle bulk have severe limitations when they desire a lean face that is well defined in

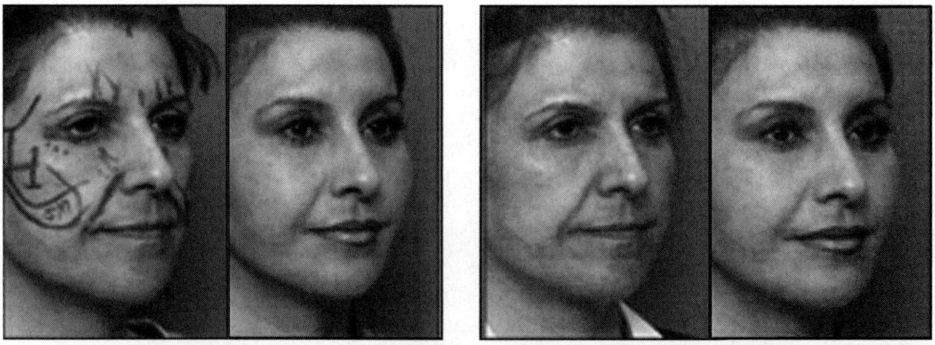

Figure 16 A 56-year-old female with significant benefit of upper midface suspension, malar–submalar augmentation, and rhytidectomy techniques.

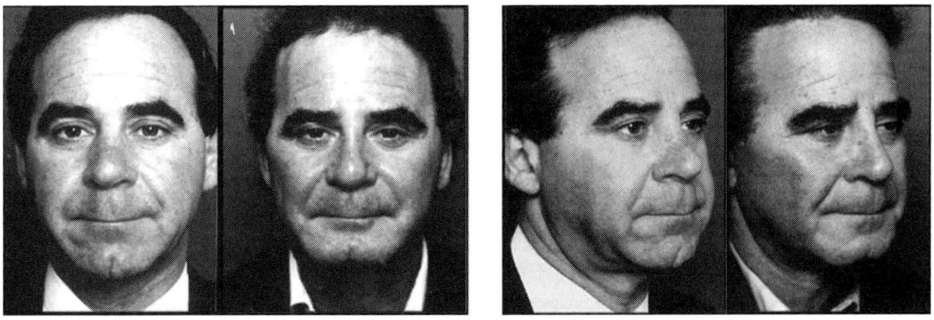

Figure 17 Example of a middle-aged male with round, full face hereditary contours, who desired a more square jaw, masculine appearance. Surgery involved malar augmentation, chin augmentation, angle of the mandible augmentation, nasal profile improvement. Postoperative views are two years following surgery.

the malar and chin/jawline regions. Only through the benefits of alloplastic augmentation can patients with full facial types enjoy modest, but often significant, alterations toward the above goal (Fig. 17). At equal disadvantage are extremely lean-faced individuals who possess a vertically long and horizontally narrow skeletal architecture and who may exhibit extreme volume-shape weakness of the malar/maxillary or chin/mandible skeleton. These patients frequently have extremely prominent nasal size profile contours. Once again, although "miracles" cannot be accomplished, modest and often significant improvements can be obtained by rearranging adjacent proportions within their facial aesthetic segments by employing alloplastic onlay techniques in the midface or mandibular regions and with or without rhinoplasty (Fig. 18).

PERTINENT ANATOMY

Understanding the fundamentals of aesthetic facial form and balance is critical for applying technical alterations to the facial skeleton, which are successful, predictable, and uncomplicated. It is imperative, therefore, that the surgeon adopt a specific method for analyzing faces, which defines both anatomic zones as well as any aesthetic segmental deficiencies of volume and mass. Relating this data about a patient's anatomy to specific goals in facial form enables alloplastic contouring to be executed with excellence and precision.

Conceptualizing the anatomy of facial form into aesthetic units and anatomic zones enables surgeons to determine which areas of the premandible, malar, and midface will respond well to augmentation and will result in contour changes which have visual and emotional impact that will benefit the patient. These anatomic zones are few in number but when augmented properly, each produces a different appearance.

The three major aesthetic segmental units of the face, upper, middle, and lower, have been discussed briefly in the previous section. Although these have been described as equal

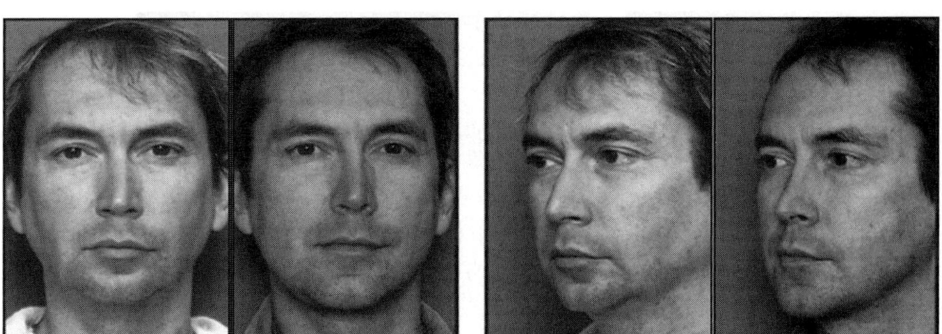

Figure 18 A 42-year-old male. Significant improvement due to augmentation of mandible with central chin implant, angle implants, and simultaneous nasal contouring technique.

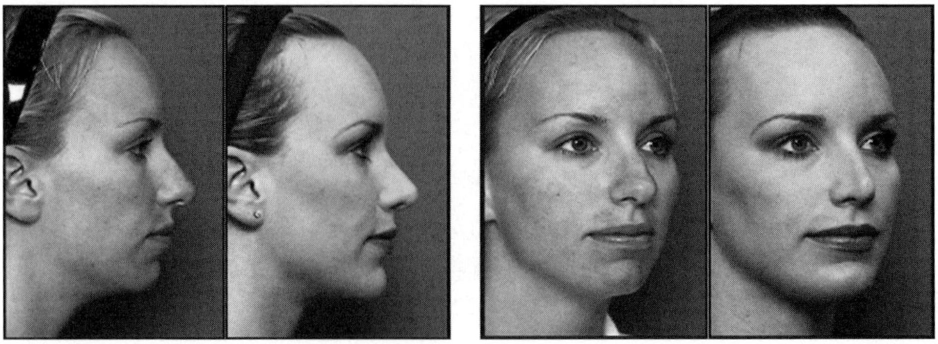

Figure 19 A deficiency in the lower third chin and jawline aesthetic segment makes the nose look more prominent. Correction with a chin implant produces facial balance in the profile. This patient, a 30-year-old female, also demonstrated the functional benefit of a minimizing mentalis movement that produces chin dimpling when a recessive central mentum segment exists.

thirds, the lower third jawline aesthetic unit is often smaller, both horizontally and vertically. This deficiency of the entire lower third of the face often makes a nose appear strong and overbearing (Figs. 19 and 20). True aesthetic deficiencies in the malar/midface region often go unobserved when there is a weak lower jawline segment. When the lower facial segment is equal to the other two aesthetic units of the face, a malar/midface deficiency is more obvious and many noses do not seem prominent but instead appear to be in balance with the rest of the face (Fig. 21).

THE MIDFACE: SIGNIFICANCE

As described previously, the upper and midface are primary regions of personality and unique personal anatomy to which another human being's attention is desired. As such, it is the most important part of the face. Yes, aging produces visible laxity of the lower face and neck and there are a considerable number of individuals who have unattractive hereditary deficiencies in the lower third aesthetic mandibular facial segment. Other publications by the author specifically discuss evaluation of premandible deficiencies and their successful treatment with alloplastic implants. Nonetheless, people mostly look at a person's eyebrows, eyes, nose, and lips. Therefore, the aesthetic appearance of the midface is first and foremost in determining aesthetic attractiveness or beauty.

As a young boy growing up, the author was drawn to certain visual images from magazines and the movies. Notable celebrities such as Rita Hayworth, Ava Gardner, Raquel Welch, and Sophia Loren attracted his attention. In the male gender Clark Gable, Kirk Douglas, and Cary Grant were men whose cheekbones and jawlines contributed aesthetic significance to their appearance and success.

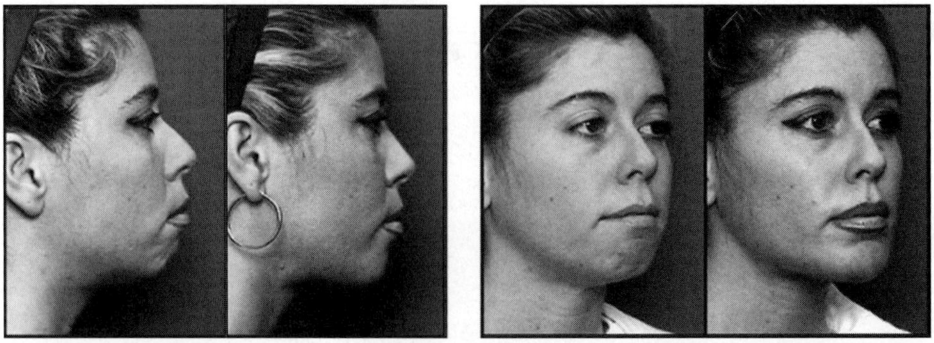

Figure 20 A deficiency of the chin contributes to increased nasal dominance. Improvement of aesthetic facial balance involves chin augmentation and dorsal nasal profile reduction.

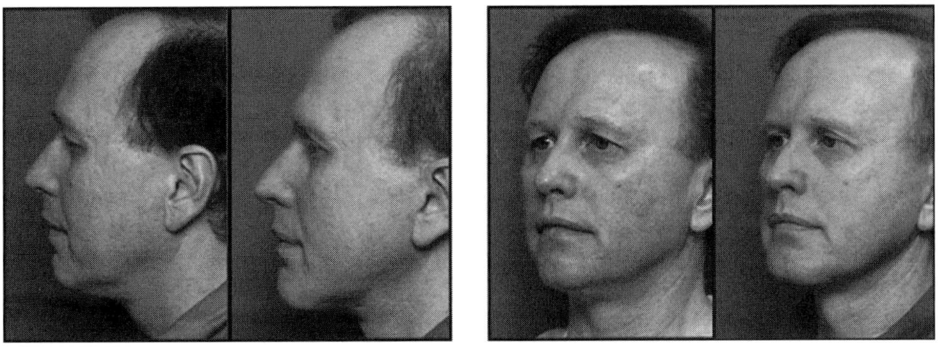

Figure 21 Example of improving facial balance by increasing the chin and jawline segment in a 44-year-old male. Note that the nose looks less prominent in the postoperative view.

The author's aspirations, therefore, as an aesthetic plastic surgeon were to not only treat the two-dimensional facial planes of skin, fat, muscle, and SMAS but also to aesthetically restructure the form of the face in three dimensions by creating alloplastic implants designed anatomically for use in both the malar/midface as well as the chin and premandible jawline regions.

ANATOMIC ZONAL ANALYSIS OF THE MALAR/MIDFACE REGION

The midface aesthetic segment comprises the entire zygomatic maxillary complex. The "malar space" is that region on the facial skeleton which when augmented appropriately, produces a beneficial aesthetic change in the contour of the midface/cheek segment. The malar space can be seen as containing five distinct anatomic zones (Fig. 22). Zone 1 is the largest subspace and includes the major portion of the malar bone. It extends from the infraorbital foramen to include the first one-third of the zygomatic arch and extends inferiorly to the lower border of the malar bone. A volume expansion of 4–5 mm in this zone increases the contour only in the upper portion of the cheek. This effect is often not suited to display a desired softness of feminine facial form. An implant in Zone 1 may appear too strong and skeletal (Fig. 23). A 3-mm volume expansion is considerably more subtle, especially when combined with midface suspension techniques (Fig. 24). Augmentation of Zone 1 by 4–5 mm is, however, frequently useful in men to create a strong, masculine "sculptured" appearance (Fig. 25).

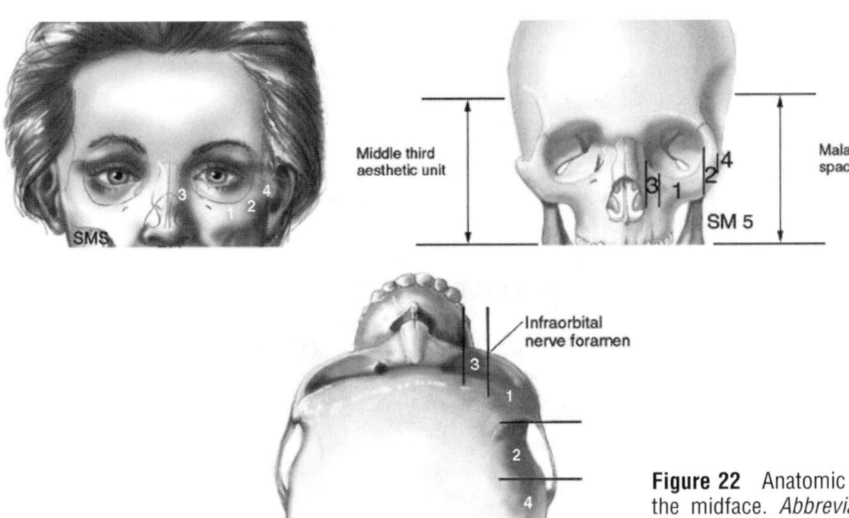

Figure 22 Anatomic facial contour zones of the midface. *Abbreviation*: SM 5, submalar Zone 5.

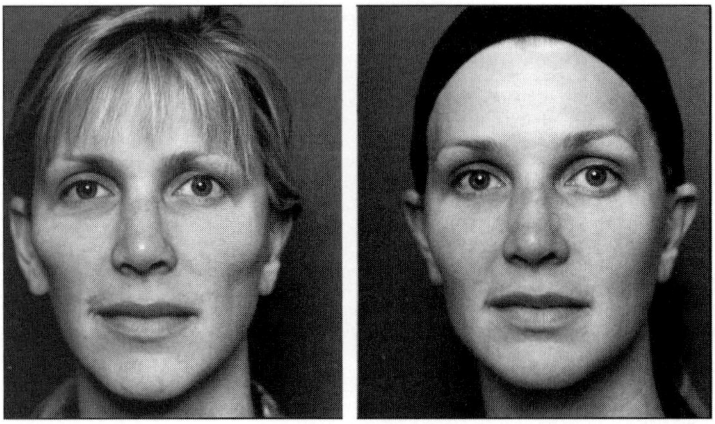

Figure 23 A postoperative appearance that is too strong and skeletal looking. Postoperative view shows significant improvement by using a generous malar shell in Zone 1 and submalar, Zone 5.

Zone 2 is of lesser aesthetic significance. It comprises the middle third of the zygomatic arch. Volume enhancement in this zone, especially in combination with Zone 1 results in a more lateral cheekbone accentuation that creates a broader dimension to the upper third of the face (Fig. 26). It is, therefore, useful in improving the appearance of patients with a narrow upper face or a "long face" syndrome.

Zone 3, the paranasal region is medial to the infraorbital foramen and nerve. Deficiency in this suborbital region can create a hollow valley appearance called a jugal-malar sulcus or "tear trough." Alloplastic implants have been specifically designed for this anatomic zone. Releasing the origins of the orbicularis oculi muscle from the medial orbit is necessary to specifically improve this suborbital hollow appearance. Due to the thin nature of the skin and subcutaneous tissues over the Zone 3 region, any alloplastic implant or transplanted tissue must be perfectly shaped and tapered to ensure invisibility (Fig. 27).

The infraorbital nerve is more sensitive to trauma than the mental nerve. Dissection around it must be gentle to prevent disabling and prolonged symptoms. Extended malar

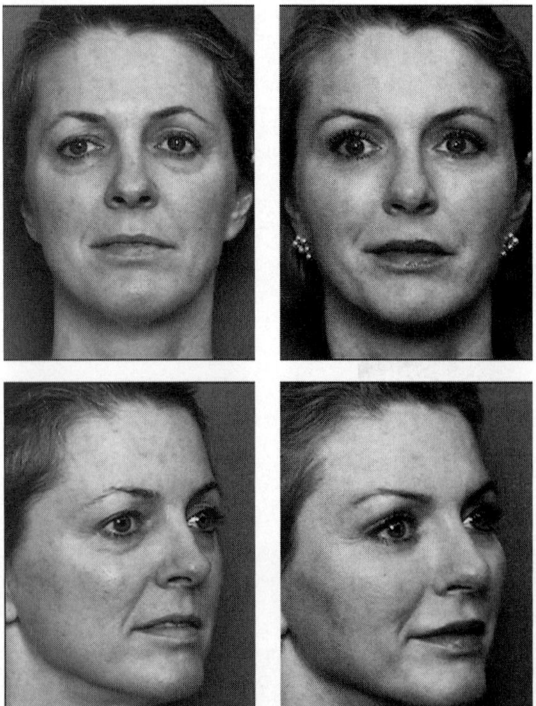

Figure 24 A subtle 3-mm volume expansion of the submalar region combined with midface suspension technology.

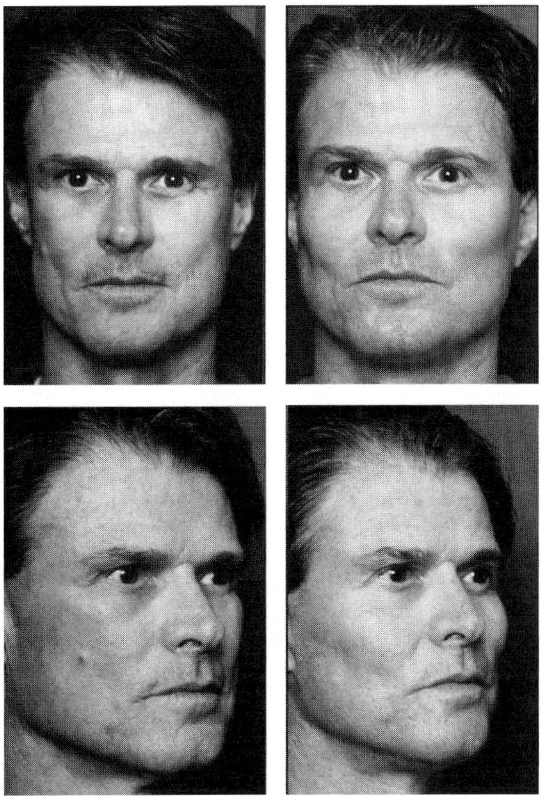

Figure 25 High malar augmentation of 4–5 mm is frequently useful to create a strong masculine sculptured appearance.

suborbital implants, which augment Zones 1, 2, and 3 comprehensively, are useful for treating people with a hereditary infraorbital maxillary bone deficiency called a negative vector "polar bear" syndrome. These specially designed implants are perhaps the most effective for minimizing or eliminating a tired, aging appearance to the lower eyelid region (Figs. 28 and 29).

Zone 4 overlies the posterior one-third of the zygomatic arch. Volume enhancement in this area is never necessary and would produce an unnatural appearance. Wrongful dissection in this zone as well as Zone 2 could produce injury either to the capsule of the temporomandibular joint or to the zygomaticotemporal branches of the facial nerve. Such injuries can produce edema, pain, temporary dysfunction of the TM joint and/or weakness of eyebrow elevation. These symptomatic deformities are rare and usually temporary.

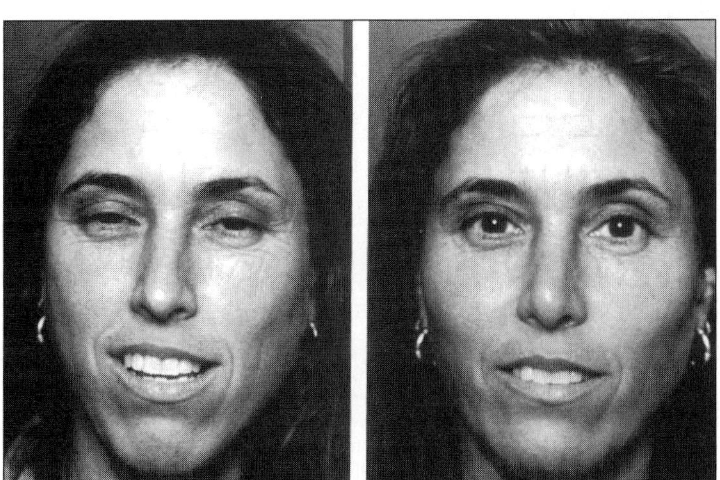

Figure 26 Malar Zone 2 augmentation and jawline augmentation are useful for improving the balance in a long, narrow face syndrome.

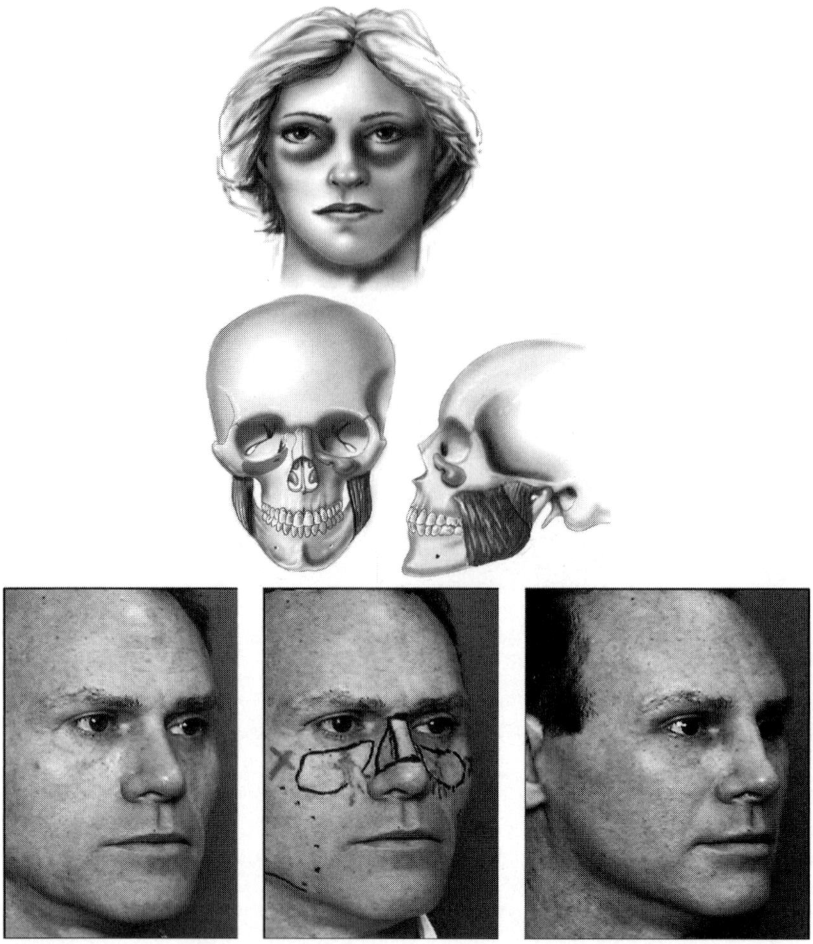

Figure 27 (*Top*) Alloplastic implants have been specifically designed for the "tear trough" sulcus. Due to the thin nature of the skin and subcutaneous tissues over this area, any implant or transplanted tissue must be perfectly shaped and tapered to ensure its invisibility. (*Bottom*) A 43-year-old male with an extreme deficiency of the suborbital maxilla causing a tired appearance. Postoperative view shows correction with a tear trough implant.

(A) **(B)**

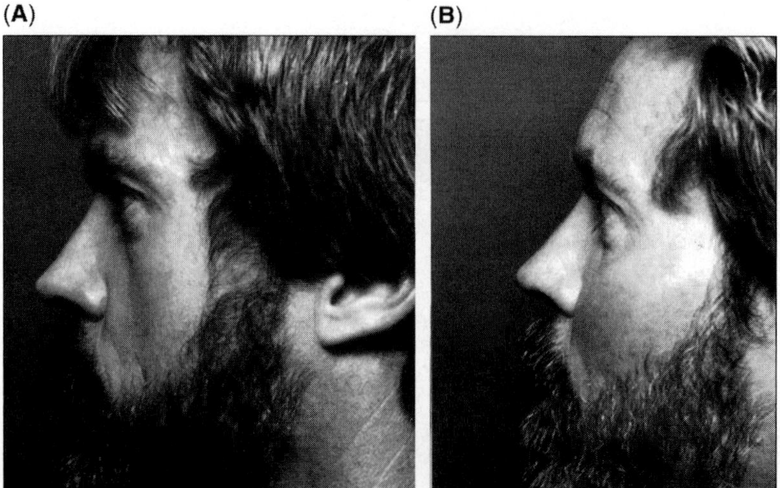

Figure 28 A 28-year-old male with "polar bear" syndrome (**A**). Extended submalar orbital implants corrected the deficiency and elevated the lower eyelid (**B**).

(A)

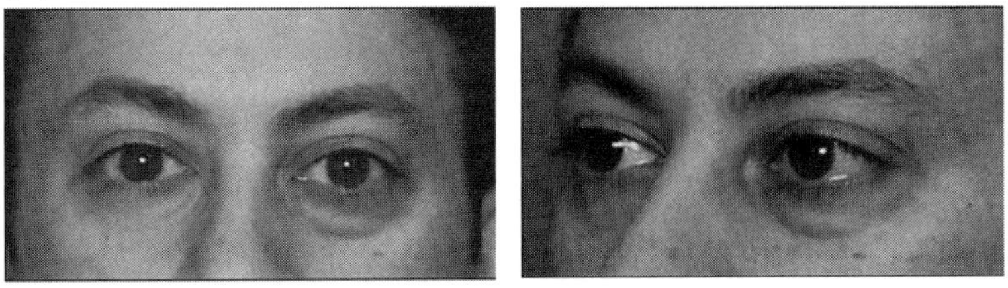

(B)

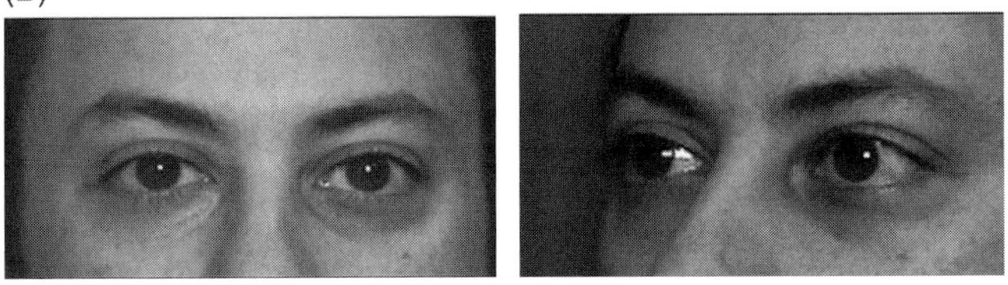

Figure 29 (**A**) A 32-year-old male with suborbital-malar deficiency. (**B**) Six months following the surgery showing correction with extended tear trough submalar orbital implant.

Zone 5 represents the submalar zonal triangle. This region of the midface has the greatest significance and requires the most frequent use of midface implants both in older and younger patients. Augmentation in this area extends midfacial fullness below the malar bone itself thereby creating a rounder, fuller "apple-cheek" contour (Fig. 30). SM Zone 5 is defined anatomically as follows: The masseter muscle and its overlying tendinous fascia are posterior. More medially the border of the masseter muscle is adjacent to the canine fossa of the maxilla.

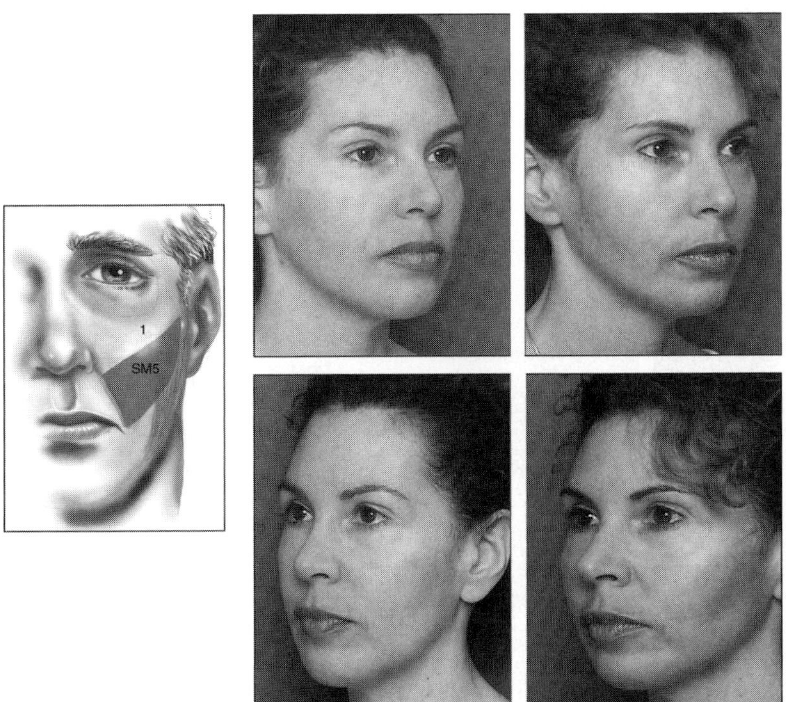

Figure 30 The submalar zonal triangle (*left*) has the greatest significance and requires the most frequent use of midface implants, both in older and younger patients. This 34-year-old patient (*right*) demonstrates the results of a submalar augmentation to restore the fullness of her face. She desired to return to her former appearance in her 20s. *Abbreviation*: SM5, submalar zone 5.

These structures serve as the floor upon which implants are placed. Its anterior soft-tissue roof consists of the overlying zygomaticus muscle groups, their origins and innervations and the SMAS. The medial limit of the submalar triangle is adjacent to the nasolabial mound. Effective alterations in this zone may often need to be extended up into the Zone 1 area to create both the illusion of a larger malar bone and to imitate soft-tissue volume as well. Sometimes an implant is indicated to augment only the submalar space. The superior boundary of the submalar Zone 5 is also the lower border of Zone 1 and constitutes the inferior bony margin of the malar eminence.

The inferior limit of the submalar zone (SM 5) is a sulcus created below the malar zone, which can be extended downward through a natural dissection plane that exists between the masseter muscle and the overlying zygomatic muscle complex. As the submalar-midface dissection and augmentation is extended lower, the fullness of the midface contour created by an implant in this location is also lowered down. No implant, however, can extend below the mucosa of the gingival buccal sulcus adjacent to the lateral commissure of the mouth.

Soft-tissue volume deficiencies in the submalar/midface region are very common. These can either be inherited or more frequently are the result of the natural aging process. Atrophy of submalar facial fat removes the soft, full contour look of youth (Fig. 31).

In many persons, midface atrophy creates a tired, drawn, and haggard appearance early in the third and fourth decades of life. Restoration of soft-tissue fullness within the submalar region is the most significant function for midface alloplastic augmentation when restoration of youthful contour is a major goal (Fig. 32).

The second most frequent need for midface contouring is comprehensive augmentation of the malar/midface region, which involves both Zone 1 and the submalar Zone 5. A large

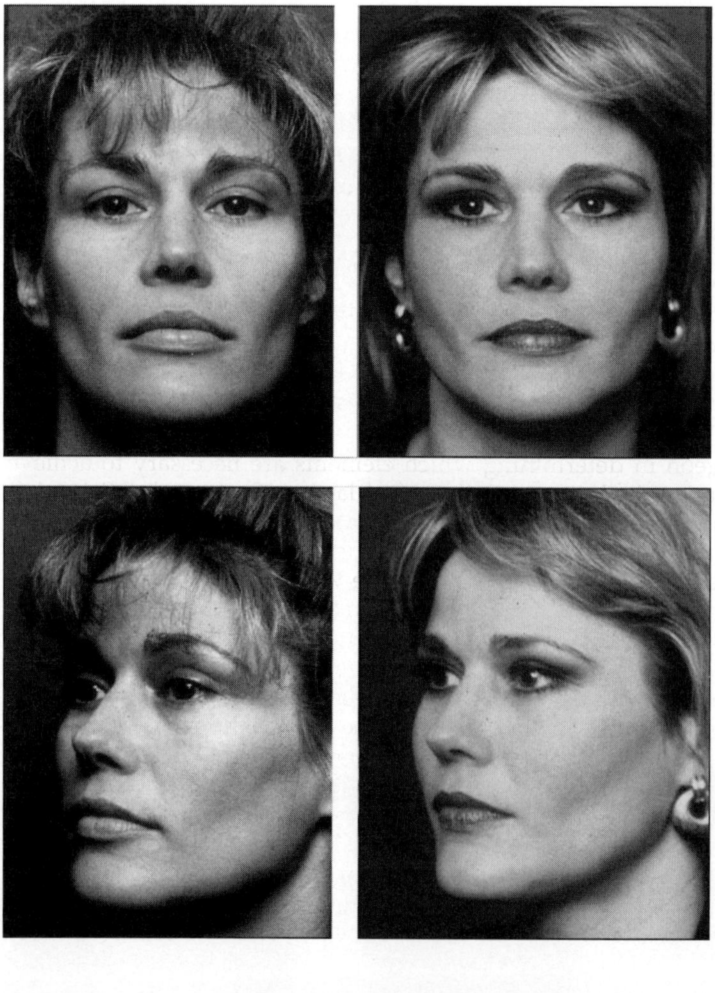

Figure 31 A 34-year-old female with inherited submalar atrophic appearance. This has been corrected by a midfacial shell to replace the soft-tissue fullness and produce an "apple-cheeked" appearance.

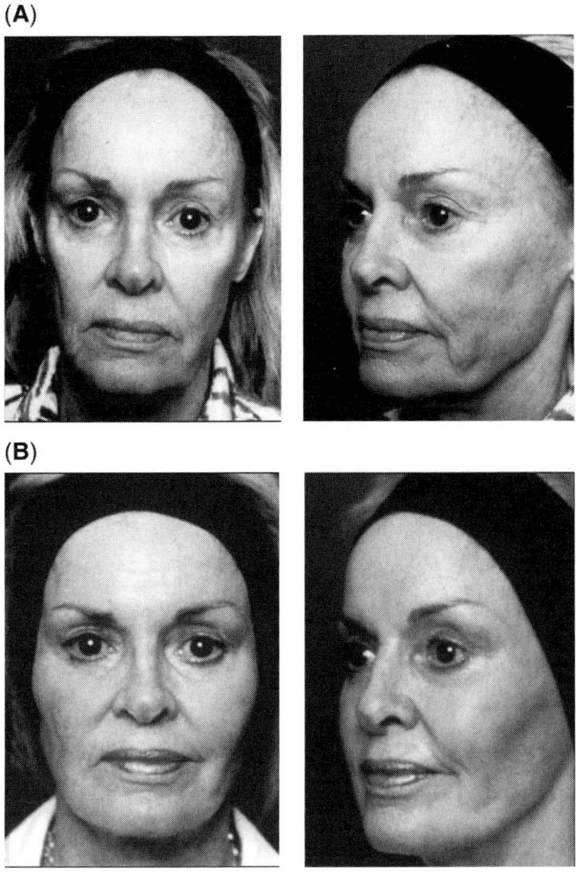

Figure 32 A 70-year-old female with aging atrophy of the submalar-midface (**A**). Following midfacial augmentation and rhytidectomy techniques, the patient developed a soft, full midface contour (**B**).

shell that augments both zonal regions mimics both midfacial soft-tissue volume in the lower aspect and bony augmentation in the more superior Zone 1 area. The design concept of a large midface shell is to augment a generous midface area with an implant that is thinly tapered at the margins to produce volume changes without being visible or palpable and without the unnatural appearance of a localized protuberance that can be produced by smaller, old-fashioned traditional oval implants (Fig. 33).

REGIONAL MIDFACIAL VOLUME DEFICIENCIES

A useful tool to assist the surgeon in determining which elements are necessary to achieve facial balance in any specific patient is the appreciation of malar/midface zonal deficiencies. Although the number of variations in facial size, shape, and contour are infinite, there are several common midfacial types that can easily be identified for the purpose of determining specific implant sizes and placement positioning. Several of these will be described.

A facial Type 1 deficiency consists of a relative contour weakness in the upper segment of the malar/midface. It encompasses Zones 1 and 2 over the malar bone and the medial third of the zygomatic arch. This represents either a bony or soft-tissue deficiency, or both. Augmentation in these zones creates upper cheek definition that simulates both bony and soft-tissue contour (Fig. 34). When a large implant is used to augment Zone 2 as well as Zone 1, the upper midface becomes broader. This shortens the appearance of a long and narrow face (Fig. 35).

A Type 2 facial regional aesthetic deficiency consists of a relatively decreased volume in the submalar (SM 5) zone. An implant placed in this location produces volume filling that also imitates both bone and soft tissues. Utilization of a large malar shell over the inferior aspect of the malar bone in Zone 1 and extending down into the submalar space creates the illusion of a round, full, apple-cheek (Fig. 36). The fat atrophy that occurs on the aging face is well corrected by implants that are placed into the submalar 5 anatomic region. This Type 2 midface

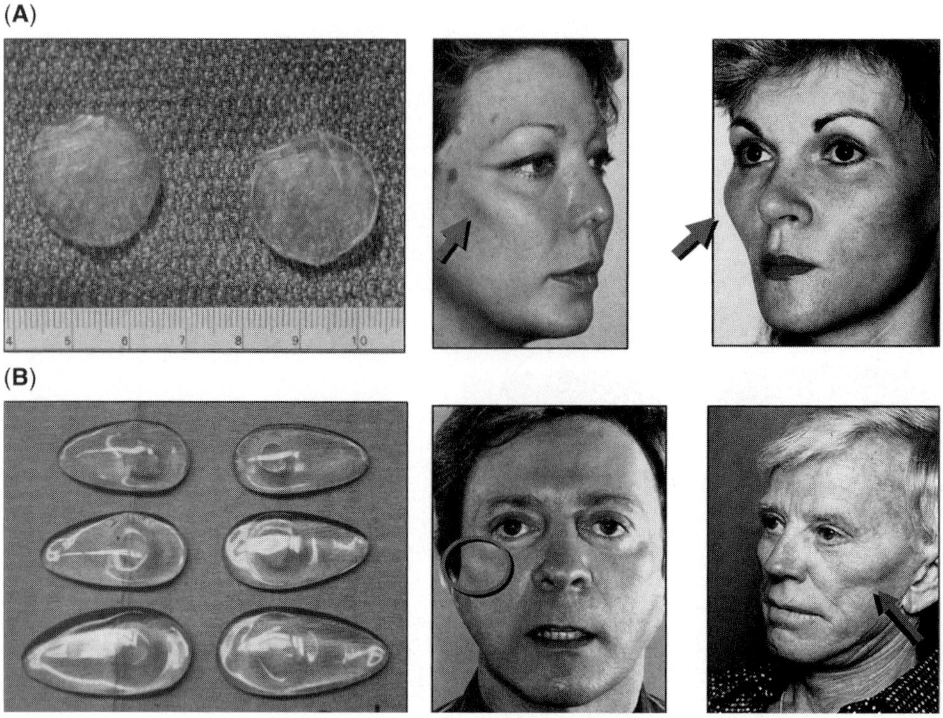

Figure 33 Old-fashioned traditional implants produce an unnatural appearance and a localized protuberance. (**A**) Hand-carved silicone implants. (**B**) Commercial silicone gel implants, circa 1971.

has adequate malar bone prominence but is specifically deficient in submalar soft-tissue volume. This can create an older, tired, haggard look. The submalar zone ends just lateral to the nasolabial smile mound. Volume filling of this space deemphasizes the appearance of the nasolabial mound and corrects the sunken or flat appearance in the midface to restore a more youthful and full appearance to the face (Fig. 37).

A Type 3 regional volume deficiency consists of a strong malar/zygomatic super structure accompanied by an extremely deficient submalar infrastructure. When this condition is

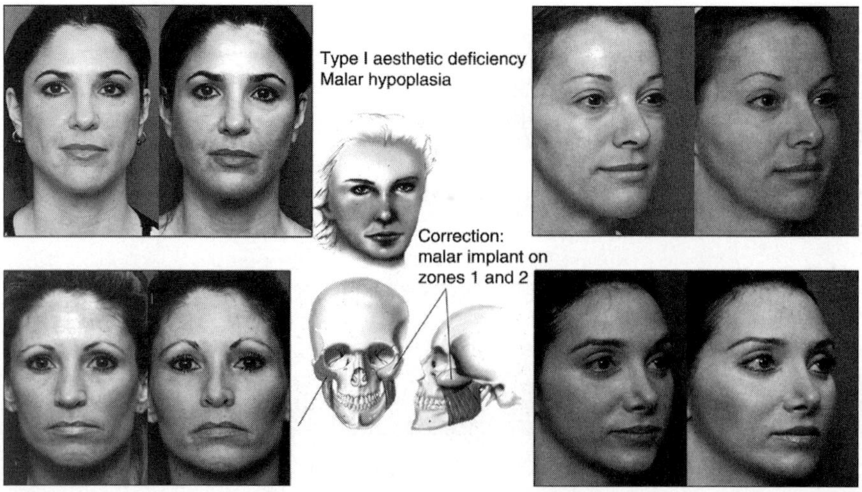

Figure 34 Four examples of Type 1 faces with relative malar deficiency. Postoperative views show attractive malar-midface contour from Zone 1, 2 malar volume enhancements.

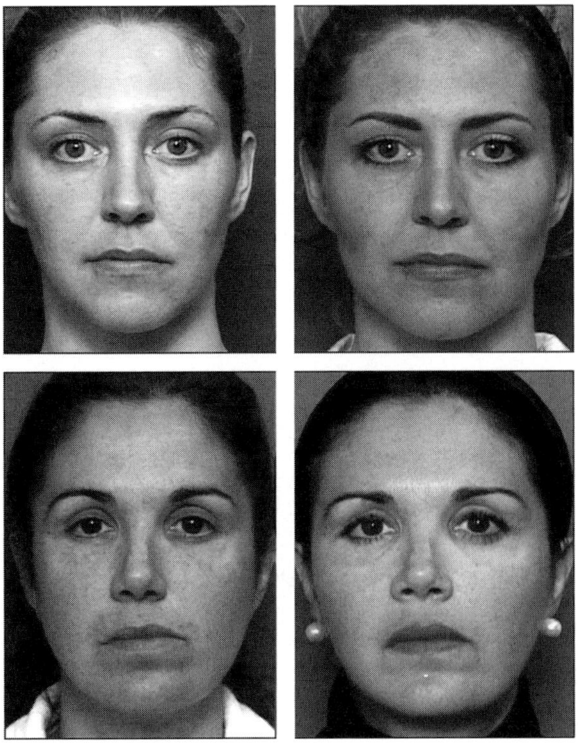

Figure 35 Augmentation within Zone 1 and 2 for a facial Type 1 deficiency creates a broadness of the upper midface and shortens the appearance of facial length. The illustration shows two patients, preoperative view (*left*), postoperative view (*right*).

accompanied by thin skin and subcutaneum, the appearance is one of emaciation atrophy and even sickness. Fortunately, unless a person has actual physical debility, this facial type is uncommon in the general population. Correction requires a generous submalar augmentation with a large surface area midface shell that may have a projection thickness of 5–7 mm (Fig. 38).

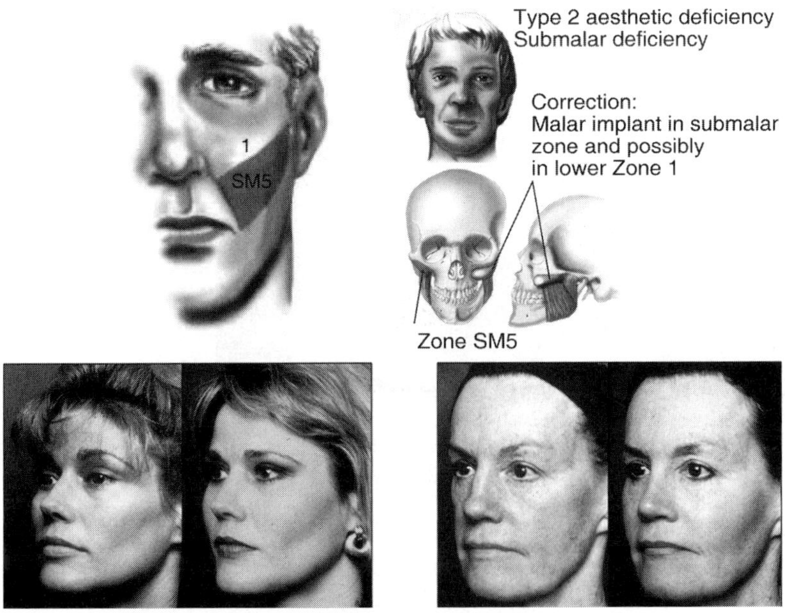

Figure 36 Fat atrophy occurs universally with the aging face. This can produce a sunken, tired, older look. When there is adequate malar bone prominence in a Type 2 or Type 3 face, a large malar shell placed in the submalar region restores a youthful fullness. Two examples of Type 2 faces with relative submalar deficiency. Post-op views show beauty enhancement using submalar shells. *Abbreviation*: SM5, submalar zone 5.

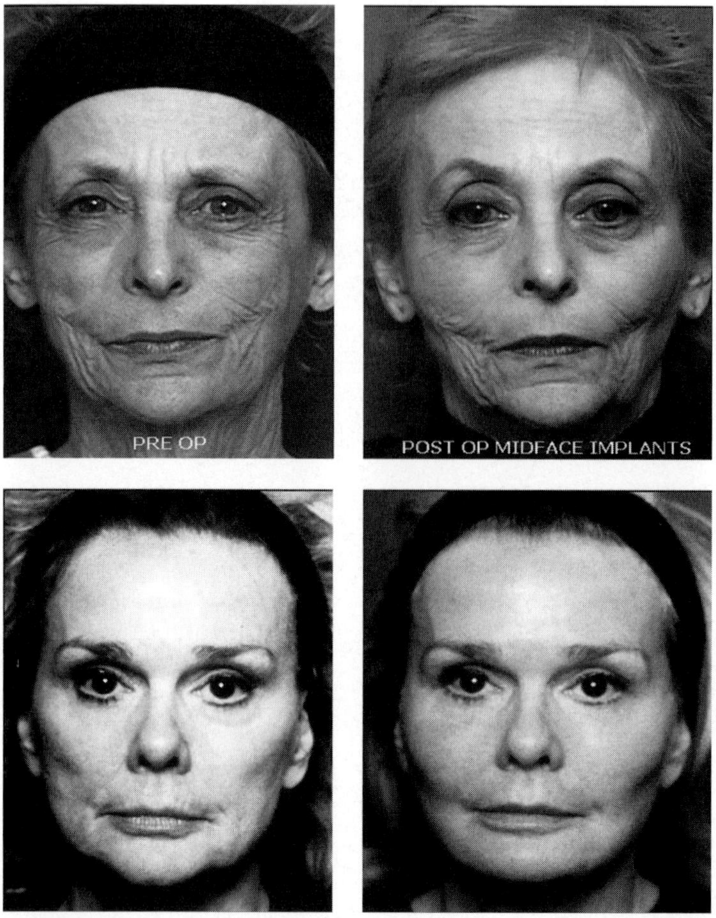

Figure 37 A Type 2 regional aesthetic deficiency is characterized by a decreased volume in submalar zone 5. Utilization of a large malar shell into the submalar space creates the illusion of a round, full apple-cheek.

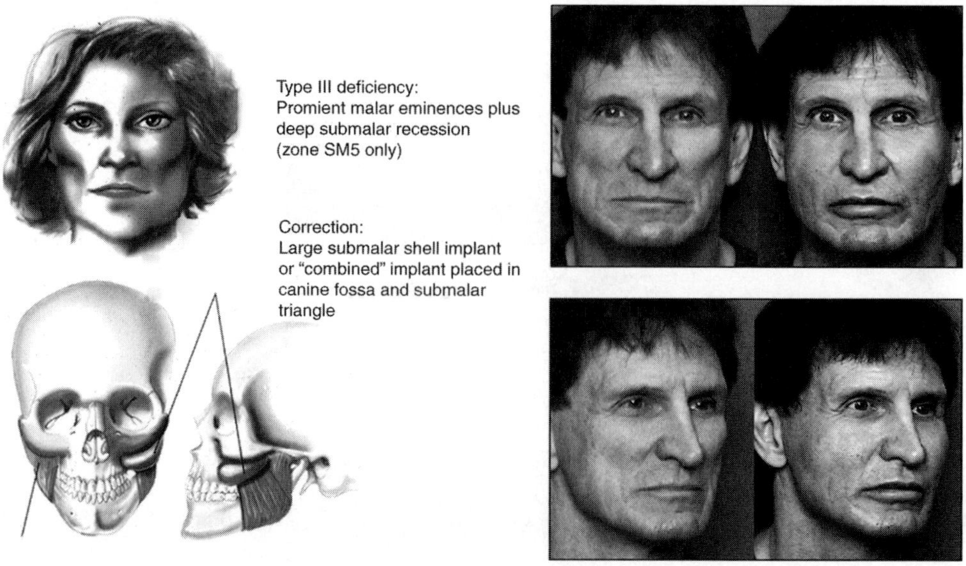

Figure 38 Submalar atrophy in an aging face produces a drawn, tired, and emaciated appearance. This 61-year-old patient demonstrates the benefits that a large submalar alloplastic shell implant produces in restoring youthful fullness to the aging face.

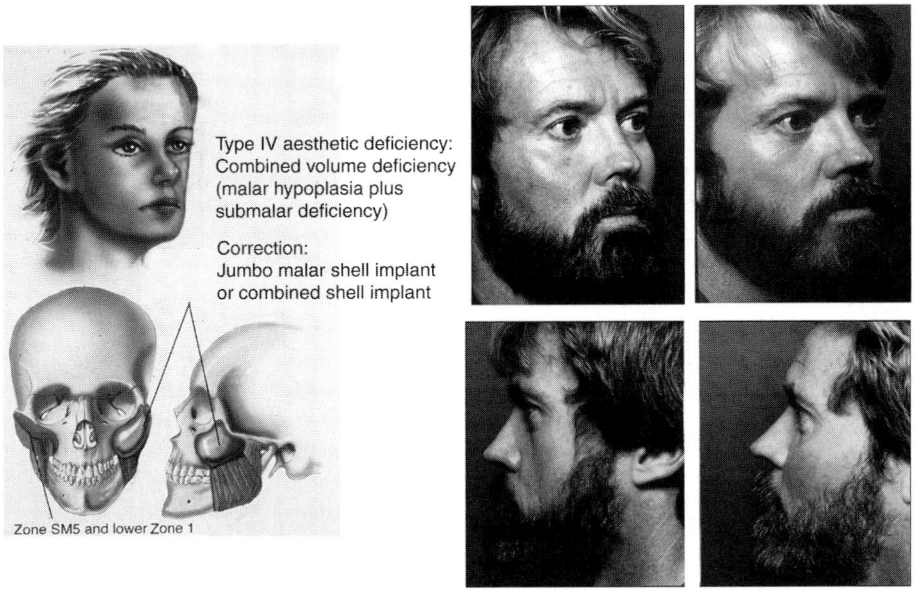

Figure 39 Before and after pictures of a patient with a Type 4 face demonstrating the improvement of an extreme volume deficiency of the entire maxilla using a comprehensive maxillary shell. This helps to correct a "flat" or "dish" face appearance.

A Type 4 face consists of extreme volume deficiency throughout the entire anterior maxillary region. This includes malar Zones 1 and 2 and the SM 5 regions; and also includes the entire orbital and paranasal Zone 3 area. This seems to be more common in men than in women (Fig. 39). It is identified by a "flat" face or "dish" face appearance. It has been described as the "polar bear" syndrome because of the deficiency recession of the inferior orbital rim, which contributes to a proptotic bulging appearance of the ocular globe. This is called a "negative vector" bony deficiency of the inferior orbital rim. It may be associated with a downward or vertical descent of the lower eyelid causing sclera show.

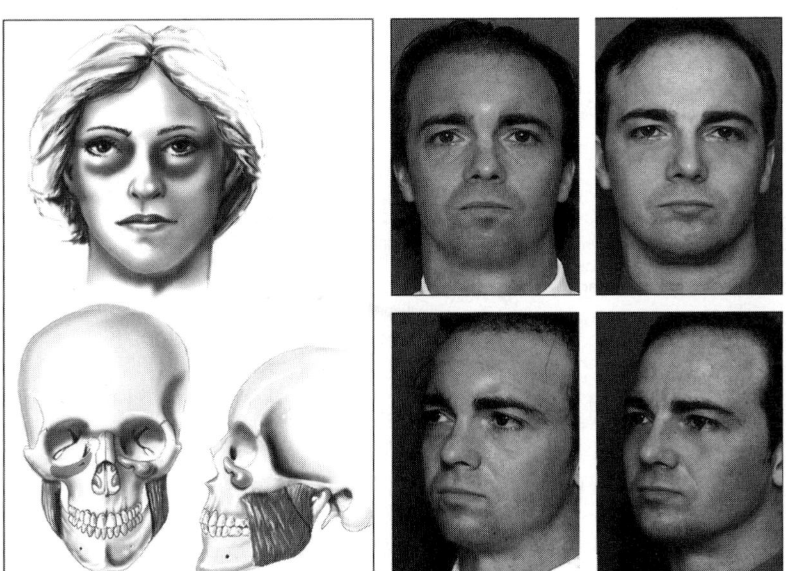

Figure 40 A comprehensive suborbital-malar extended implant contributes volume throughout the entire infraorbital and malar region. This also adds support to the lower eyelid to elevate it to a more attractive horizontal position.

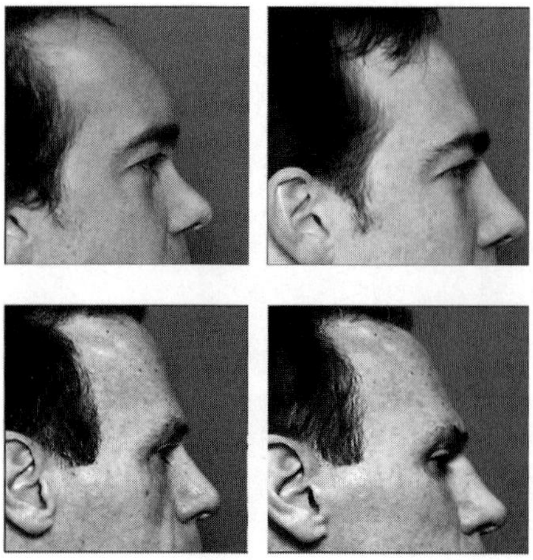

Figure 41 The use of a uniquely designed suborbital-malar implant extending from the medial canthus to beyond the lateral orbital rim considerably improves a Type 5 deficiency. Autogenous tissue transplants of fat, muscle, etc., placed into this area are also successful, but their permanence is controversial.

Significant improvement in this Type 4 aesthetic imbalance occurs by placement of a comprehensive shell implant or suborbital-malar extended implants that contribute volume in all of these midface zones including the infraorbital region. This implant also adds support to the lower eyelid and elevates it to a more attractive horizontal position (Fig. 40).

Lateral canthopexy techniques are often necessary to correct the descent of the lower eyelid which is common with this facial type and to prevent its worsening after malar surgery. This represents both an aesthetic and a functional correction.

A Type 5 aesthetic regional deficiency represents a specific weakness of skeletal structure in the inferior orbital and medial tear trough region. This contributes to a tired, hollow appearance around the eyes, which occurs following the deflation-atrophy of the periorbital tissues with aging.

A uniquely designed suborbital-malar implant extends from the medial canthus beyond the lateral orbital malar rim. It considerably improves this appearance (Fig. 41). Autogenous tissue transplants of fat, muscle, galea, and temporalis fascia placed into this area are also successful but their persistence and complication rate is still controversial. Fat grafting along the inferior orbital rim has been considered by some to be advantageous. In general, the author's experience is that all autologous soft-tissue grafting manifests unpredictable shrinkage and may produce irregularities or result in negligible improvement.

Over the past five years there has been strong interest in a subperiosteal elevation of all soft-tissue layers from the maxilla followed by a suspension of them in an upward direction to provide greater volume filling in the inferior orbital rim area. This midface suspension can be

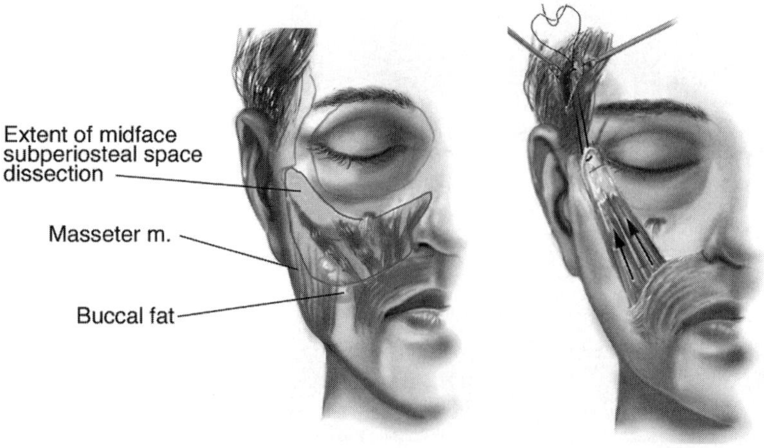

Figure 42 A subperiosteal upper and midface suspension, especially in the presence of an underlying malar-midface implant, will provide greater volume filling in the inferior orbital rim and malar region.

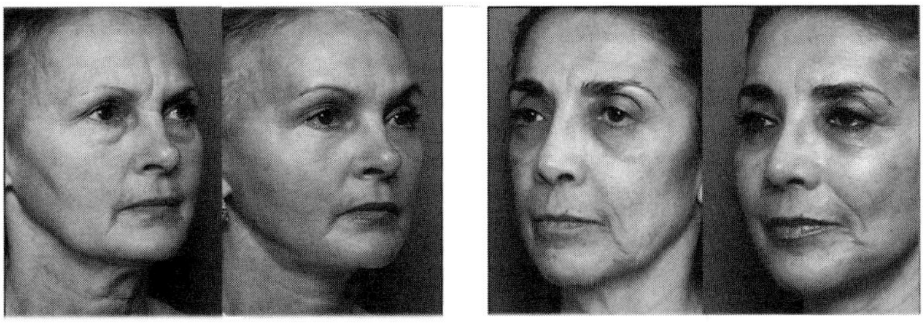

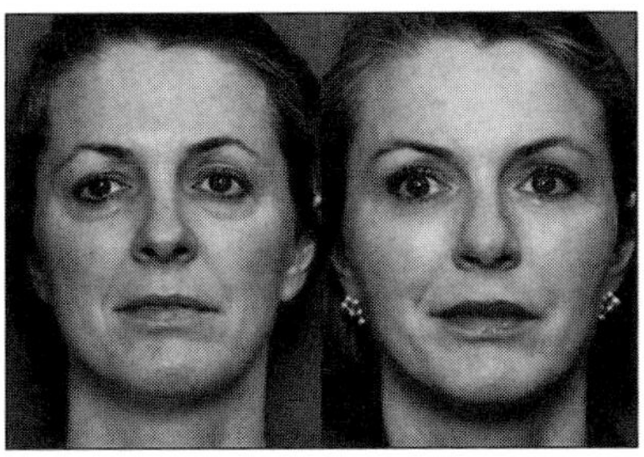

Figure 43 Here are three examples, before and after surgery, of patients who had subperiosteal upper and midface suspension accompanied by midface implants with improvement in midface contour and suborbital hollowness treated by fat transposition.

accompanied by inferior orbital fat rearrangement over the inferior orbital rim. This is done after severing the origins of the orbicularis muscle and disrupting the arcus marginalis and underlying SOOF tissues in the medial tear trough area (Fig. 42).

Subperiosteal midfacial suspension alone without the addition of alloplastic implants is a technique that is still new enough to require the test of time to evaluate long-term persistence of volume correction and three-dimensional improvement of the suborbital hollow appearance and malar–submalar shape (Fig. 43).

A Type 6 midface deficiency exists in the perinasal premaxillary region. Volume deficiency or the appearance of retrusiveness in this aspect of the skeleton is common in certain ethnic groups, especially Asians and Western Indians in the Americas. It also exists as a congenital hereditary trait, which can be mild or severe and which may require complicated orthognathic surgery using maxillary LeForte bony advancement techniques.

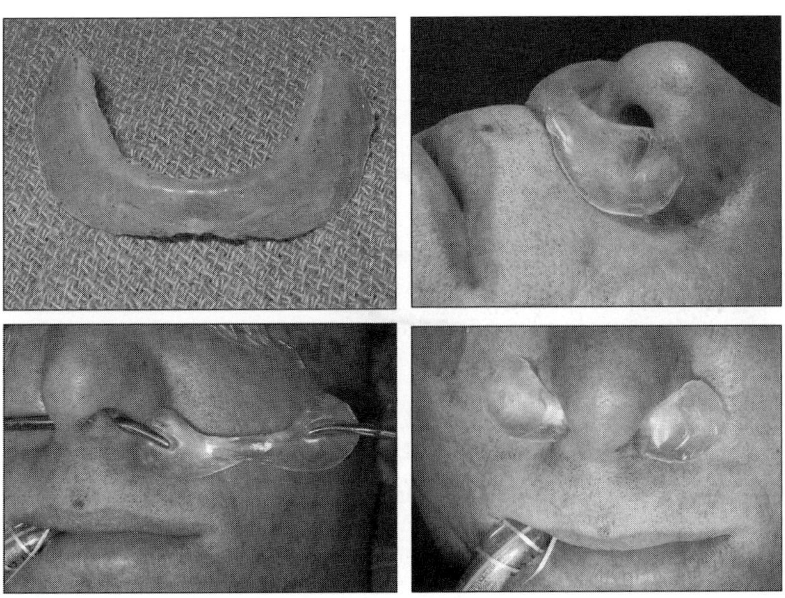

Figure 44 A peripyriform implant is a successful new implant design that can improve premaxillary retrusion volume contour deformities.

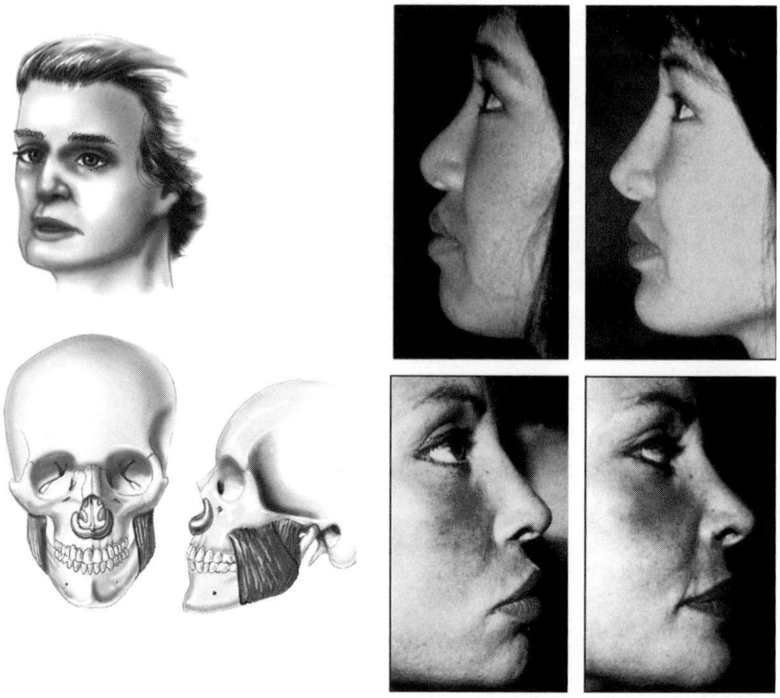

Figure 45 Example of two patients in whom premaxillary retrusive contour deformities were corrected using a peri-pyriform premaxillary contemporary design implant. Preoperative photos are on the left.

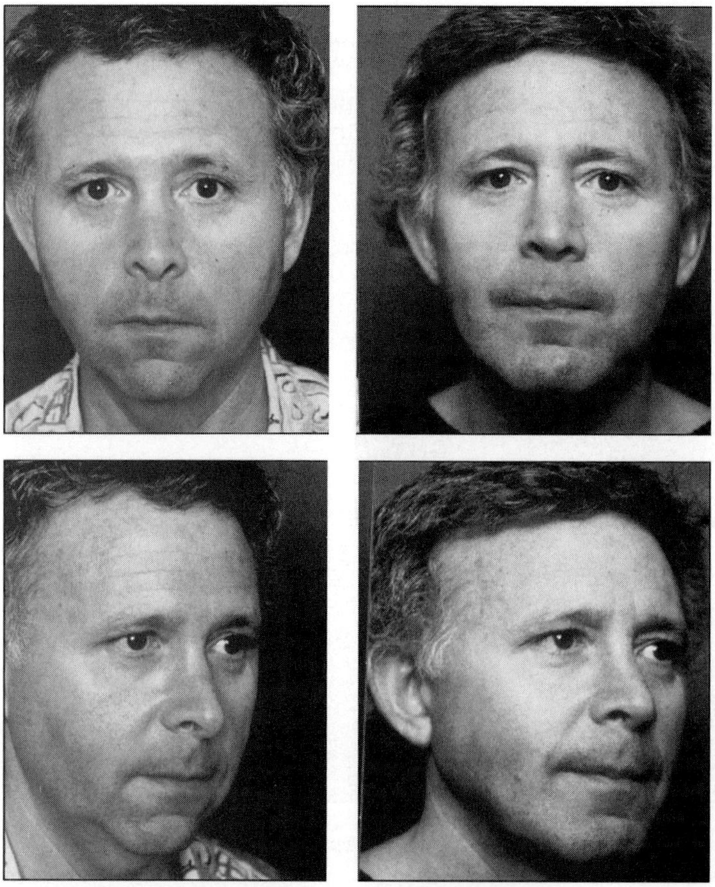

Figure 46 Alterations of the premandible space or lower third aesthetic facial segment are essential in producing a facial balance, which enhances an attractive appearance. This 56-year-old male demonstrates improvement from a rhytidectomy and a large anatomic premandible implant to augment the central mentum and midlateral zones.

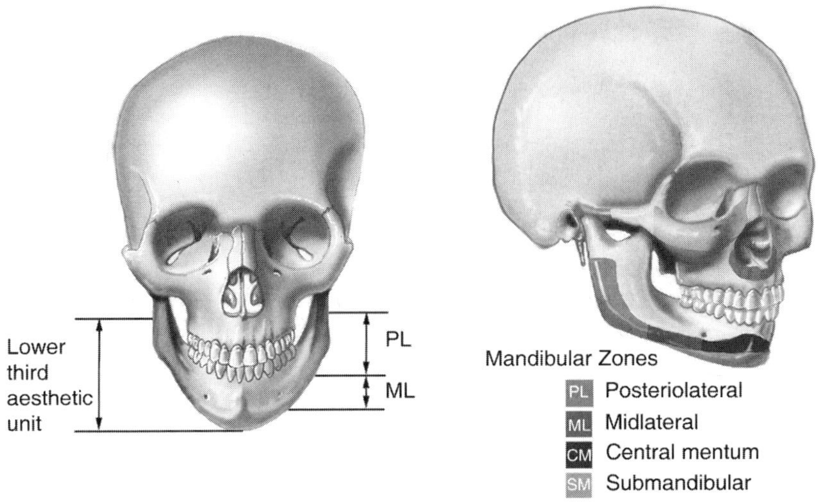

Figure 47 There are four anatomic zones within the premandible space that can be augmented to correct specific regional contours for the lower aesthetic mandibular facial segment.

Alloplastic augmentation can improve mild to moderate premaxillary deficiency to produce significant aesthetic changes. There are several implant designs and sizes of silicone rubber implants, which have been used successfully over the years to alter nasolabial and premaxillary relationships (Fig. 44). Although other materials such as alloderm, autologous fat, Gore-Tex, collagen, and other injectibles are used in the nasolabial and perioral sulcus, these materials have only resulted in temporary augmentations. Alloplastic augmentation is permanent. Type 6 peripyriform and premaxillary volume deficiencies are common. They are frequently overlooked by aesthetic surgeons. They are usually of lesser magnitude than the greater volume/mass interrelationships of the malar/midface, jawline, and nose. Therefore, they do not command as much attention during an initial aesthetic facial contour consultation unless the patients themselves are focused on their deficiency (Fig. 45).

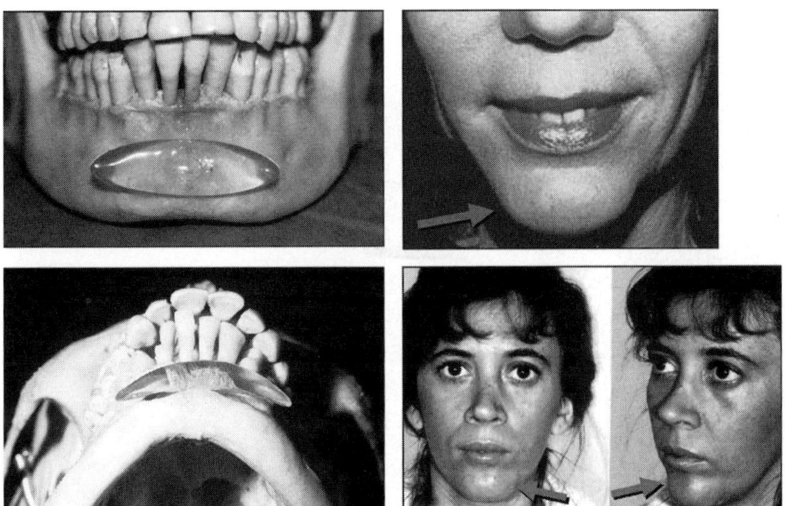

Figure 48 Traditional chin implants have been placed centrally between the mental foramina. This often produces a nonattractive, central abnormal, rounded protuberance.

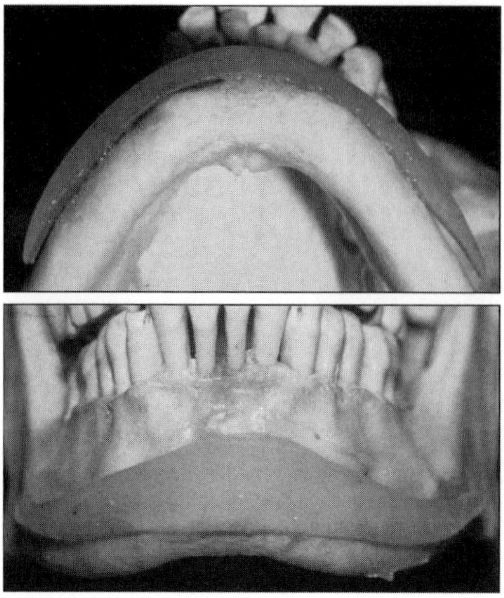

Figure 49 Anatomic design implants are contoured posteriorly to securely fit the bony surface like a glove.

ZONAL ANATOMY OF THE PREMANDIBLE JAWLINE AESTHETIC FACIAL SEGMENT

Assessment of the lower third facial aesthetic segment is also necessary to comprehensively evaluate facial aesthetic balance that improves appearance. The "premandible space" is, therefore, that anatomic region and its zones which, when variously augmented, produces attractive changes to the shape and volume characteristics of the lower third of the face and jawline (Fig. 46).

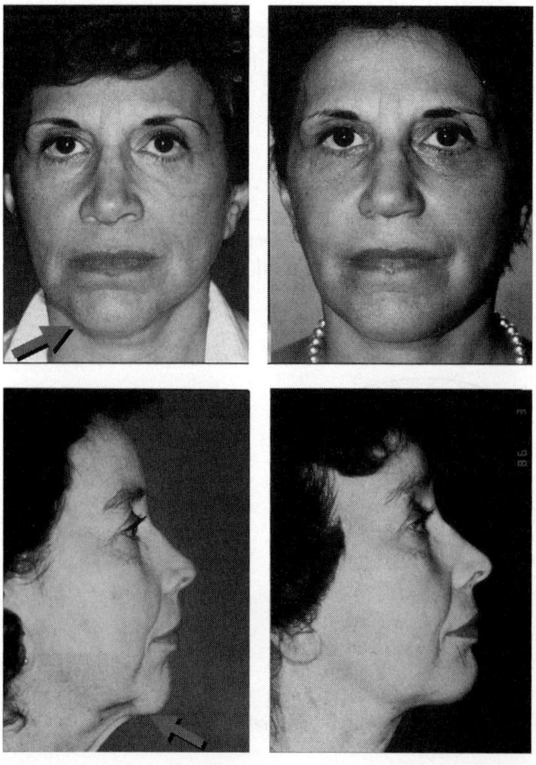

Figure 50 Abnormal contours from traditional central implants can be corrected by using extended anatomic chin implants designed by the author.

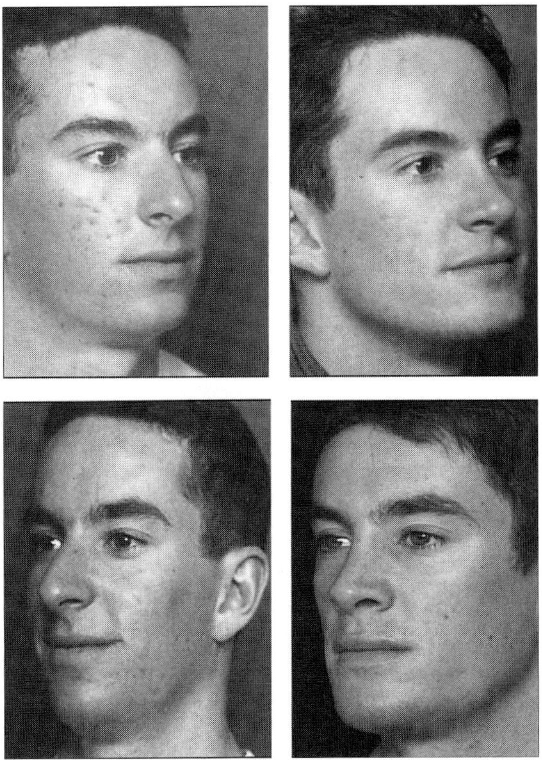

Figure 51 A dramatic example of a 22-year-old male who achieved a more aesthetic, attractive facial balance from rhinoplasty, chin, and angle of jaw augmentation.

Within the premandible space, four anatomic zones may be defined (Fig. 47). These zones enable the surgeon to analyze and correct relative volume deficiencies in the premandible jawline. Correction of such deficiencies by alloplastic implants can create specific contours for the lower face according to the patient's needs and preferences.

The central mentum (CM) is the area between the mental foramina where traditional chin implants have been placed for over 40 years. Implants placed under this central segment alone, without lateral extension, produce an unattractive contour with an abnormal central rounded protuberance that accentuates the appearance of a prejowl sulcus or "valley" in the area of the anterior mandibular ligament just below the mental foramen (Fig. 48). The floor of the CM zone is the surface of the central mandible, which includes the midline mental tubercle. Recent design implants are contoured posteriorly to securely fit this bony surface "like a glove" (Fig. 49). They correct abnormal central chin contours from traditional implants (Fig. 50). They, therefore, provide an entirely natural looking augmented jawline (Fig. 51).

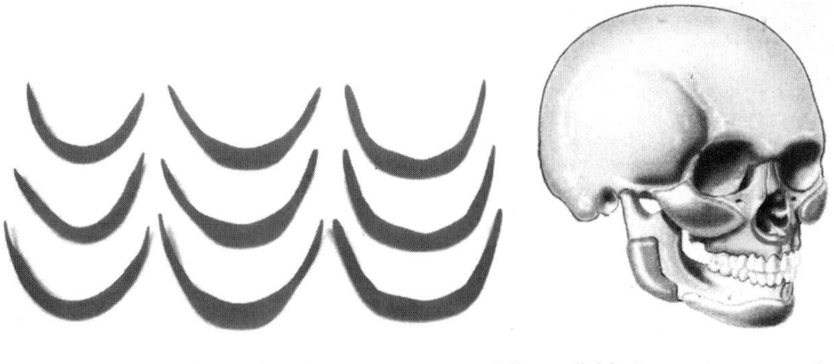

Figure 52 Anatomic implants are now commercially available to create many external contours. They produce a natural-looking augmented jawline.

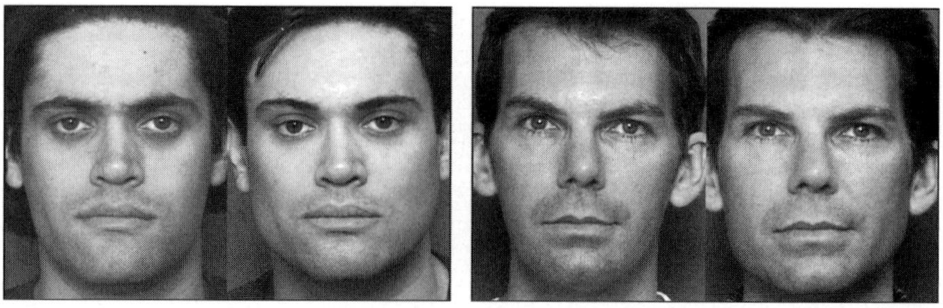

Figure 53 Jawline enhancement is frequently requested by men. (*Left*) Before and after placement of angle of jaw implant, central chin implant, tear trough implant, and eyebrow and palpebral shape contouring. (*Right*) Before and one year postoperative placement of angle of jaw implant.

The ML zone of the mandible extends from the mental foramen posterior to the oblique line of the horizontal ramus. The anterior limit of this zone is at the mental nerve and foramen. The posterior limit is the oblique ridge of the mandible. Its superior boundary is the upper border of the horizontal mandible. The lower extent is the inferior border of the mandible. The mandibular branch of the facial nerve exits through the mental foramen 8–10 mm above the inferior border of the mandible. The "roof" of overlying soft tissues in the mid jawline contains the platysma, the SMAS, the anterior facial vein and artery, and the marginal branch of the facial nerve as it crosses the mandible to enter the depressor muscles of the lower lip. Implants can augment the ML zone and widen the appearance of the lower jawline segment while at the same time increasing the anterior-posterior dimension of the CM. The author has designed a variety of implants that have differing shapes and volumes and which can alter both the central projection, the vertical length of the mandible, and the ML zone of the horizontal ramus. All these implants are available commercially (*) (Fig. 52).

Jawline changes are frequently requested by men (Fig. 53). These requests are rapidly increasing every year. They mainly relate to the PL zone of the mandible (Fig. 54). This zone includes the posterior one-third of the horizontal ramus extending back from the oblique line and includes the angle of the mandible and the lower 4 cm of the ascending ramus. Its boundaries are as follows: (*i*) the floor is the mandible itself, (*ii*) the roof is the overlying masseter muscle, (*iii*) the superior border is limited by the sigmoid notch of the mandible, (*iv*) the posterior and inferior borders are limited by strong, fibrofascial insertions of the masseter muscle.

These must be completely released to expand the space around the bony borders of the mandibular angle. This release is necessary to allow the curved borders of the commercially available angle implants to extend around the inferior and ascending posterior mandible margins to secure these implants into position (Figs. 55 and 56).

Avoidance of a traumic dissection when releasing the masseter muscle from the bone is necessary so that neither the mandibular branch of the facial nerve (VII) nor the fragile posterior jugular veins or anterior facial vein and artery are harmed. When damaged these vessels can bleed profusely.

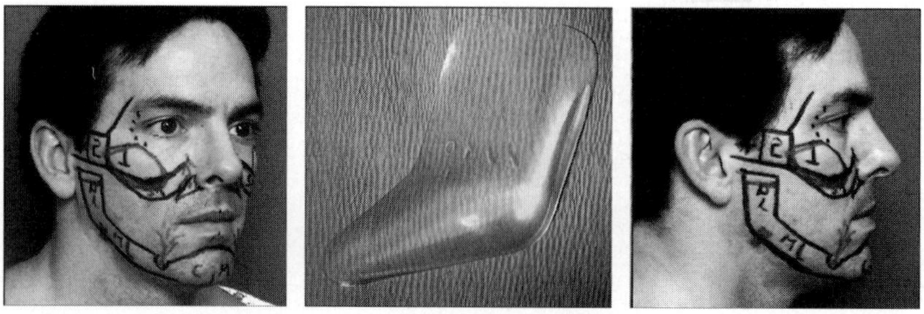

Figure 54 Preoperative markings are used prior to placement of mandibular angle implants into the posterolateral zone.

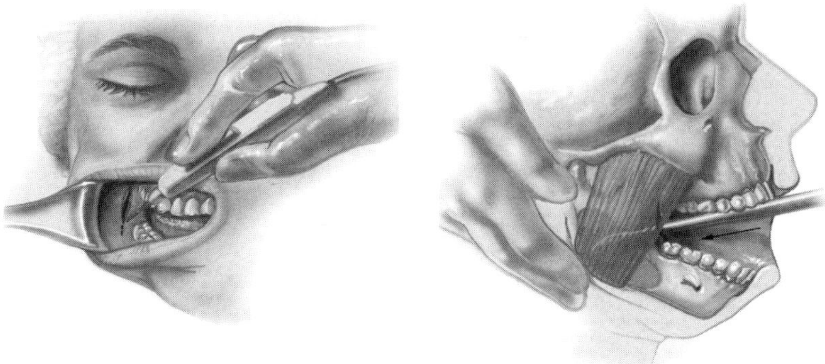

Figure 55 Artist's illustration, demonstrating a 3-cm intraoral incision just posterior to the molar teeth. A subperiosteal space is created, disinserting the masseter from the inferior posterior border and angle of the mandible, as well as on its anterior surface extending up the ascending ramus.

Variable augmentation of the angle can be produced to produce a strong posterior jawline contour with excellent angle definition (Fig. 57). Implants are available commercially that either widen this PL segment in a lateral direction or extend it downward in an inferior direction. Extending the posterior mandible down creates a less obtuse and more acute posterior mandibular angle that gives the lower mandibular border more horizontal definition.

The fourth, final, and very important jawline region is the submandibular (SM) zone. This zone is defined as "that region in the lower facial jawline/mandible aesthetic segment where volume-mass alloplastic alterations will produce variable lengthening of the vertical dimension of the face" (Fig. 58).

Traditional alloplastic chin implants do not and cannot increase the vertical height to lengthen the lower third aesthetic segment. Osteotomies with interpositional bone grafting or autologous fat transplant techniques are currently methods chosen by most plastic surgeons to accomplish this important contour change. For the novice and ordinarily trained plastic surgeon orthognathic genioplasties are technically complicated, imprecise, and have significant complications (5–10%) such as nerve damage, asymmetries, and "step-off" irregularities.

A unique vertical extension implant was developed by the author in 1986 to wrap around the inferior bony margin of the mandible and increase the vertical distance from the lower lip to the inferior chin. It extends 4 mm down and also laterally augments this SM zone (Fig. 59). This implant adds volume to the anterior mandible segment and to the prejowl sulcus or marionette groove at the origin of the anterior mandibular ligament. Implants in the submandibular zone improve or correct a witch's chin deformity, as well the anterior mandibular prejowl sulcus (Fig. 60).

Augmentation of the SM zone involves complete disinsertion of the muscular origins along the lower mandibular border. At the present time, the submandibular implant affords only 4 mm of projection. There are times when additional projection necessitates placement of a second implant on the anterior surface of the central mentum.

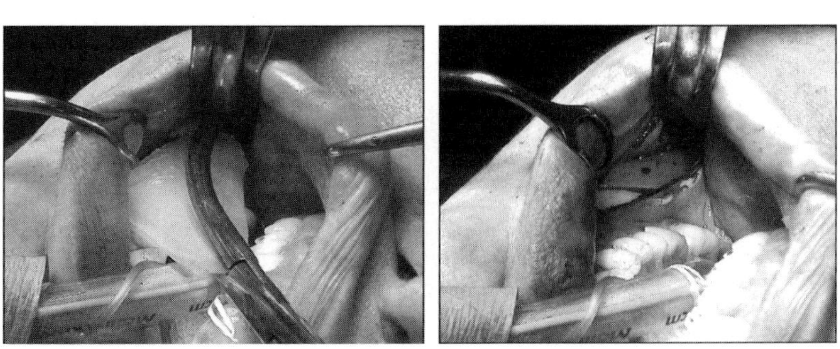

Figure 56 Photographs of a mandibular angle implant insertion using a curved clamp and placing it in an upward and posterior position over the mandibular angle and ascending ramus.

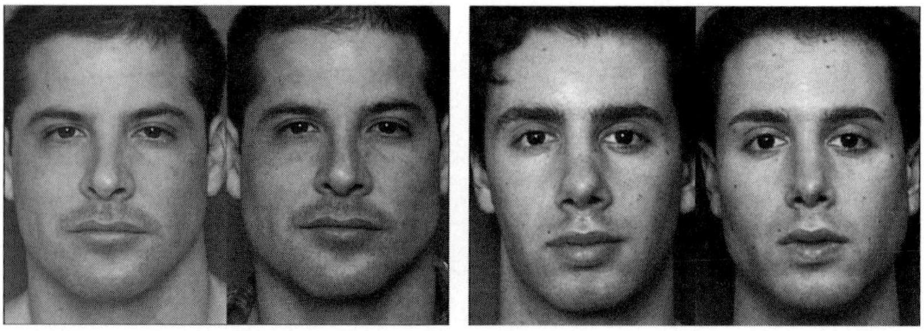

Figure 57 Examples of mandibular augmentation. (*Left*) Preoperative and six months' postoperative mandibular angle augmentation. (*Right*) Preoperative and one year after placement of mandibular angle implant.

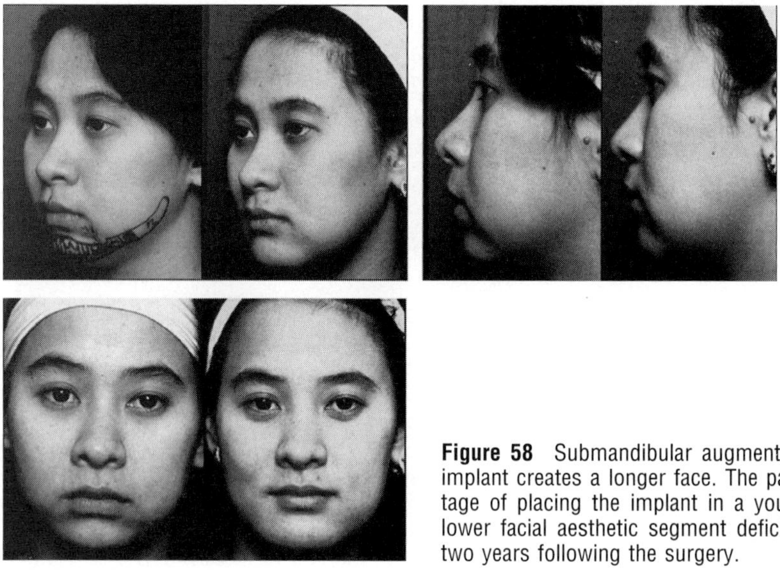

Figure 58 Submandibular augmentation with a vertical extension implant creates a longer face. The patient demonstrates the advantage of placing the implant in a young woman who has a severe lower facial aesthetic segment deficiency. Postoperative views are two years following the surgery.

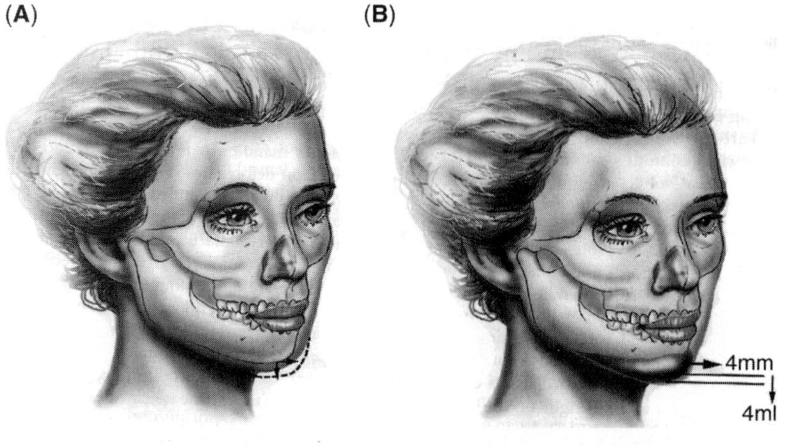

Figure 59 Illustration showing the position of a vertical extension submandibular implant and its dimensions, which produce augmentation of 4 mm of anterior and downward projection.

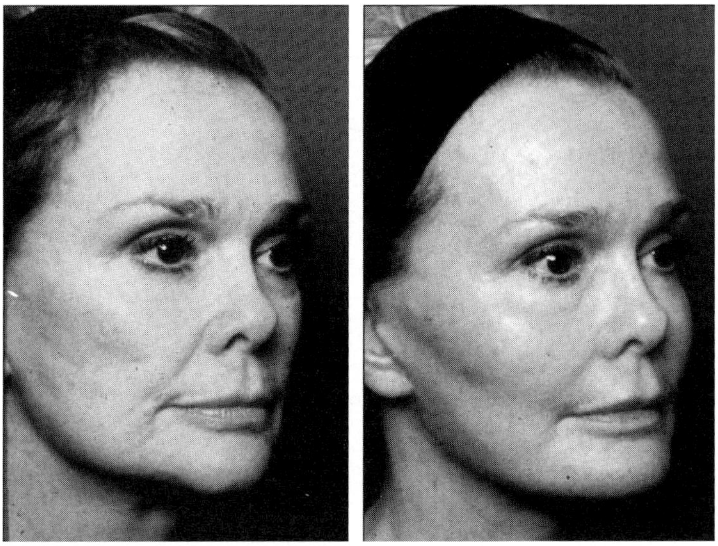

Figure 60 A vertical extension implant can improve a "witch's chin" deformity and augment the prejowl sulcus. This patient demonstrates a rhytidectomy, a malar–submalar volume augmentation, and a prejowl augmentation using a vertical extension implant to correct the aging, tired appearance of her face. Postoperative view is at one year.

Just as volume augmentation changes are specific for each zonal area of the malar/midface middle third facial segment, contour changes can be differentially produced in the lower third premandible jawline. The correct choice of implant size, shape, and positioning when properly selected are the key steps to achieving specific predictable results.

Nasal contour-volume alterations are frequently requested. These procedures also contribute greatly to overall aesthetic facial balance (Fig. 61), especially as they relate volumetrically to the profile balance of the mandible chin aesthetic segment.

POTENTIAL COMPLICATIONS

Midface

Midface complications can arise from too vigorous a dissection over the middle third of the zygomatic arch when a malar implant placement into Zone 2 is desired to create a broader face. The overlying facial nerve branch to the frontalis muscle may be damaged temporarily or permanently.

Branches of the zygomaticus muscle groups, as well as those that extend up into the inferior lateral orbicularis muscle, can be traumatized during dissection into the malar Zone 1 and submalar Zone 5 areas. This may result in transient or permanent lagophthalmus and impaired ability to elevate the nasolabial area during smiling and facial animation (Fig. 62).

Dissection in the Zone 3 medial suborbital maxilla area exposes the infraorbital nerve to harmful damage when introducing alloplastic tear trough implants or during midface suspension techniques.

When a subperiosteal malar space is created over the lateral aspect of the orbital rim but the dissection space is not opened inferior enough on the maxilla to permit a malar shell to reside approximately 4 mm below the orbital rim, the implant can be positioned high, overlap the lateral rim, encroach on the orbit, and produce lower eyelid vertical descent or ectropion. This is particularly common when implants are introduced through the subcilial lower eyelid approach.

Premandible

During premandible dissections, trauma to the mental nerve is common but symptoms are usually transient. Dissecting gently along the inferior border of the mandible and sweeping upward gently to observe and protect the mental nerve helps to avoid these symptoms.

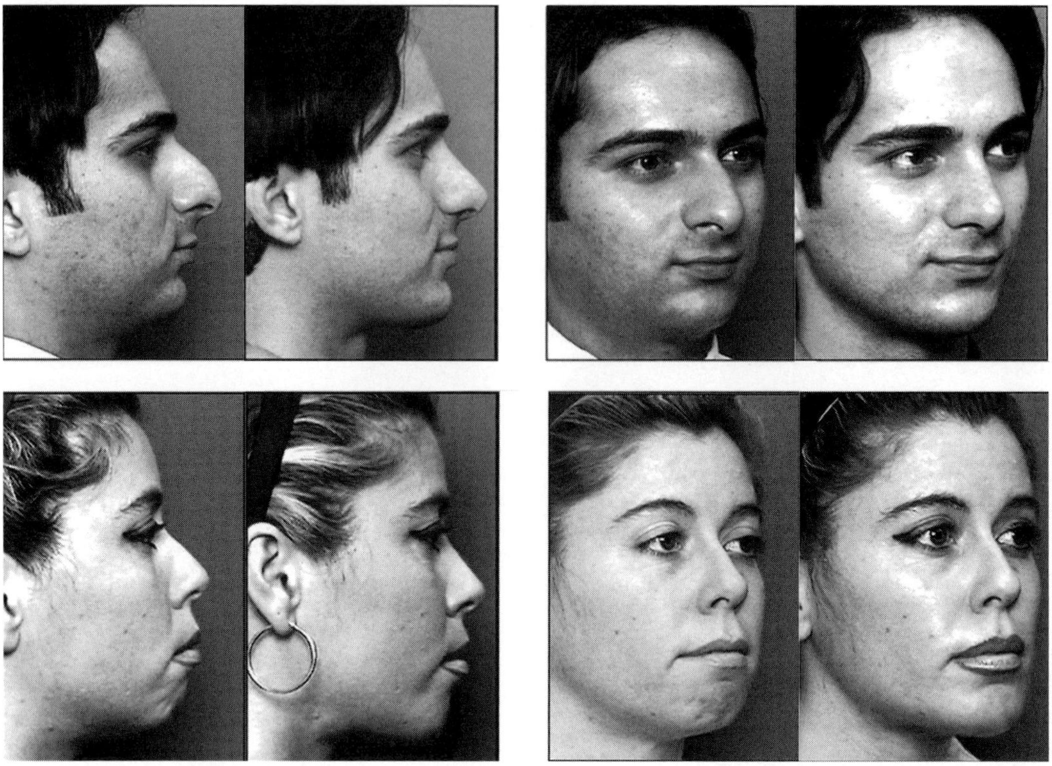

Figure 61 These two patients demonstrate the advantages of chin augmentation in profileplasty with or without nasal contour refinement. Both postoperative photographs are taken 12 to 16 months following surgery. Note the significant improvement in mentalis muscle dimpling in the female patient after giving anatomic structural support to the central chin region.

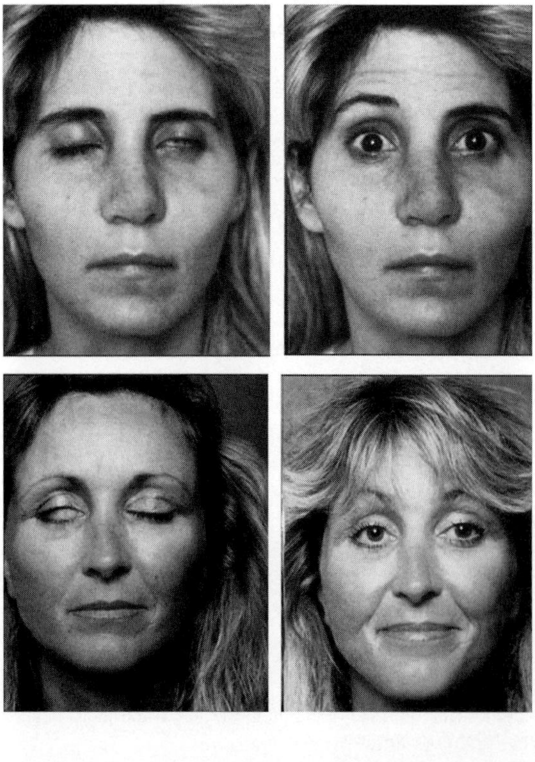

Figure 62 Nerve complications following facial implants occur in less than 1% of patients. Most nerve injuries are temporary. One typical injury involves facial nerve branches to the frontalis and orbicularis oculi muscle. Both patients experienced complete recovery at six to eight weeks following surgery.

Dissecting and degloving the muscles along the inferior mandibular border are an absolute necessity for ML zone augmentation. However, during this dissection the marginal mandibular branch of the facial nerve can be injured to produce a lower lateral lip dysfunction (Fig. 63).

Dissecting in the PL mandibular zone by degloving the entire posterior region of the inferior border and ascending ramus of the mandible can, if great care is not taken, produce injury to the jugular vessels posterior to the ascending ramus. This could conceivably create profuse and dangerous bleeding. To avoid this complication care must be taken during the posterior dissection.

A forceful upward dissection into the area of the sigmoid notch and coronoid process of the mandible could produce troublesome temporomandibular joint symptoms. These are usually transitory and less than a week in duration. Trismus is an uncommon sequela of posterior angle augmentation. In the author's experience it has always been extremely brief and short lived, at most 7–10 days.

THE CONSULTATION INTERVIEW

In the author's practice, patient education begins with the requirement that patients who desire facial contour alterations must describe not only verbally, but also in writing, the specific details of their desired contour changes. This must include their perception of the contour deficiencies, which they feel they possess. This written statement must be accompanied by standard professional photographs of the patient in five views: frontal, two profile and two oblique views. These facilitate analyzing their perceived contour deficiencies and are used along with photographs they choose from magazines and other sources to demonstrate the "ideal scene" they would like the surgery to create. Photos of the patients taken at earlier times of life are also requested (Fig. 64).

Before a face-to-face consultation with the surgeon, other educational tools are used. The Confirm Program CD on facial implants, which the American Society of Plastic Surgery requested the author to do in 1995, serves as an excellent instructional tool to explain concepts of facial balance as they relate to the basic interrelationship of the three major promontories: the malar/midface, the nose, and the chin/jawline. The author also uses other videos and photos which demonstrate him drawing the malar zygomatic and premandible zones of the facial skeleton on the patient's face and their magazine photo "ideal scenes" to show how specific "positioning of various size and shape implants alters the third dimension of the midface in different ways" (Fig. 65).

Computer imaging is an invaluable tool to assist the surgeon. Not only can changes be made that simulate desired volume and shape alterations but these can also be compared using a side-by-side pre- and postimage of the patient's presurgical image (Fig. 66). When used cautiously and conservatively, the final result of surgery one year postoperatively is

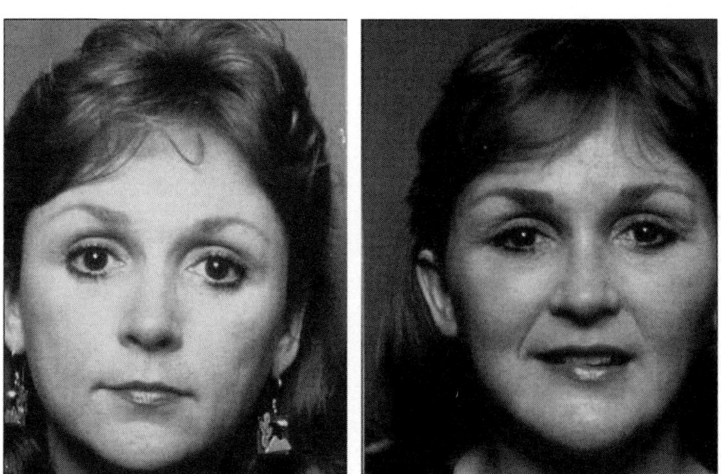

Figure 63 Chin augmentation can be accompanied by damage to the marginal mandibular branch of the facial nerve. Complete resolution almost always occurs by 6 to 10 weeks following surgery.

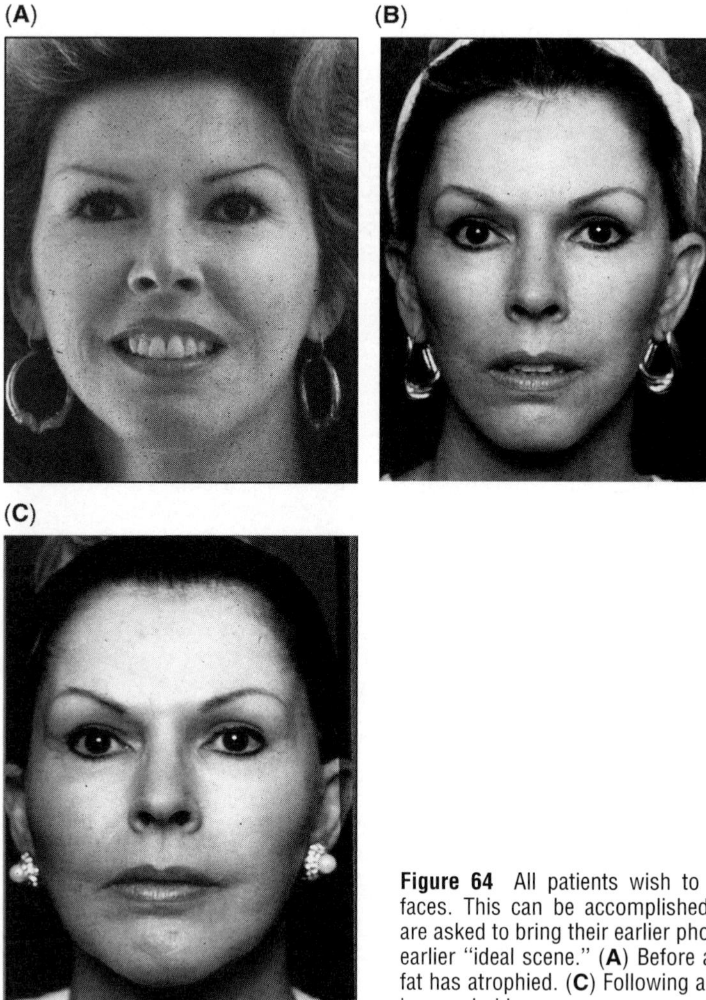

Figure 64 All patients wish to have youthful fullness return to their faces. This can be accomplished by alloplastic augmentation. Patients are asked to bring their earlier photographs in order to try to recover their earlier "ideal scene." (**A**) Before any surgery, age 29. (**B**) Age 40, facial fat has atrophied. (**C**) Following alloplastic volume replacement in cheek, jaw, and chin.

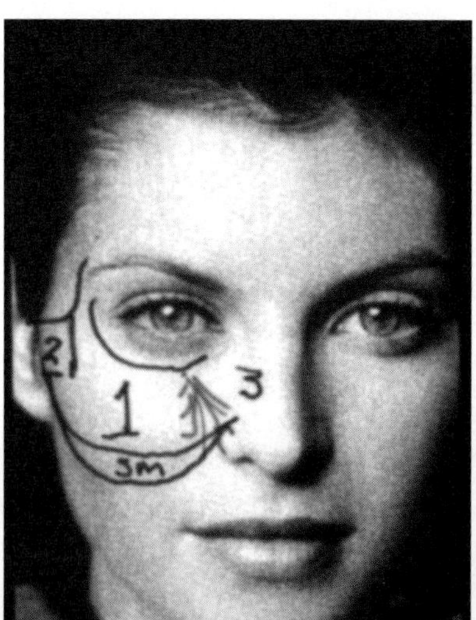

Figure 65 Zonal anatomy is drawn on both the patient's face and the magazine photos of their "ideal scene" to demonstrate how specific positioning of various size and shape implants alters the third dimension of a face in various ways.

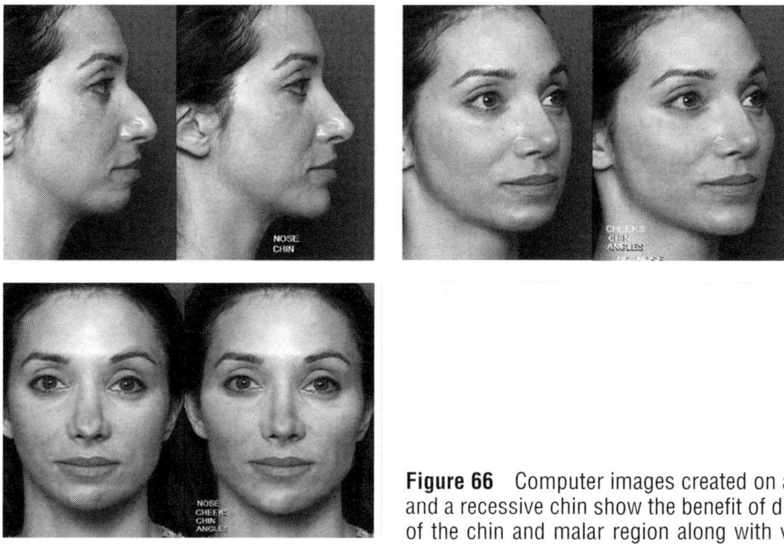

Figure 66 Computer images created on a patient with a prominent nose and a recessive chin show the benefit of differential volume augmentation of the chin and malar region along with volume reduction of the nose.

photographically superior to the image alterations made in the examining room during the consultation (Fig. 67).

Final planning is done on the morning of surgery before the patient is taken to the operating room or given any form of preoperative medication. The surgeon sits with the patient before the image computer and with the selected magazine photographs brought by the patient. Markings are made on the patient's face to outline the borders of the bony architecture and designate the facial zones of the midface and premandible regions (Fig. 68). Similar markings can be made on the magazine photographs. An interactive process then occurs, whereby the patient is asked to identify the specific zones that need to be altered by looking at the magazine photo drawings and their own facial markings in a mirror. Then, the implant size, surface area, and projection are discussed with the patient by placing implant "sizers" on the patient's cheek over the skin markings of the anatomic zone or zones, which the patient has selected. This way, the patient assists in the decision about which zone area and implant size is most suitable to accomplish his "ideal scene." The implications of various sizes and thicknesses of implants and how they would achieve subtle, conservative, or more dramatic appearances are also discussed with the patient.

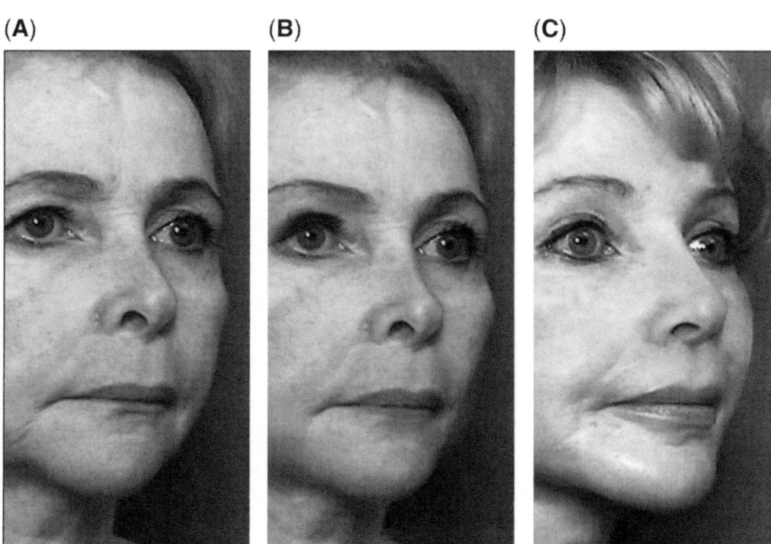

Figure 67 The final result of surgery one year post-op is superior to image alteration data on the computer. (**A**) Preop, (**B**) the computer image, and (**C**) one year post-op.

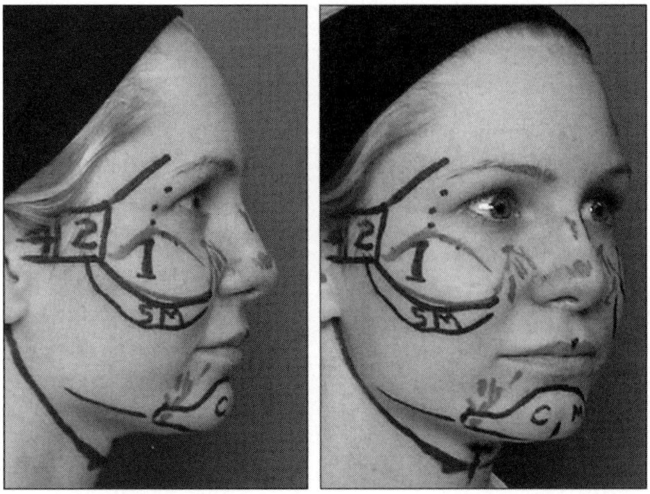

Figure 68 Preoperative markings are made on all patients' faces the morning of surgery to outline their zonal anatomy and bone structure.

A similar patient-doctor communication session with the computer and magazine images is used when augmenting the lower third of the face, chin, and jawline.

Once an implant is selected, the outline of its margins are drawn with red ink on the patient's face overlying the facial zone to be altered. During the surgical procedure, the inside anatomic skeletal landmarks are compared to the outside surface markings. This allows the surgeon to place implants precisely and is a method of ensuring much greater accuracy than any other means that the author has used. This type of preoperative assessment, evaluation, and patient education provides a greater precision and accuracy to the art of alloplastic facial augmentation than any other method. It applies equally in either primary or secondary procedures. Whether this regimen will continue to be the final and best in the future remains to be seen.

PHYSICAL EXAMINATION

In the author's practice physical examination is done with the aid of computer imaging to provide a more objective analysis of the patient's anatomic contours. Utilization of a mirror held by the patient is also necessary. One of the most important points in the physical examination is to identify precisely the various asymmetries that the patient's face has, as well as bone and soft tissues. It is imperative to get the patient to understand the severe limitations in correcting them (Fig. 69).

A fundamental and critical element in a consultation is to accurately define the patient's desires and goals. This is done by asking them to precisely describe changes they are looking for and in which anatomic regions. The surgeon must then be able to relate the patient's remarks to the anatomic zonal analysis data previously described. Patients are required to bring: (*i*) two sets of standard medical facial photos and (*ii*) most importantly, examples of contour ideals they want to emulate. This is done by having them choose images from magazines. It cannot be overemphasized that the selection and placement of implants is determined by directly comparing the anatomic zonal contours from their choice of images to the patient's own face.

ANESTHESIA

It has been learned from several thousand facial implant procedures that anesthesia is a critical factor in determining the safety and precision with which they can be accomplished (Table 2).

Two basic principles must be followed: First, the subperiosteal plane, as well as the subcutaneous layers must be infiltrated generously. A solution of dilute lidocaine and epinephrine is used. The epinephrine concentration is 1/800,000 and the lidocaine concentration is 0.125%. This is prepared by mixing 250 mL of 0.5% lidocaine containing 1/200,000 adrenaline with 750 mL of sterile normal saline (total volume 1000 cc).

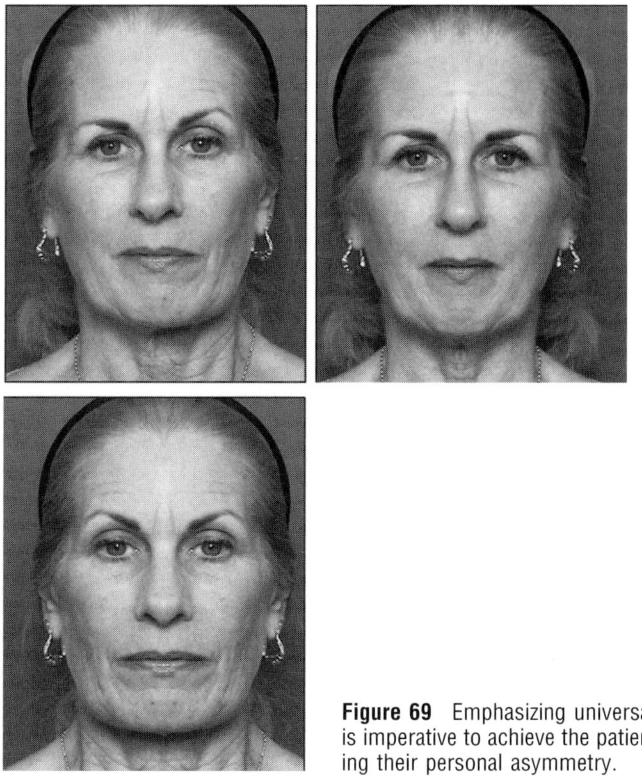

Figure 69 Emphasizing universal asymmetry on each and every patient's face is imperative to achieve the patient's understanding of the limitations in correcting their personal asymmetry.

Generous tumescent infiltration of up to 30 or 40 mL of this dilute lidocaine/epinephrine solution appears to create an increased interstitial pressure at the capillary level, which contributes to optimum hemostasis.

Secondly, all procedures are performed under general anesthesia making certain that the blood pressure is maintained at a systolic level of 90–110 mm of mercury. It can be consistently and predictably demonstrated that elevation of the blood pressure over this limit results in significant troublesome oozing and bleeding.

INCISION PLACEMENT

Incisions to approach the malar/midface and premandible regions are as follows:

There are several surgical approaches for augmenting the malar/midface space: (*i*) intraoral, (*ii*) lower blepharoplasty (subcilial), (*iii*) rhytidectomy, (*iv*) transcoronal, and (*v*) transconjunctival.

Intraoral route—The most traditional and commonly used approach for midface augmentation is the intraoral route. A 1.5-cm incision is made only through the mucosa. The excision is extended in an oblique upward direction over the anterior buttress of the maxilla just above the canine tooth (Fig. 70).

Table 2 Ideal Anesthesia for Alloplastic Facial Contouring

General anesthesia
Maintain blood pressure at 90–100 systolic
Clonidine, 2 mg orally preoperatively
Local anesthesia
Lidocaine solution 0.2%
Adrenalin 1:800,000
Generous tissue infiltration into malar or premandible space (20–30 mL each)

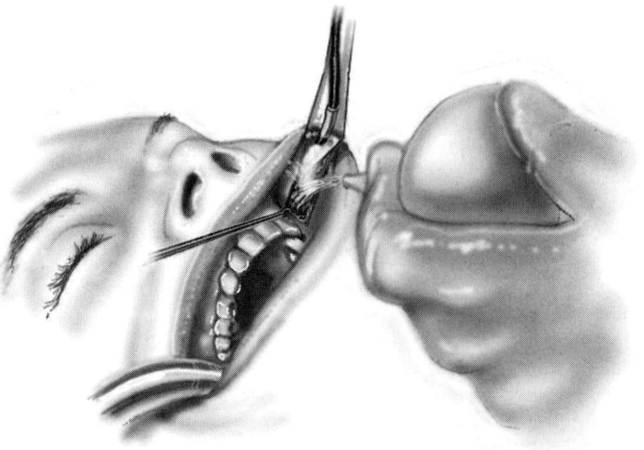

Figure 70 The intraoral approach to malar augmentation involves an oblique and a horizontal 1.5-cm incision just over the maxillary buttress and only through mucosa. Only dissection is subperiosteal. The dissection is through the lower border of the incision beneath the muscles and always remains on bone.

It is connected with another 1.5-cm horizontal incision made 1 cm above the gingival buccal sulcus, which is extended posterior to the premolar tooth. The dissection is initiated onto the bone only through the lower border of the incision and always remains on the bone.

A lower blepharoplasty incision can also be used by dissecting beneath a skin muscle flap onto the lower orbital bony margin and penetrating the SOOF layer in the lateral aspect of the orbit down to the bone. The midface Zone 1 area can be dissected subperiosteally from that location (Fig. 71).

If a rhytidectomy insertion is intended, a small penetration is made through the soft tissues over the lateral aspect of the malar bone at the junction with the zygomatic arch. This provides entrance into the subperiosteal malar space easily and in an area where no major facial nerve branches are endangered (Fig. 72).

When midface implants accompany a vertical subperiosteal midface suspension procedure the approach is variable and individualized. Sometimes only a subcilial incision is made and sometimes only an intraoral approach. For greater ease of access and implant placement, the surgeon may choose to use both approaches. Either way, the dissection must be extended

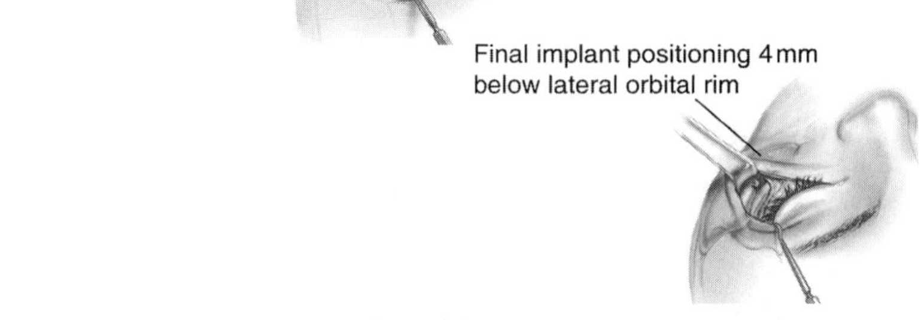

Figure 71 A subcilial lower eyelid incision is performed using a skin muscle flap down to inferior orbital bony margin and penetrating the periosteum and SOOF layer 4 mm below the orbital rim.

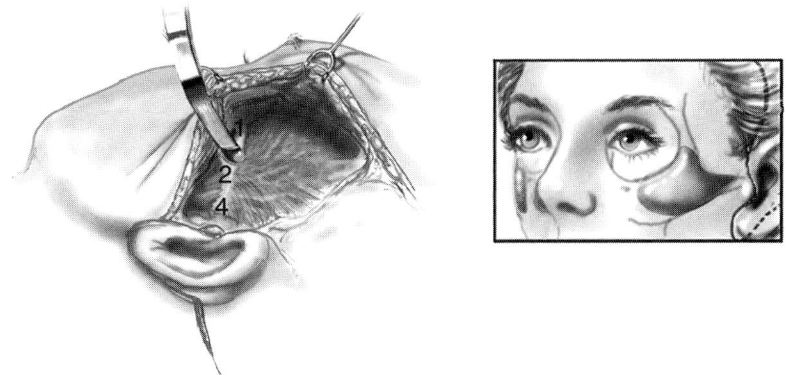

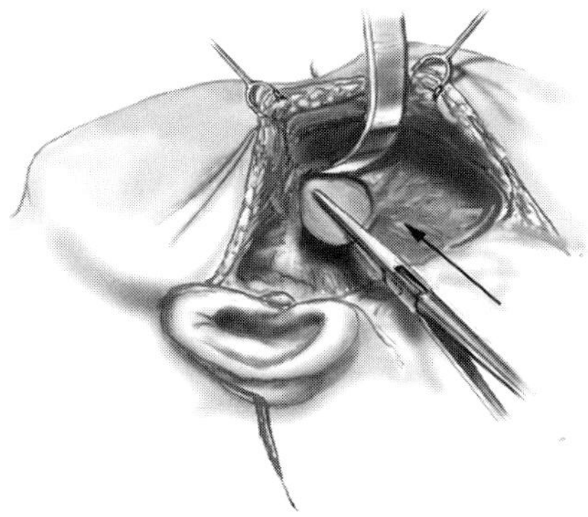

Figure 72 A rhytidectomy insertion of a malar implant is performed by penetrating the soft tissues at the lateral margin of Zone 1 and the medial margin of Zone 2 over the malar-zygomatic junction. The dissection is routinely performed on the subperiosteal plane. No facial nerve branches are endangered.

down into the submalar space all the way to the buccal fat pad and the gingival buccal sulcus (Fig. 73). This submalar extension gives a better cosmetic result by providing an increased ability to lift the midface by 2.5–3.5 cm (Figs. 74 and 75).

Premandible augmentation involves two types of incisions: (*i*) to augment the angle of mandible and (*ii*) to create the central mentum space for insertion of a central implant with

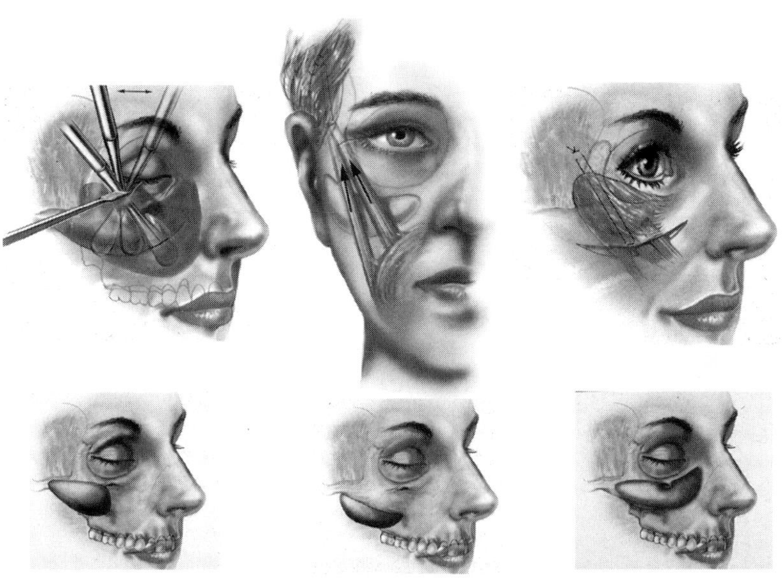

Figure 73 Vertical subperiosteal midface suspension. The surgical dissection involves degloving not only the maxilla but down over the masseter muscle to the buccal fat pad and the gingival buccal sulcus. Implants are easily positioned to improve deficiencies in Zones 1, 2, 3, and SM 5.

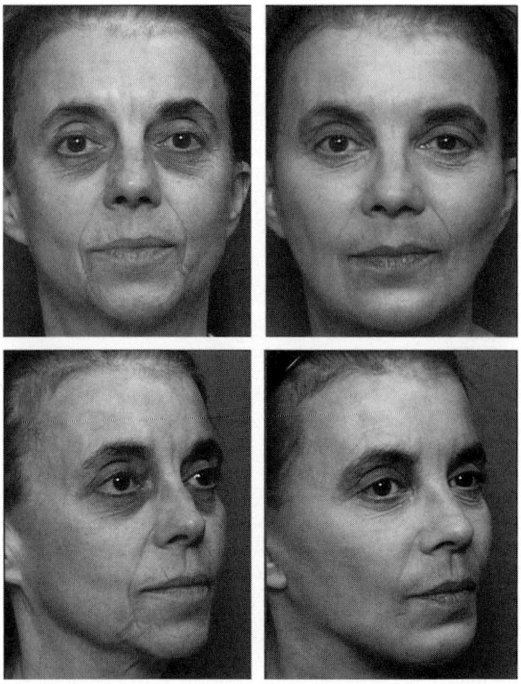

Figure 74 A 60-year-old female who underwent upper and midfacial suspension with malar augmentation, chin augmentation, and lower face and neck rhytidectomy. Photos on right are one year postoperative.

lateral anatomic extensions. The central mentum space can be approached from the intraoral route or with an incision in the submental crease. The submental crease incision is preferred whenever there is dissection into the neck either to remove fat or to manipulate and tighten the platysma muscle or both. This incision is approximately 2.5 cm in transverse length and penetrates directly down onto the lower border of the mandible. From that location a subperiosteal dissection is accomplished laterally in both directions (Fig. 76).The intraoral incision is a transverse mucosal incision of 2 cm only. This is placed 1 cm superior to the gingival labial

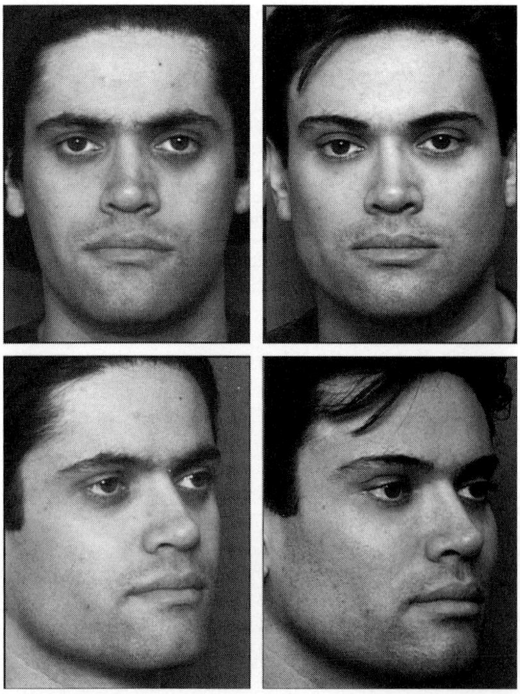

Figure 75 A 34-year-old male entertainer who underwent upper midface suspension along with malar, chin, mandibular angle augmentation, and lateral canthopexies to give him an eye shape which he desired. Right photos are one-year postoperative.

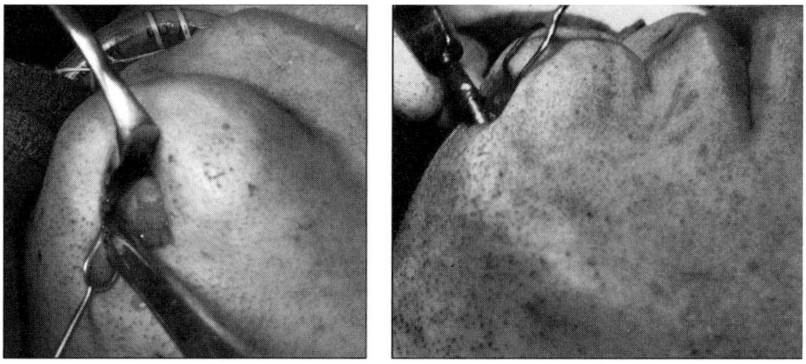

Figure 76 A submental incision is preferred for a generous jawline augmentation in the central mentum and midlateral zone. Dissection is along the lower border of the mandible below the margin of the mental nerve. It is subperiosteal.

sulcus. A vertical penetration is then made between the two pillars of the mentalis muscle. The mentalis muscle should never be transected because this maneuver can produce weakening and ptosis of the central chin mound. By dissecting vertically between the muscles and then developing the subperiosteal space inferior to them, the muscular support of the soft tissues chin mound is maintained.

In either dissection, the mental nerve should be located and identified. It generally is situated 8 to 12 mm above the inferior border of the mandible and between 2.5 and 3.5 cm from the midline of the central mandible. Extreme variations of these distances are reported although rare.

The posterior mandibular angle space is created by an incision made 1 cm anterior to the molar teeth in the gingival buccal sulcus and extending it laterally 3 cm. A sturdy 1-cm layer of mucosa and muscle must be preserved to enable a secure closure. The dissection is then immediately directed onto the bone. The soft tissues elevate very easily from the inferior border and ascending ramus of the mandible. At the angle itself, there may be tendinous attachments of the masseter muscle, especially in male patients. These may need lysis with an electrocautery needle to enable the muscles to be disinserted from the angle and posterior border of the mandible.

It is critical, however, to disinsert the fibrous attachments at the angle and the posterior border completely so that the implant will seat correctly in position. The masseter muscle itself

Implant Choices Malar–Midface Augmentation, Regional Volume–Mass Deficiencies, Anatomic Zone Augmentation Size

Facial type	Anatomic augmentation zone	Size (depends on skull size)
1	1 and 2	3 or 4 mm (occasionally 5 or 6 mm)
2	SM 5	4 or 5 mm (possibly a combined shell)
3	SM 5	5 or 6 mm (Large or extra large)
4	1, 2, SM 5	5 or 6 mm malar shell (Large or extra large)
5	3	Tear trough implant (small, medium or large)
6	Premaxilla	Various premaxilla implants brink implant[a]

Implant Choices Premandible Augmentation, Regional (Zonal) Volume–Mass Deficiencies

Zone	Implant[a] (depends on face size)
Central mentum (CM)	Anatomic or styles 1 and 2 4–9 mm
Posteriolateral (PL)	Mandibular angle implants 8–12 mm lateral projection
Midlateral (ML)	Lateral bars 4–6 mm to widen lateral jawline
Submandibular (SM)	Vertical extension implant 4 mm implant inferior and anterior projection

[a]Implantech Corporation, Ventura, California, U.S.A.

is quite thick and strong and will hold it in proper position without fixation. Malpositions and extrusions are rare when the PL space is dissected properly (Fig. 46).

A long, curved clamp is placed on the implant to facilitate the posterior and upward placement of the implant.

A peripyriform premaxillary implant is inserted through a single 4- to 5-mm nasal floor incision, although one on each side may be used if necessary. An intraoral incision in the superior labial sulcus is to be avoided because it may predispose to implant erosion through that area. The plane of dissection is developed deep to the orbicularis oris muscle to create a subperiosteal pocket for the implant.

FACIAL SKIN MARKINGS

On the morning of surgery, markings are made with ink on either the midface or the lower facial segment or both, depending in which location alloplastic augmentation will be performed. The markings are made to outline the borders of the malar bone and zygomatic arch and to demonstrate the five zones of the midface, including the submalar zone. Similar markings are made in the lower jaw area to completely outline the mandible centrally and posteriorly. Once again the three bony zones of the mandible and the submandibular zone are outlined.

The implant size and shape is then chosen by the surgeon and the patient together. It is placed on the skin overlying the exact anatomic zonal region that has been selected to augment. The implant is outlined in red marking ink so that the surgeon may compare the internal anatomy to the external anatomy during surgery as the implant is being positioned.

Tear trough implants can be placed through an external subcilial blepharoplasty incision, a transconjunctival incision, or an intraoral route. The most important consideration is to carefully dissect around the infraorbital nerve under direct visualization to prevent nerve trauma and subsequent disabling symptoms. The tear trough implant is placed after cutting out a segment, which allows it to surround the main trunk of the infraorbital nerve. If desired, it can be secured by one or two stitches to the medial orbicularis muscles or to the inferior orbital rim.

POSTOPERATIVE CARE

Postoperative care for facial implants is straightforward and uncomplicated. Perioperative oral antibiotics are utilized. At the present time cephalosporins are favored. Prior to the start of surgery 1 g of Ancef is given intravenously by the anesthesiologist. Decadron (10 mg) is also given intravenously during the surgery to control postoperative edema. During the postoperative period a five-day diminishing course of steroid in the form of a Medrol dose pack is taken orally. For the first 12 hours cold compresses are applied intermittently to the operative site either in the midface or premandible region. No bandages are used. Removal of intraoral mucosal and external subcuticular sutures is unnecessary. A soft diet is maintained for 10 days. It is highly recommended that the patient recline at a 45° angle and in the supine position for at least one week. Vigorous physical activity is not permitted for four weeks, after which patients may engage in any and all types of exercise activities.

TECHNIQUE ESSENTIALS

1. Always perform the anatomic space dissection directly on the bone and beneath the periosteum.
2. Maintain the dissecting elevator on bone at all times.
3. Never push the tip of an elevator into adjacent soft tissues. This can create severe trauma to the facial nerve, infraorbital nerve, and/or zygomaticus muscles disturbing facial expression in the malar/midface region. In the perioral and mandibular regions traumatic dissection into the soft tissues can produce mental nerve or marginal mandibular nerve damage, and even mimetic muscle dysfunction. Potential dangers in posterior angle dissections involve trauma to a large retromandibular vein behind the posterior border of the mandible or to the anterior facial artery just adjacent to the inferior border of the mandible. Disruption of these would produce profuse hemorrhage.

4. External palpation of the lower mandibular border with the index finger facilitates an accurate and controlled dissection beneath the mental nerve as well as protecting the inferior soft tissues and marginal branch of the VII nerve.
5. Manual palpation externally over the malar region facilitates a precise dissection of the malar space beneath the external preoperative ink markings on the midface skin. A small hockey-stick incision with 1.5-cm limbs will facilitate a wide midfacial premaxillary and submalar dissection. Once again, the entry point should be beneath the muscles and onto the bone of the anterior maxillary buttress.
6. The intraoral chin space dissection should be done vertically between the mentalis muscle pillars to go beneath the muscle and onto the bone without transecting or damaging the mentalis muscle, which can produce central chin ptosis.
7. All intraoral incisions should have a secure muscle and mucosal closure to prevent entrance of bacteria or wound dehiscence.
8. Intermittent irrigations with copious amounts of antibiotic solution should be performed inside the anatomic zonal spaces during the surgery.
9. A "no-touch" technique should be meticulously enforced when inserting implants. This is done by placing a clamp on the implant and immersing it in a Betadine and antibiotic solution before inserting it gently into the soft-tissue anatomic space aperture.
10. Implants should be inserted as gently and atraumatically as possible. Finger manipulations are to be avoided. Silicone rubber implants have the advantage of being extremely flexible and therefore easily insertable or removable.

SUMMARY

Alloplastic augmentation of the facial skeleton produces three-dimensional soft tissue and skeletal contour "balance" which represents the final chapter in *Asthetic Surgery of the Face.*

REFERENCES

1. Guerrerosantos J, . The role of the platysma muscle in rhytidoplasty. Chin Plast Surg 1978; 5:29.
2. Hamra ST, . The zigorbicular dissection in composite rhytidectomy: an ideal midface plane. Plast Recontr Surg 1998; 102(5):1646–1657.
3. Hinderer U. Malar implants for improvement of the facial appearance. Plast Reconstr Surg 1975; 56:157.
4. Hester TR, Codner MA, McCord CD. The centrofacial approach for correction of facial aging using the transblepharoplasty subperiosteal cheek lift. Aesthetic J Spring 1996:52–57.
5. Jelks GW, Jelks EB. Chapter 5. In: Complications and Problems in Aesthetic Plastic SurgeryPeck GCGower Medical PublishersLondon1992.
6. Lilla JA, Vistnes LM, Jobe RP. The long-term effects of hard alloplastic implants when put on bone. Plast Reconstr Surg 1976; 58:14.
7. Pitanguy I. Augmentation mentoplasty. Plast Reconstr Surg 1968; 42:441.
8. Ramirez OM. The subperiosteal rhytidectomy: the third generation face lift. Ann Plast Surg 1992; 28:218.
9. Serman NJ. Differentiations of double mental foramina mandibular nerve: anatomic study. Dental Med 1987; 5(3):20–21.
10. Terino EO. Complications of chin and malar augmentations. In: Complications and Problems in Aesthetic Plastic SurgeryPeck GGower Medical PublishersNew York1991.
11. Terino EO. Alloplastic facial contouring: surgery of the fourth plane. Aesth Plast Surg 1992; 16:195–212.
12. Terino EO. Unique mandibular implants including lateral and posterior angle implants. Facial Plast Surg Clin N Am 1994; 2(3):311–328.
13. Terino EO. Three-dimensional facial contouring: utilizing upper-midface suspension technology and alloplastic augmentation. Facial Plast Surg 2003; 2:19.
14. Terino EO. Three-dimensional facial contouring: alloplastic augmentation of the lateral mandible. Facial Plast Surg Clin N Am 2002; 10:249–264.
15. Tolleth H. Concepts for the plastic surgeon from art and sculpture. In: Facial Aesthetic Surgery: Art, Anatomy, Anthropometrics and Imaging. Clin Plast Surg 1987; 14(4):585–598; Philadelphia: WB Saunders, 1987:585–598..

2 Facial Cosmetic Surgery: Personal Contributions

Ivo Pitanguy
Department of Plastic Surgery, Pontifical Catholic University of Rio de Janeiro and The Carlos Chagas Institute of Post-Graduate Medical Studies, Rio de Janeiro, Brazil

INTRODUCTION

Beauty is intrinsically related to the search for harmony, and is a powerful means of achieving intimate well-being. Throughout the history of mankind, great value has been given to beauty in objects and people. Self-esteem is enhanced when an individual feels he or she externalizes an image of youthfulness, vitality, and health. Inevitably, aging brings about changes that are undesirable. The face, due to its exposure and expression and the constant action of gravity, is frequently the main focus of anxiety in individuals who have attained a certain age. Patients will seek the plastic surgeon to correct these anatomical alterations.

Senescence brings about skin flaccidity, marked lines of expression, and loss of fat deposits. These are the typical objective factors that lead the patient to desire a facial rejuvenation procedure. Anatomy of the aging face should be examined carefully, each area separately and as a whole, so as to allow for a personalized treatment plan.

On the other hand, motivations for surgery for the aging face are generally deeply hidden, and may include aspects in the personal, social, and professional realms. Experience is necessary to investigate and appreciate these subjective motivations. This evaluation requires both empathy and openness toward the patient.

Facial aesthetic surgery witnessed enormous progress in the second half of the last century. Consequently, expectations have increased considerably on the part of the patients. The surgeon must be knowledgable in details of different surgical approaches and variations thereof to attain the best result for each individual case. A satisfactory outcome of an aesthetic facial procedure is obtained when signs of an operation are undetectable and anatomy has been preserved.

The author's personal approach to surgical treatment of the aging face will be presented in this chapter, citing principles that have offered consistent and satisfactory results in over 40 years of experience. Patient assessment is discussed and technical aspects detailed and illustrated. Emphasis is given to the correct traction applied to the facial flaps (the "round-lifting" technique) and the forehead ("block" lifting), assuring that all anatomical landmarks are precisely preserved. Finally, complementary surgical procedures that may be useful are presented, with a brief discussion of indications (1–21).

THE ROUND-LIFTING TECHNIQUE

Rhytidoplasty is one of the most frequently performed surgeries in the author's private practice. A total of 7868 personal consecutive cases have been analyzed to date (Fig. 1). More recently, a noticeable increase in male patients has been noted. In the 1970s, men represented 6% of face-lifting procedures; in the 1980s, approximately 15%; currently, 20% of face-lift patients are men (Fig. 2).

After appropriate intravenous sedation and prepping, local infiltration is performed. The standard incision is demarcated, beginning in the temporal scalp, and proceeds in the preauricular area in such a way as to respect the anatomical curvature of this region. The incision then follows around the earlobe, in a curving fashion, and finishes in the cervical scalp (Fig. 3). (This S-shaped incision creates an advancement flap that prevents a step-off in the hairline, allowing the patient to wear her hair up without revealing the scar.)

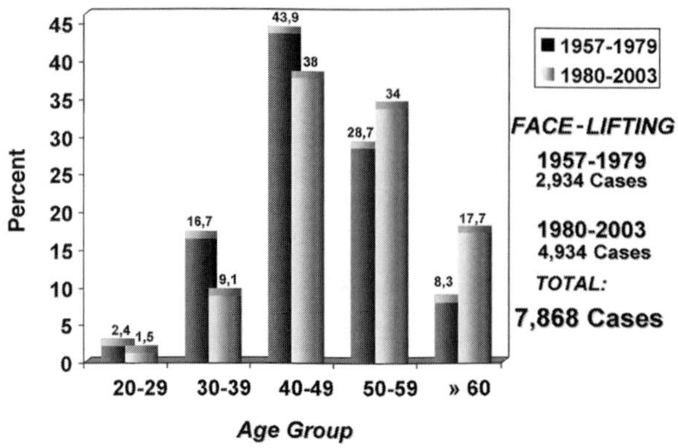

Figure 1 Age distribution of face-lift patients in the Ivo Pitanguy Clinic, 1951–2003.

Secondary rhytidoplasties require variations of this incision, which are chosen depending on each case, with the following goals in mind: treatment of specific regions with redistribution of skin flaps, resection of previous scars, and maintenance of anatomical landmarks. An earlier publication has established the indications and advantages of each different incision.

Undermining of the facial and cervical flaps is performed in a subcutaneous plane, the extension of which is variable and individualized for each case. A danger area lies beneath the non–hair–bearing skin over the temples, which we have called "no man's land," where most of the temporofrontal branches of the facial nerve are more frequently found. Dissection over "no man's land" should be superficial, and hemostasis carefully performed, if at all. Larger vessels should be tied (Fig. 4).

The treatment of the very heavy, fatty neck requires that the dissection proceed all the way to the other side under the mandible. With the advent of suction-assisted lipectomy, submental lipodystrophy is mostly addressed by liposuction, in a crisscross fashion (Fig. 5). Sometimes this is still done with direct lipectomy using specially designed scissors, defatting the submental region, as has been described historically. Following this, treatment of medial platysmal bands is carried out under direct vision. Approximation of diastasis is done with interrupted sutures, plicating down to the level of the hyoid bone.

Undermining of the facial flaps is extended over the zygomatic prominence to free the retaining ligaments of the cheek. Dissection of the deeper elements of the face has evolved over the past 20 years. Almost no treatment was advocated before the publications that first described the superficial muscle-apponeurotic system (SMAS). Approach to this structure has been a topic of much discussion. It is our preference to determine whether to dissect or simply plicate the SMAS after subcutaneous dissection has been completed. Pulling of the SMAS is done, noting the effects on the skin.

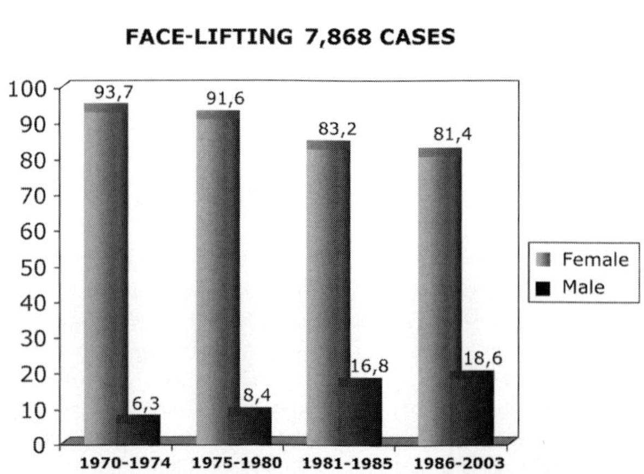

Figure 2 Distribution of face-lift patients, by gender, in the last three decades, in the Ivo Pitanguy Clinic.

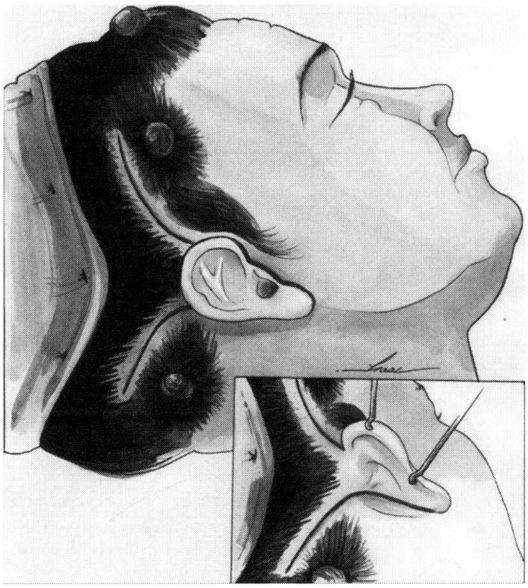

Figure 3 The classical incision, as described for the round-lifting, curves around the anatomical landmarks, and finishes in a sinuous italic S in the cervical scalp.

We have noticed that, although extensive undermining of the SMAS was performed in an earlier period, plication of this structure in the same direction as the skin flaps, with repositioning of the malar fat pad, has given a more satisfactory and natural result (Fig. 6). The durability of this maneuver is relative to the individual aging process. Tension on the musculoaponeurotic system allows support of the subcutaneous layers, corrects the sagging cheek, and reduces tension on the skin flap.

Techniques that treat the pronounced nasolabial fold include either the traction of skin flaps, SMAS, or fascial fatty layer, with variable results. Filling with different substances may also be done at the end of surgery, either with fat grafting or other material. Direct excision of the nasolabial fold is reserved for the older male patient. This technique gives a definite solution to the nasolabial fold, with a barely noticeable scar that mimics the nasolabial fold itself.

The direction of traction of the skin flaps is a fundamental aspect of the "round-lifting" technique. In this manner, the undermined flaps are rotated rather than simply pulled, acting in a direction opposite to that of aging, and assuring a repositioning of tissues with preservation

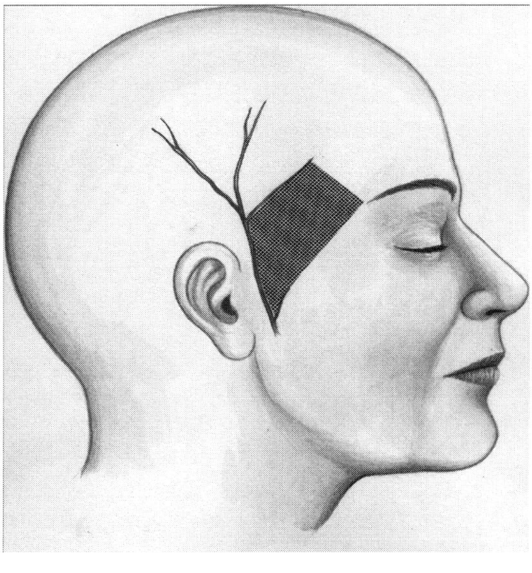

Figure 4 The variation in the anatomical distribution of the frontal branch of the facial nerve determines an area called "no man's land," where this nerve is particularly vulnerable to lesion by electrocoagulation.

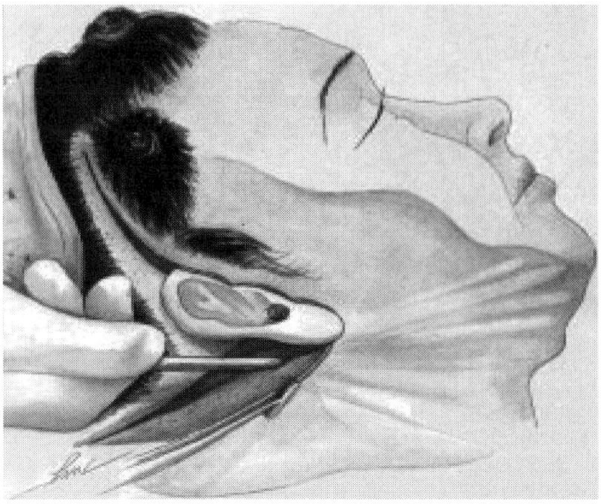

Figure 5 Liposuction has been useful to complement a face-lift and permits the removal of fatty tissue from the cervical region. This maneuver should be done in a criss-cross fashion to assure an even plane of subcutaneous tissue.

of anatomical landmarks. A second advantage in establishing a precise vector of rotation is that the opposite side is repositioned in the exact manner.

This vector connects the tragus to Darwin's tubercle for the facial or anterior flap. A Pitanguy flap demarcator is placed at the root of the helix and, following precise traction, point *A* is marked on the skin flap (Fig. 7). The edge of the flap is then incised along a curved line crossing the supra-auricular hairline so that bald skin, not pilose, is resected. A key suture is located here.

Likewise, the cervical flap should also be pulled in an equally precise manner, in a superior and slightly anterior vector, to avoid a step-off of the hairline. Key stitches are placed to anchor the flap along the pilose scalp at point B so that there is no tension on the thin skin at the peak of the retroauricular incision.

Only when the temporary sutures have been placed will excess facial skin be resected. Skin is accommodated and demarcated along the natural curves, with no tension whatsoever (Fig. 8). Final scars are thus not displaced or widened. The tragus is preserved in its anatomical position, and the fine skin along its edge is trimmed so as to perfectly match the region.

When performing a brow-lift, placing these key sutures at points A and B is mandatory before any traction is applied to the forehead flap, essentially "blocking" the facial flaps (Clinical Cases 1–5; Figs. 9–13).

The effects of the "round-lifting" technique have been studied by analyzing the mechanical forces applied and the displacements produced. The Method of Finite Elements was

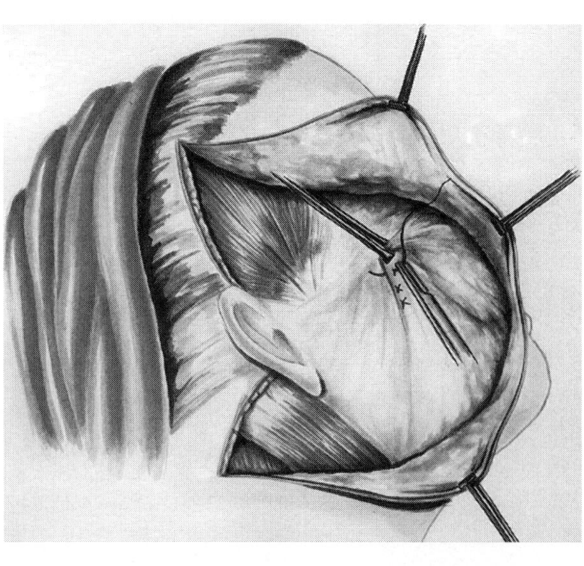

Figure 6 Repositioning of the malar pad is done after subcutaneous dissection has been completed.

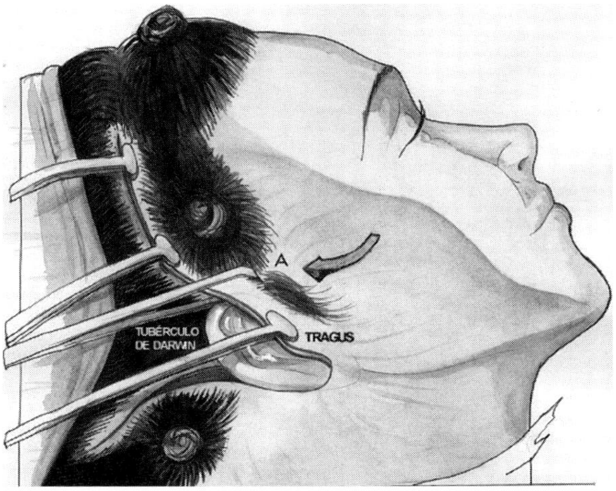

Figure 7 The direction of traction of the anterior or facial flap follows a vector that connects the tragus to Darwin's tubercle. Excess tissue is marked with a Pitanguy flap demarcator.

employed and, by means of computers, the relevant equations were defined. Human skin was modeled as a pseudo-elastic, isotropic, noncompressible, and homogeneous membrane, and a computational study of the fields of displacement and the forces applied to the flaps during a rhytidoplasty demonstrated that the direction of traction creates areas of tension, which can be either negative or positive. These forces ultimately result in the correction of signs of aging. The vectors described in the "round-lifting" technique address both the main features that suffer distortion with aging and maintaining anatomical parameters. Although there were limits due to the variety of factors involved because of the complexities of human skin (basic properties and individual variations) the study holds a close parallel to a real surgical procedure.

FOREHEAD-LIFTING

Aging in the upper face becomes evident with a descent in the level of the eyebrow and the appearance of wrinkles and furrows, sometimes from an early age. These are a direct consequence of muscle dynamics, responsible for the multitude of expressions so characteristic of man, and loss of skin tone. Elements of the upper face that must be considered preoperatively for any procedure are: the length of the forehead and the elasticity of the skin; muscle force and wrinkles; the position of the anterior hairline; and the quality and quantity of hair.

An important decision to be made regarding a brow-lift is the placement of incisions. There are basically two classical approaches: the bicoronal incision and limited, prepilose incisions. The first allows for treatment of all elements that determine the aging forehead while

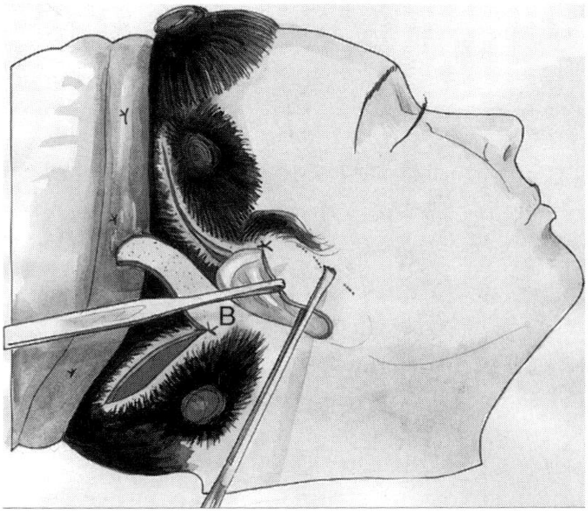

Figure 8 The posterior flap has been rotated and fixed at point B, with a strong suture placed behind the ear. Excess facial skin is demarcated with no tension on the flap.

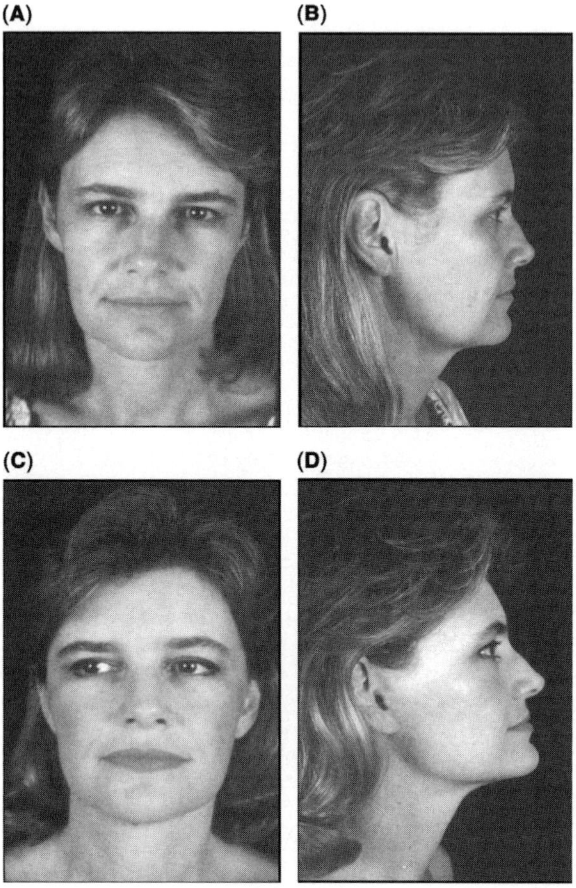

Figure 9 A round-lifting procedure was performed on this 41-year-old woman, with a simple plication of the SMAS. (**A**, **B**) The patient is seen preoperatively. (**C**, **D**) The patient is seen at 18 months follow-up.

hiding the final scar within the hairline. Certain situations, however, preclude this incision. Patients with a very long forehead or those that have already been submitted to previous surgery will have an excessively recessed hairline if the forehead is further pulled back. The final aspect will be displeasing giving the patient a permanent look of surprise.

The second approach is the juxtapilose incision, performed when the patient presents with ptosis of lateral eyebrow and scant lines of expression of the forehead itself. The short distance required to reach the eyebrow region is easily performed by subperiosteal blunt dissection.

Endoscopical instrumentation has permitted treatment of the brow through minimal access, and has proved useful in select cases.

Major advantages of the bicoronal approach are a wide exposure of the forehead flap, which allows for weakening the muscles that act in this region by a method of multiple incisions, freeing the muscle fibers. The entire upper third of the face is undermined in a subgaleal plane until the orbital ridges are reached. In patients where the aging process has resulted in a drooping nose, the nasal tip and the membranous septum can be manipulated by dissecting with a long scissors in a subcutaneous plane, starting at the root of the nose. A rotation of the scissors tip will section the dermocartilaginous ligament of the nose. This structure, described by the author, tends to hold the nasal tip downward. Once it has been interrupted, the tip of the nose assumes a slightly more superior position.

For the release of the supraorbital region, when correction of a ptotic eyebrow is indicated, the periosteum is incised along the supraorbital rim and blunt dissection is carried over the rim for approximately 1 cm, preserving the supraorbital neurovascular bundle.

The "frontalis-procerus-corrugator aponeurotic expansion" is a structure that spreads over the entire upper third of the face, uniting the frontalis, procerus, and corrugator muscles, as described by the author. By dividing its fibers, weakening of the forehead is obtained,

(A) (B)
(C) (D)

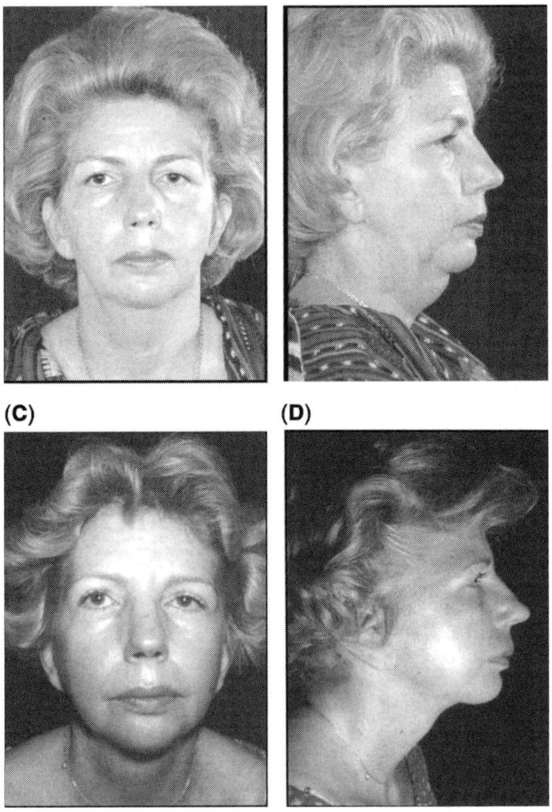

Figure 10 Submental lipectomy was a primary concern in this 58-year-old patient. This was done by ample liposuction, together with a round-lifting technique to reposition facial and cervical tissues. (**A**, **B**) The patient is seen preoperatively. (**C**, **D**) The patient is seen at two years' follow-up.

(A) (B)

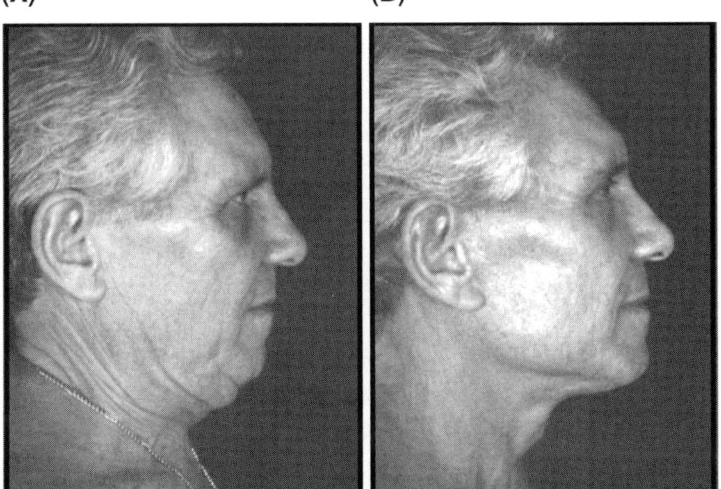

Figure 11 Male patients are seen more frequently in the office of the plastic surgeon, and many seek rejuvenation procedures. This 63-year-old man was submitted to a face-lift with blepharoplasty, with special attention given to correction of platysmal bands. (**A**) The patient is seen preoperatively. (**B**) The patient is seen at two years' follow-up.

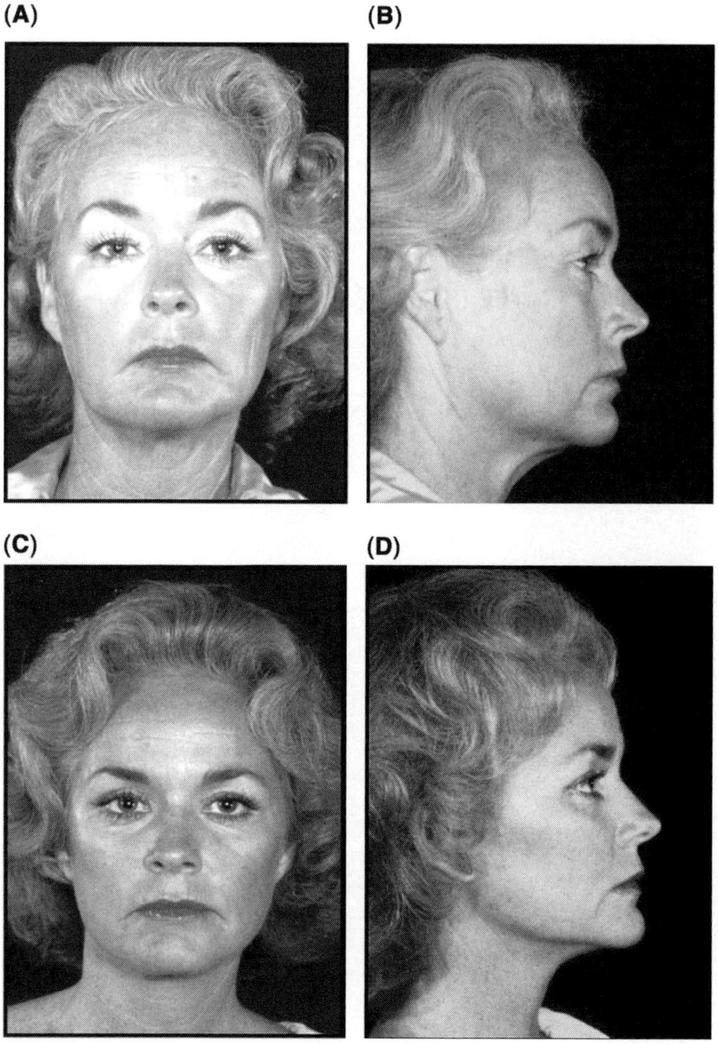

Figure 12 This 66-year-old patient presented with cervicofacial flaccidity and furrows of the upper face. She was submitted to a round-lifting technique with treatment of platysmal bands, and a forehead-lifting. Notice that the height of the forehead was not increased. (**A**, **B**) Preoperative view. (**C**, **D**) The patient is seen at one year follow-up.

smoothing the lines of expression. This is done in a crisscross fashion, without excision of tissue, so as to avoid surface irregularity.

Having "blocked" the facial flaps at points A and B, as described above, the forehead may be pulled in any direction, either straight backwards, or more laterally (Fig. 14). The amount of scalp flap to be resected is determined by the length of the forehead and the effect that traction causes on the level of the eyebrow. The midline is positioned, demarcated, incised, and blocked with a temporary suture. Sometimes no traction is necessary and no scalp is removed in the midline. Two symmetrical flaps are created, and lateral resection can now be performed allowing the eyebrow to be raised as necessary (Fig. 15).

Ptosis of the eyebrow is an element that may cause aging of the upper third of the face. Correction of the level of the brow to a more elevated position has classically been undertaken by a large, bicoronal incision, as described previously. A less aggressive approach is the reduced prepilose lateral incision or juxtapilose incision, performed when the patient presents with ptosis of lateral eyebrow and scant lines of expression on the forehead itself. The short distance required to reach the eyebrow region is easily performed by subperiosteal blunt dissection (Fig. 16).

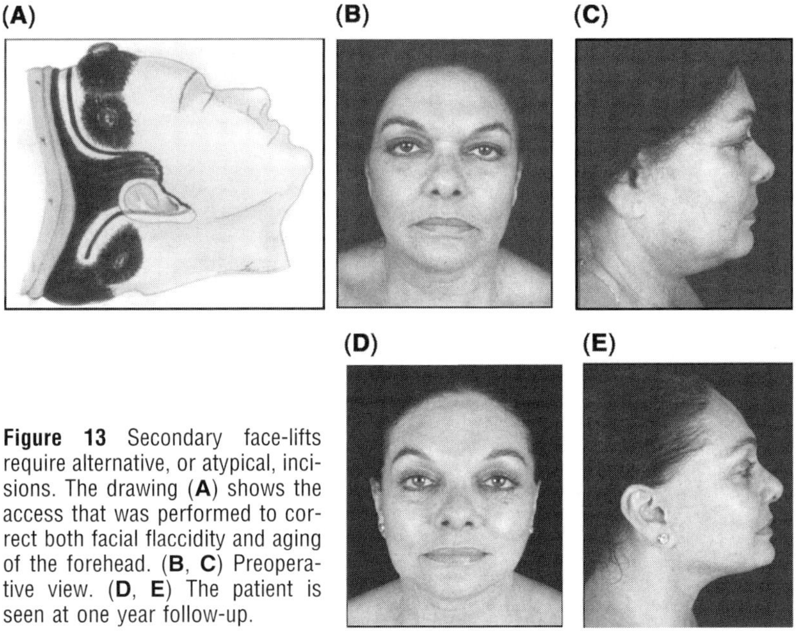

Figure 13 Secondary face-lifts require alternative, or atypical, incisions. The drawing (**A**) shows the access that was performed to correct both facial flaccidity and aging of the forehead. (**B**, **C**) Preoperative view. (**D**, **E**) The patient is seen at one year follow-up.

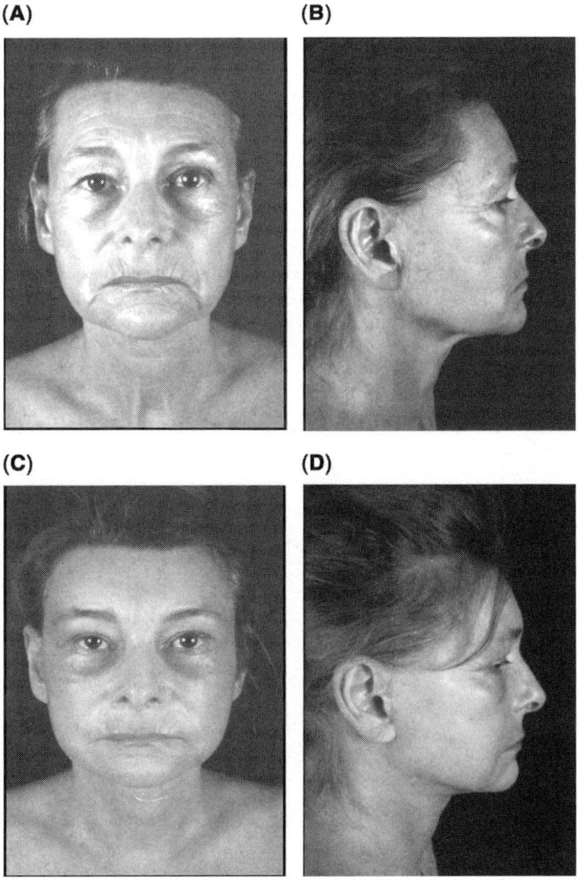

Figure 14 Correction of the aging face was done together with elevation of the lateral third of the eyebrow, through a juxtapilose incision. This 50-year-old patient is seen before and one year following the surgical procedure. (**A**, **B**) Preoperative view. (**C**, **D**) Postoperatively.

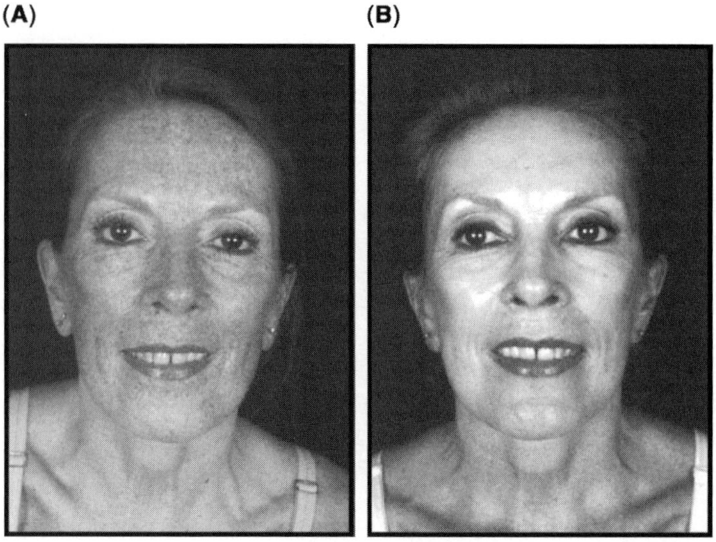

Figure 15 Laser skin resurfacing is an excellent adjunct to face-lifting, or can be indicated as a single procedure. Laser resurfacing was done on this 59-year-old patient; she is seen before (**A**) and one year following the procedure (**B**).

Complications in rhytidoplasty are infrequent, yet can bring great distress to the patient and to the surgeon. It is essential to eliminate patients who continue to smoke, as the risk for skin slough is greatly increased. Smoking must be stopped completely at least two weeks in advance. In the immediate postoperative period, blood pressure must be constantly monitored by the nursing staff, to prevent hypertension and consequently hematoma formation. If an expansive hematoma is diagnosed, the surgeon may initially attempt to drain the collection at the bedside. Early identification and treatment of large hematomas is essential to prevent sequela. Nerve injuries, dehiscence and other complications are infrequent and should be treated conservatively.

ANCILLARY PROCEDURES

Several surgical techniques are part of the armamentarium that a surgeon should have to enhance the result of a rhytidoplasty. These procedures may be complementary to the face-lift, or may be indicated by themselves. Three of the more frequently performed procedures will be summarized.

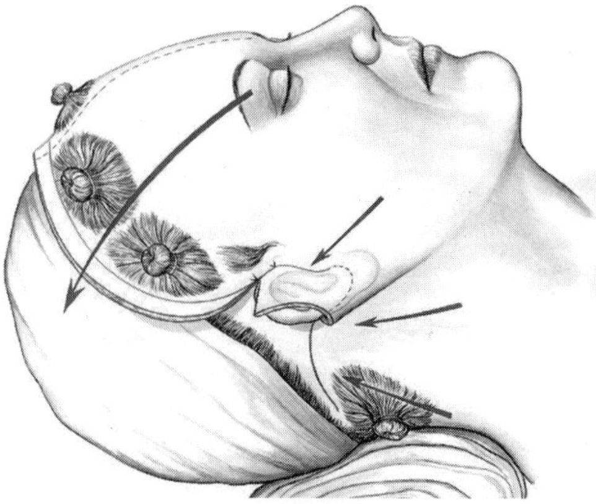

Figure 16 Positioning of the forehead flap is only done after the facial flaps have been rotated and "blocked." This avoids excessive elevation of the facial tissues and alteration of the hairline.

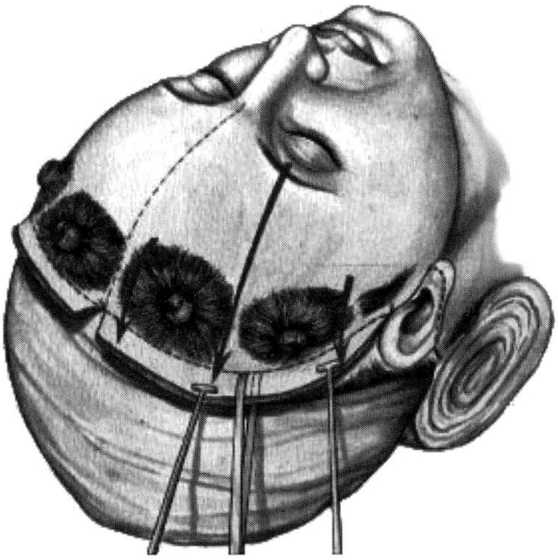

Figure 17 The midline of the forehead flap is fixed, and each lateral flap is tractioned according to the amount of correction required.

Blepharoplasty

Although changes around the eyes generally accompany the aging process of the face, it is not uncommon to observe younger patients with excess skin and baggy lower lids. There are several important points that should be emphasized regarding surgical technique. Final scars should be well hidden, lying in the supratarsal fold in the upper lids, and along the ciliary margin in the lower lids. The incision should never extend beyond the orbital rim because of the difference in thickness between these two regions. Because of the advent of laser resurfacing, there has been an increase in the transconjunctival access for removal of fat pads of the lower lids.

When associated with a face-lift and/or forehead-lift, as is generally the case, treatment of the palpebral region is done only after the face and the brow have been "blocked," as traction of the flaps may alter the amount of excess skin that needs to be removed. The shape of the incision is tailored to each patient, matching the individual's anatomical features, and correcting for asymmetry when this is present. Both sides are demarcated before any infiltration is performed.

Fat pouches are treated by clamping excess pads as they bulge out spontaneously. Care should be taken to avoid removing too much fat, because this will result in a sunken appearance. Cutaneous resection of the lower eyelids must be parsimonious. Skin is readapted, rather than removed, after undermining. The surgeon should not hesitate in reinforcing the lower eyelid with a canthopexy procedure if there is any looseness, which might result in scleral show.

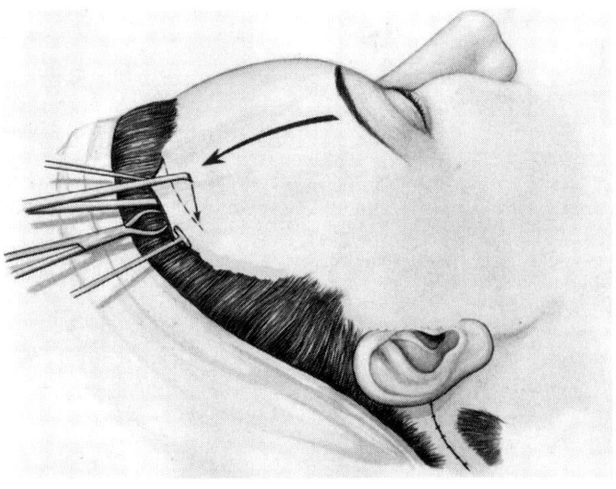

Figure 18 Correction of the level of the brow to a more elevated position may be done by the juxtapilose incision, with a subperiosteal blunt dissection.

The Aging Lip

The full, sensuous lip is a much desired feature of a young face. Loss of vermilion definition denotes aging, as does lengthening of the upper lip and the presence of radial lines. These aspects require specific attention, as they are not corrected by traction of facial flaps. Traditional methods include planing of the skin, and surgery for increasing of the vermilion and shortening of the height of the upper lip.

Elimination of skin rhytids along the upper lip remains a challenge. Peeling with chemical substances has been favorably reported by other authors. Laser resurfacing offers good results, yet mechanical abrasion should not be abandoned. Dermabrasion has the following advantages: it is a relatively simple procedure, requiring unsophisticated equipment, and causing few postoperative restrictions.

Enlargement and definition of the vermilion is achieved by resection of skin above the mucocutaneous border, and results in a scar that softens with time. Repositioning of the vermilion also decreases the vertical length of the upper lip. Although less frequent, the same procedure may be performed on the lower lip.

Laser Resurfacing

Laser resurfacing is a safe and efficient procedure, when performed by an experienced medical team and when all clinical and technical aspects are understood. The depth of peeling must be absolutely controlled by the surgeon, and this requires training and experience. Laser peeling is an ancillary procedure that enhances surgery for the aging face. In some cases, resurfacing by laser alone may produce tightening of the skin and elimination of rhytids with very satisfactory results. It is important to mention that laser resurfacing requires a long absence of social activities due to prolonged erythema, and the patient should be made aware of this limitation.

ACKNOWLEDGMENT

The author is grateful to Henrique N. Radwanski, M.D., for his close collaboration in the preparation of this chapter.

REFERENCES

1. Pitanguy I, Ramos A. The frontal branch of the facial nerve: the importance of its variation in the face-lifting. Plast Reconstr Surg 1966; 38:352–356.
2. Pitanguy I. Ancillary procedures in face-lifting. Clin Plast Surg 1978; 5:51–69.
3. Pitanguy I. Frontalis-procerus-corrugator aponeurosis in the correction of frontal and glabellar wrinkles. Ann Plast Surg 1979; 2:422–427.
4. Pitanguy I. The aging face. In: Carlsen L, Slatt B, eds. The Naked Face. Ontario: General Publishing, 1979:27.
5. Pitanguy I, Ceravolo MP, Dègand M. Nerve injuries during rhytidectomy: considerations after 3,203 cases. Aesth Plast Surg 1980; 4:257–265.
6. Pitanguy I, Ceravolo M. Hematoma post-rhytidectomy: how we treat it. Plast Reconstr Surg 1981; 67:526–528.
7. Pitanguy I. Indication for and treatment of frontal and glabellar wrinkles in an analysis of 3,404 consecutive cases of rhytidectomy. Plast Reconstr Surg 1981; 67:157–166.
8. Pitanguy I. Les Chemins de la Beauté. In: Un maitre de la chirurgie plastique témoigne. Paris: J.C. Lattes, 1983.
9. Pitanguy I. The face. In: Aesthetic Surgery of Head and Body. Berlin: Springer Verlag, 1984:165–200.
10. Pitanguy I. Forehead lifting. In: Aesthetic Surgery of Head and Body. Berlin: Springer Verlag, 1984:202–214.
11. Pitanguy I, Salgado F, Radwanski HN. Submental liposuction as an ancillary procedure in face-lifting. FACE 1995; 4(1):1–13.
12. Pitanguy I, Brentano JMS, Salgado F, Radwanski HN, Carpeggiani R. Incisions in primary and secondary rhytidoplasties. Rev Bras Cir 1995; 85:165–176.
13. Pitanguy I, Pamplona DC, Giuntini ME, Salgado F, Radwanski HN. Computational simulation of rhytidectomy by the "round-lifting" technique. Rev Bras Cir 1995; 85:213–218.
14. Pitanguy I, Amorim NFG. Treatment of the nasolabial fold. Rev Bras Cir 1997; 87:231–242.
15. Pitanguy I, Pamplona DC, Weber HI, Leta F, Salgado F, Radwanski HN. Numerical modeling of the aging face. Plast Reconstr Surg 1998; 102:200–204.

16. Pitanguy I, Radwanski HN. Rejuvenation of the brow. In: Matarasso SL, Matarasso A, eds. Dermatology Clinics. Philadelphia: W.B. Saunders, 1998:623–635.
17. Pitanguy I, Radwanski HN, Amorim NFG. Treatment of the aging face using the "round lifting" technique. Aesth Surg J 1999; 19:216–222.
18. Pitanguy I, Soares G, Machado BH, de Amorim NF. CO_2 laser associated with the "round-lifting" technique. J Cutan Laser Ther 1999; 1:145–152.
19. Pitanguy I. The Round-lifting technique. Facial Plast Surg 2000; 16(3):255–267.
20. Pitanguy I. Facial cosmetic surgery: a 30-year perspective. Plast Reconstr Surg 2000; 105:1517–1529.
21. Pitanguy I, Amorim NFG. Forehead lifting: the juxtapilose subperiosteal approach. Aesth Plast Surg 2003; 27:58–62.

3 Aesthetic Surgery: Some Personal Thoughts and Contributions

Ivo Pitanguy

Department of Plastic Surgery, Pontifical Catholic University of Rio de Janeiro and The Carlos Chagas Institute of Post-Graduate Medical Studies, Rio de Janeiro, Brazil

INTRODUCTION

The search for beauty is universal and has been one of man's eternal quests. This is reflected in how much time and energy people dedicate to the search for physical beauty as a means of achieving intimate well-being. Furthermore, competition and success, in social and professional circles, are intimately related to how a person reflects, in his or her physical appearance, this inner harmony. Basically, aesthetic surgery achieves this by correcting deformities that are experienced as psychologically uncomfortable or undesirable.

In the last few decades, the number of patients requesting plastic surgery has increased significantly. Personal, social, and, especially, professional aspects have greatly influenced the search for a youthful appearance or a more leaner, athletic profile. Myriad different surgical and nonsurgical procedures have been developed to meet the aesthetic requirements of these patients, offering a natural and harmonious result.

The approach to meeting these expectations involves a thorough analysis of the patient's desires, body anatomy, and knowledge of the available techniques. In this way, a personalized treatment may be performed with satisfactory results with no stigma of a surgical procedure or distortion of important anatomic landmarks. The author's contributions and perspectives on aesthetic plastic surgery are presented in this chapter, outlining the general principles, important aspects of assessment and management, and the landmark techniques developed over the years.

Consistently successful outcomes require absolute respect for surgical principles and the adoption of a fundamentally conservative approach. Overly aggressive techniques tend to cause greater trauma, without significantly increasing results. In the author's experience, as outlined in this overview, covering more than four decades in the treatment of aesthetic deformities, the reader will appreciate the emphasis on sound principles and the importance of careful assessment and postoperative management.

THE PATIENT'S PROFILE

The increasing number of people seeking aesthetic surgery reflects the psychological, social, and cultural evolution of our society. Plastic surgeons have witnessed a distinct change in the profile of both males and females seeking aesthetic surgery.

Gender differences tend to follow general patterns. A psychological profile of the male patient presenting for an aesthetic procedure often reveals the fear of losing self-identity and usefulness in today's competitive society, and this helps him to overcome the apprehension of surgery and its risks, postoperative discomfort, and the cost of treatment. Consequently, the social and psychological barriers have diminished, and men now seek these procedures more liberally. In our experience, male patients may have a higher prevalence of personality disorders, a lower threshold for pain, greater expectations, and an increased tendency to question a technically faultless outcome.

Women, on the other hand, are more inclined for an aesthetic procedure, either surgical or nonsurgical. Throughout history, different peoples have adopted innumerous techniques to enhance the female face and body. Anatomical changes throughout a woman's lifetime are more evident than in men. There are also markers that affect women to a greater degree: the transition from adolescence to adulthood; societal pressures for wedding and breeding; the changes that arise from motherhood; and skin looseness and loss of muscle tone in the senior age. The female patient is also more tolerant of discomfort and pain, and tends to be more cooperative.

Although the aesthetic ideals for males and females are somewhat different, the satisfactory result is dependent on obtaining a sound relationship between surgeon and patient, accurate planning, correct indication, and knowledge of the vast array of existing procedures. Together, these elements allow for an overall improvement of physical appearance and hence self-esteem.

PATIENT SCREENING

Appropriate screening determines the successful outcome of any operation. Patient's expectations must be carefully investigated, as this is probably the single greatest cause of postoperative frustration. Factors such as anxiety regarding anesthesia and pain, the aspect of the first weeks, the final outcome, peer pressure to return to work as soon as possible, and the tendency to disregard postoperative instructions have been cited as possible obstacles to a favorable outcome. In selected cases, surgery may be considered even in emotionally unstable patients, as long as they are carefully assessed and receive intensive counseling before and after surgery.

Motivation is closely related to patient satisfaction. Highly motivated individuals tend to have less pain, a better postoperative course, and a higher level of satisfaction regardless of the outcome. The ideal candidate possesses an internal motivation to improve his self-image. Patients desiring surgery due to external factors (such as the need to please others or to save a deteriorating relationship) are often dissatisfied with the results and are not ideal cases.

A detailed medical history is fundamental to glean for any previous problems or untoward effects from any medication. Clinical assessment should screen out patients with cardiovascular disease and heavy tobacco and/or alcohol abuse, which consequently increase the rate of postoperative clinical complications. For example, it is known that men have a greater tendency for transoperative and postoperative bleeding following a face-lift so appropriate measures are required. The anesthesiology team should avoid fluctuation in blood pressure throughout the procedure and during the first 24 hours postoperatively. Hemostasis is particularly important, and the possibility of hematoma must be anticipated. Control of pain, both during and after surgery, is a fundamental aspect of patient care; an aesthetic procedure should not be identified with anything greater than reasonable discomfort.

Preoperative blood tests are always requested, as well as a clinical checkup with our own general physician. It is our practice that all surgical procedures performed in our clinic have the assistance of the anesthesiology department to assure adequate sedation and pain control. Many operations are now performed under local anesthesia with endovenous sedation; yet sometimes general anesthesia is preferred, especially when combining two or more procedures.

PERSONAL CONTRIBUTIONS

The principal contributions to aesthetic plastic surgery that I have established over the years is covered in this chapter, giving a brief description of the main elements of each technique, which have permitted for reliable, safe, and efficient results.

Rhytidoplasty

Face-lifting is one of the most frequently requested procedures, and the aim of this operation is to reposition facial tissues, with removal of flaccid skin and excess fat deposits, so as to bring a younger appearance. In more than 40 years of experience, over 8000 cases have been performed by the author. Interestingly, an increase in male patients has been noted. In the 1970s, male patients represented 6% of face-lifting procedures; in the 1980s, approximately 15%; and currently, almost 20% of face-lift patients are men.

The standard incision is demarcated, beginning in the temporal scalp, proceeding in the preauricular area in such a way as to be "broken" by anatomical curves. A straight incision is unsightly and will call attention to the scar. The incision then follows around the earlobe, and, in a curving fashion, finishes in the cervical scalp.

In patients who have previously undergone this operation (i.e., secondary rhytidoplasties), variations of this incision are chosen depending on each case, with the following goals in mind: treatment of specific regions, resection of previous scars, and maintenance of anatomical landmarks. Advantages of each different incision have been mentioned in previous publications. These so-called atypical incisions should be carefully planned to maintain hair-bearing flaps in the appropriate position and avoid other anatomical distortions.

Undermining of the facial and cervical flaps is performed in a subcutaneous plane, the extension of which is variable, individualized for each case. Attention has been called to a danger area that lies beneath the non–hair-bearing skin over the temples, called "no man's land," where the most frequent variation of the facial nerve, the temporofrontal branch, is particularly vulnerable. Dissection over "no man's land" should be superficial, and hemostasis carefully performed.

Often the dissection proceeds all the way to the other side under the mandible to treat very heavy, fatty necks. With the advent of suction-assisted lipectomy, lipodystrophy is mostly addressed by liposuction, in a crisscross fashion. Sometimes, this is associated with direct lipectomy using specially designed scissors, to defat the heavy submental region. Following this, treatment of loose neck bands (platysmal bands) is carried out under direct exposure.

Dissection of the deeper elements of the face has evolved over the past 20 years. We currently favor the undermining of the facial flaps over the zygomatic prominence to free the retaining ligaments of the cheek. Approach to the superficial muscle-apponeurotic system (SMAS) has been a topic of much discussion. It is our preference to determine whether to dissect or simply plicate the SMAS after subcutaneous dissection has been completed, by pulling it and noting the effects on the skin flap.

Although extensive undermining of the SMAS has been performed by me in an earlier period, plication of this structure in the same direction as the skin flaps, with repositioning of the malar fat pad, has given equally satisfactory results in most cases. The durability of this maneuver is relative to the individual aging process. Tension on the musculoaponeurotic system allows support of the subcutaneous layers, corrects the sagging cheek, and reduces tension on the skin flap.

The direction of traction of the skin flaps is a fundamental aspect of what I have termed the "round lifting" technique. This implies that the undermined flaps are rotated rather than simply pulled. This vector of traction acts in a direction opposite to that of aging-and assures a repositioning of tissues with preservation of anatomical landmarks. A second advantage in establishing a precise direction of rotation is that the opposite side is repositioned in the exact manner. This direction is determined by a vector that connects the tragus to Darwin's tubercle of the ear. Likewise, the cervical flap should also be pulled in an equally precise manner, in a superior and slightly anterior vector, to avoid a step-off of the hairline.

After key stitches have been placed to anchor the flaps along the pilose scalp, excess skin in front of the ear is estimated with no tension whatsoever; the flap is positioned over the tragus, and the natural curvature of this region is delineated and then excised.

Ptosis of the eyebrow is an element that may cause aging of the upper third of the face. Correction of the level of the brow to a more elevated position has classically been undertaken by a large, bicoronal incision. A less aggressive approach is the prepilose or juxtahairline incision. This reduced incision, placed just inside of the temporal hairline, is performed when the patient presents with ptosis of lateral eyebrow and scant lines of expression on the forehead itself. A subperiosteal undermining is done to free the lateral brow, and is relatively easy due to the short distance required to reach the eyebrow region. Elevation is achieved by traction and removal of a wedge of excess scalp.

Rhinoplasty

Due to its central position, the shape and projection of the nose strongly influences facial aesthetics. In ancient cultures, the similar anatomy between the nose and the male genital organs gave the former a symbolic sexual importance, and long noses were considered a sign of masculinity and virility. In fact, both organs tend to develop during adolescence and possess erectile tissue. Therefore, a patient who demonstrates dissatisfaction with his nose (giving excessive importance to discrete deformities) may, in fact, be concealing difficulties related to emotional relationships or dissatisfaction of a sexual nature.

The key for planning a rhinoplasty is to obtain an accurate diagnosis (both objective and subjective) of the particular deformity. The unique anatomy of the nose, composed of cartilage, bone, and soft tissues, is organized in such a way that minimal change in one of the elements can cause an alteration of the whole. In a mixed population, such as in Brazil, patients may request a change of profile to decrease racial prejudice; this is acceptable, yet facial harmony should always be maintained. Finally, functional complaints must be adequately evaluated, so as to perform correction of nasal obstruction concomitantly with the aesthetic procedure.

Our approach to rhinoplasty is through the closed incision, although this is the access that demands the most of the surgeon: during a closed rhinoplasty, most of the maneuvers have to be "seen" through the skin, adding to the difficulty, especially for the inexperienced plastic surgeon. Psychologically, the absence of an external scar keeps the mystery that an operation was performed at all. Infrequently, an open approach is chosen, usually for the correction of trauma or congenital deformities.

Technical details are the key to an aesthetic long-lasting result. In general, reduction of size should be conservative, with contouring of the supporting framework without excessive resections of the dorsum. Concavity and too much opening of the nasolabial angle cause an obvious and artificial aspect. Resection of cartilage, to reshape the nasal tip, is also done conservatively, and always maintaining the mucoperichondrial flap attached to the remaining cartilage. This avoids postoperative retraction of tissues. The use of delicate cartilaginous grafts, and the placement of fine sutures, are useful adjuncts to enhance tip projection.

After adequate treatment of the osteocartilaginous nasal framework, the lower third of the nose may retain a residual "supratip" deformity marked by convexity of the tip region. This may be corrected by identifying and resecting the dermocartilaginous ligament, which was first described in 1965 and is routinely sectioned during primary rhinoplasty. This structure, also called the Pitanguy ligament, connects the middle third of the nose to the two medial crura (extending anteroposteriorly into the membranous septum), and has been identified in various ethnic groups. A system of classification has been established and has proven useful to determine its thickness.

In recent years, we have seen a greater number of patients seeking secondary rhinoplasty. Complaints may range from small alterations in nasal profile to severe deformities of form and function. The correct management of these patients consists in an individual analysis of each case, precise diagnosis, and a personalized surgical approach.

Of the approximately 9000 cases operated in my clinic, primary cases still represent the majority. In the last 10 years, a growing rate of secondary procedures has been noted, accounting for almost 30% of cases. The most common cause of secondary rhinoplasty is excessive nasal tip reduction with loss of projection and detail. In order to correct these deformities, the use of autogenous grafts is always recommended, and various different shapes may be carved to support the columella and define the nasal tip. The use of a swallow wing–shaped cartilaginous graft has shown excellent results in these cases.

Otoplasty

The preferred technique involves creating and projecting an island of cartilage anteriorly in the antihelical area to define the antihelical fold. This approach contrasts with most other techniques, because we are actually building a fold, instead of merely bending the cartilage. This results in a permanent antihelical projection, with almost no cases of recurrence. When applicable, the concha should be reshaped by rotation (and fixated to the mastoid) instead of excision because the latter may result in unsightly skin folds in the conchal skin. Excessively protruding earlobes may be corrected by triangular or bow-shaped excisions of skin between the lobe and the concha or by dissecting out the cauda helices and fixating it to the concha.

Finally, the ears should be carefully examined at the end of the operation. They should not be laid too far back, and the angle between the ear and the head at the antihelix level should be preserved, ensuring a natural and aesthetically pleasing result.

Breast Hypertrophy

In our population, breast hypertrophy represents one of the most common contour deformities. Women in Brazil are more concerned about being slim over the chest, and this has cultural explanations. When considering a surgical technique for the correction of the enlarged breast, certain aspects that are unique to this structure must be emphasized, such as its psychosocial importance, the primary sensual connotation of the breast, the embryological origin, and the lactiferous function of the mammary gland. The principal aspects of my personal approach have been maintained in over 40 years of experience in treating diverse aesthetic breast deformities.

Reduction mammaplasty must preserve function and maintain sensitivity, while limiting the extension of the scars. The Pitanguy technique is indicated in cases of large hypertrophies. In cases of moderate hypertrophy or ptosis, when less tissue is to be resected, the Pitanguy rhomboid technique (also called the Arié-Pitanguy technique) is well indicated, finishing in a single vertical scar. In both approaches, glandular resection is restricted to the inferior pole of the breast, respecting the principle of avoiding large dissections. Resection varies according to the firmness of breast parenchyma and may be straight when the parenchyma is composed mainly of fatty tissue, or can resemble an inverted "ship's keel," if the breast tissue is more glandular. This may be stated as an adjustment of the container (skin envelope) to its content (remaining breast parenchyma).

The feasibility of both techniques is further emphasized when considering the results obtained at the Santa Casa General Hospital (a public charity hospital) where senior residents under the supervision of the author and his assistants have performed over 5500 breast reductions. The predictability and safety of these procedures are demonstrated by noting that the final results are comparable between the two groups of patients, at the Ivo Pitanguy Clinic (almost 4000 cases) and at the public institution.

Breast Augmentation and Nipple Deformities

The approach that is personally preferred for the placement of a breast implant or for resection of breast tissue in gynecomastia is the transareolar incision. This incision respects the very anatomy of the nipple-areolar complex (NAC). The NAC is divided transversally along its equator, permitting a very good exposure of the entire pectoral region, while at the same time preserving the innervation of this structure. Except in rare cases, where the NAC is considered too small, this approach has proven useful over the many years since it was first described.

This incision is equally valuable when correcting the inverted nipple. Through the transareolar approach, the retaining fibers that hold the nipple inwards are resected, and the final scar is imperceptible. Finally, a simple means of reducing the hypertrophic nipple, which may be called the flip-over technique, consists in resecting one-half of the nipple, and suturing the remaining tissue over itself.

Body Contouring: Trunk and Limbs

The voluptuous figures that were idealized by artists in the past have, today, been substituted by slimmer forms. Until recently, the obese body was mostly hidden under heavy clothing or was reluctantly accepted. Medical advances in the past century have permitted safe and efficient surgical correction of contour deformities. Furthermore, current fashion trends generally promote body-revealing attire, and the media frequently encourages fitness and good health, linking these qualities with youthfulness and beauty. The subliminal as well as overt message is that these are necessary and desirable requirements for social acceptance and professional success.

On the other hand, with the advent of gastroenterological techniques that greatly reduce the patient's weight, we are experiencing a return of many of the techniques that we have previously advocated, but that fell into disuse.

"Body contouring" is a term coined by ourselves, and denotes surgery that corrects excessive tissues of the trunk and limbs. Excisional surgery for correction of contour deformities of the abdomen and trunk, and the upper and lower limbs, has evolved over the years. Extensive scars that were considered indispensable to treat large lipodystrophies of the trunk and upper and lower limbs have been generally replaced by the advent of suction-assisted lipectomy in the 1980s.

Contour deformities of the abdomen cause variable aesthetic and/or functional alterations, and are caused by different conditions. A personal approach to abdominal deformities was described in the American literature in 1967, where attention to both function and aesthetics was emphasized. The principles of the author's technique in abdominoplasty have remained, such as reinforcement of the muscle aponeurosis through plication without opening of the fascia. Placement of scars has changed according to the model of beach attires, and currently places the incision immediately above the pubic area with a horizontal lateral extension, curving upwards. There may be a certain variability, dictated by the patient's preference for bathing suits. Finally, a small but important detail of the postoperative dressing is that we still place a plaster cast over the abdomen, to exert a gentle and uniform pressure over the entire abdominal flap; this cast is left in place for the first 48 hours.

As mentioned, dermolipectomies of the arms and lower limbs are again demanded of the plastic surgeon, especially by patients who have undergone great loss of weight. We have described techniques that correct flaccidity of the arm, either by itself or associated to excessive tissues of the thorax and breast (the thoracobraquial dermolipectomy). The riding breeches deformity, which was corrected by excisional surgery until the 1970s, was then treated by liposuction. We currently see some cases where this procedure is again indicated, such as in the massive weight-loss patient or for correction of gross irregularities and skin excess, following liposuction of the thighs.

Combined Procedures

Contour alterations, which involve multiple body regions, may be approached either through serial operations or can be treated by a combination of procedures done simultaneously. As a general rule, any type of aesthetic surgical combination can be performed, provided that it is technically feasible. There are a number of advantages to the patient: a one-stage operation allows the correction of two or more deformities; multiple anesthesias and hospital admissions are avoided, as well as a long postoperative recovery. In addition, the patient has a considerable psychological benefit in addressing his or her deformities in one setting. The main disadvantage lies in the extent of surgical trauma, with all that this entails.

The surgeon should be particularly careful in indicating these combined procedures. The age and condition of the patient are two decisive factors. A personal methodology has been developed that makes it possible to execute two or more simultaneous aesthetic operations, being both expeditious and safe. However, only years of training and constant preparation give the surgeon sufficient dexterity and ability to be successful in combined surgery. This demands that the surgeon possess a teaching mind and also requires a perfect and functioning surgical team.

FURTHER READING

Books

Pitanguy I. Aesthetic Plastic Surgery of the Head and Body. Berlin: Springer-Verlag, 1981.
Pitanguy I. El arte de la Belleza. Barcelona, Spain: Ediciones Grijalbo S.A., 1984.
Pitanguy I. Imparando Con la Vita. Milano: Mediamix, 1996.
Pitanguy I. Le vie Della Bellezza. Milano, Italy: Rizzoli, 1984.
Pitanguy I. Les Chemins de la Beauté: un Maitre de la Chirurgie Plastique Témoigne. Paris: J.C. Lattès, 1983.

Articles

The Face

Pitanguy I. La ritidoplastia: soluzione eclética del problema. Minerva Chir 1967; 22(17):942–947.
Pitanguy I. Ancilary procedures in face lifting. Clin Plast Surg 1978; 5(1):51–69.
Pitanguy I. Frontalis-procerus-corrugator apponeurosis in the correction of frontal and glabellar wrinkles. Ann Plast Surg 1979; 2(5):422–427.
Pitanguy I. The aging face. In: Carlsen L, Slatt B, eds. The Naked Face. Ontário: General Publishing, 1979:27.
Pitanguy I. Indication for and treatment of frontal and glabellar wrinkles in an analysis of 3404 consecutive cases of rhytidectomy. Plast Reconstr Surg 1981; 67(2):157–166.
Pitanguy I. Eyelid surgery and temporal lift. Fourth Annual Multispecialty Oculoplastic Surgery Symposium, Sept 3–5. Lexington: Ophtalmology Center, Humana Hospital, 1988:96.
Pitanguy I. Aging face surgery. In: Stucker FJ, ed. Plastic and Reconstructive Surgery of the Head and Neck. Philadelphia: B.C. Decker, 1991:145.
Pitanguy I. Aging face surgery. Aesthetic Surgery of the Aging Face 1993. Symposium A Mayor Course of the American Academy of Facial Plastic & Reconstructive Surgery, March 3–7. Indianópolis: William H. Beeson (Diretor do Curso), 1993.
Pitanguy I. Surgery for the correction of the ageing face [abstr]. First Middle East Conference on Head & Neck Aesthetic and Reconstructive Surgery, State of Kuwait, Kuwait Society of Plastic Surgeons, 01 a 04 de dezembro de, 1996:43.
Pitanguy I. The round-lifting technique. Facial Plastic Surg 2000; 16(3):255–267.

Pitanguy I. Facial cosmetic surgery: a 30-year perspective. Plast Reconstr Surg 2000; 105(4):1517–1526.
Pitanguy I, Ceravolo M. Hematoma postrhytidectomy: how we treat it. Plast Reconstr Surg 1981; 67(4):526–528.
Pitanguy I, Radwanski HN. Rejuvenation of the brow. Dermatol Clin 1994; 15(4):623–634.
Pitanguy I, Ramos A. The frontal branch of the facial nerve: the importance of its variations in the face-lifting. Plast Reconstr Surg 1966; 38(4):352–356.
Pitanguy I, et al. Nerve injuries during rhytidectomy: considerations after 3203 cases. Aesth Plast Surg 1980; 4:257–265.
Pitanguy I, et al. Blepharoplasty: personal experience with 4564 consecutive cases. Ophtalmic Plastic Reconstr Surg 1985; 1(1):9–22.
Pitanguy I, et al. Rhytidoplastik: perioperative richtlinien. Laryng Rhinol Otologie 1987; 66:586–590.
Pitanguy I, et al. Treatment of sequels of rhytidoplasty. Rev Soc Bras Cir Plast Est e Reconstrutiva 1994; 9(1):31–42.
Pitanguy I, et al. Incisions in primary and secondary face-lifting. FACE 1994; 5(2):49–61.
Pitanguy I, et al. Numerical modeling of facial aging. Plast Reconstr Surg 1998; 102(1):200–204.
Pitanguy I, et al. Treatment of the aging face using the "round-lifting" technique. Aesth Surg J 1999; 19(3):216–222.
Pitanguy I, et al. CO_2 laser peeling associated with the "round lifting" technique. J Cutan Laser Ther 1999; 1:145–152.
Pitanguy I, et al. Laser resusfacing as an adjunct to the "Round Lifting" technique. In: Simunovic Z, ed. ecoord. Laser in Surgery and Dentistry. European Medical Laser Association, Rijeka, Croatia: Vitagraf, 2001:347.

The Nose

Pitanguy I. Management of alar cartilage defects. Am J Surg 1958; 95(2):331–33.
Pitanguy I. Of the presence and importance of a dermocartilaginous ligament in globous noses. Rev Lat Am Cir Plastica 1965; 9(3):228–237.
Pitanguy I. Surgical importance of a dermocartilaginous ligament in bulbous noses. Plast Reconstr Surg 1965; 36(2):247–253.
Pitanguy I. The Negroid Nose. 1st International Symposium Reconstruction Surgery of Face and Neck, USA, 1972:136.
Pitanguy I. Dermocartilaginous ligament of the nose: its surgical importance in different ethnical group. In: Hinderer UT, ed. Plastic Surgery. Amsterdam: Excerpta Médica, 1992:439–440.
Pitanguy I. Revision rhinoplasty. Am J Cosmetic Surg 1994; 11(3):183–187.
Pitanguy I. Revisiting the dermocartilaginous ligament. Plastic Reconstr Surg 2001; 107(1):264–266.
Pitanguy I, Ceravolo M. Secondary rhinoplasty. Aesth Plast Surg 1982; 6:47–54.
Pitanguy I, Treciak H. Operative therapie bei nasenspitzenläsionen. Aesth Medizin 1969; 18(12): 233–234.
Pitanguy I, et al. The surgical importance of the dermocartilaginous ligament of the nose. Plast Reconstr Surg 1995; 95(5):790–794.
Pitanguy I, et al. Lesões nasal e palatina provocadas por cocaína. Rev Bras Cir 1995; 85(6):245–252; Bol Cir Plástica 1995: 148.
Pitanguy I, et al. Surgical treatment of hemangiomas of the nose. Ann Plastic Surg 1996; 36(6):586–593.

The Ear

Pitanguy I. Dysplasia auricularis. 4th International Congress of Plastic and Reconstructive Surgery, Roma 1967:660.
Pitanguy I. Total ear reconstruction. 1st International Symposium Reconstruction Surgery of Face and Neck, USA, 1972; 256.
Pitanguy I, Fleming I. Plastiche Eingriffe an der Ohrmuschel. Stuttgart: Springer Thieme Verlarg, 1976.
Pitanguy I, Fleming J. Plastic operations on the auricle. In: Naumann H, ed. Head and Neck Surgery. Vol. 3. New York: Verlag 1982:1–69.
Pitanguy I, Rebello C. Ansiform ears correction by island technique. Acta Chir Plast 1962; 4(4): 267–277. (Em russo p.235–245).
Pitanguy I, et al. Prominent ears: Pitanguy's island technique long-term results. Head Neck Surg 1985; 7(5):418–426.
Pitanguy I, et al. The treatment of prominent ears: a 25 year surgery of the Island technique. Aesth Plast Surg 1987; 11:87–93.

The Breast

Pitanguy I. Beitrag zur technik der hautüberflanzun zwecks verbesserung das hypertrophies der bruste. Aesth Medizin 1962; 11(3):65–74.
Pitanguy I. Une nouvelle technique de plastic mammaire: estude de 245 cas consecutifs et presentation d'une technique personelle. Ann Chir Plastique 1962; 7(3):199–208.
Pitanguy I. Breast hypertrophy: contribution to its treatment. Rev Lat Am Cir Plástica 1963; 7(3):162.
Pitanguy I. Contribuition au traitment des plastics mammaires. Ann Chir Plastique 1964; 9(3):236.

Pitanguy I. Breast hypertrophy. 2nd Int Soc Plast Surgeons Londres, 1965:509–512.
Pitanguy I. Contribution to the technique of free grafting for the repair of the large mammary hypertrophies. Plast Reconstr Surg 1965; 36(1):135.
Pitanguy I. Transareolar incision for gynecomastia. Plast Reconstr Surg 1966; 38(5):414–419.
Pitanguy I. Surgical treatment of breast hypertrophy. Brit J Plast Surg 1967; 20(1):78–85.
Pitanguy I. Breast Hypertrophy. 5th International Congress of Plastic and Reconstructive Surgery, Austrália: Butterworths, 1971:1180.
Pitanguy I. Personal preferences for reduction mammaplasty. In: Goldwyn RM, ed. Plastic and Reconstructive Surgery of the Breast. 2. Boston: Little Brown, , 1976; 167–179.
Pitanguy I. Transareolar incision for augmentation mammaplasty. Aesth Plast Surg 1978; 2(4): 363–372.
Pitanguy I. Inverted nipple. Aesth Plast Surg 1978; 2(1):53–64.
Pitanguy I. Breast reduction and ptosis. In: Georgiade N, ed. Aesthetic Breast Surgery. Baltimore: Williams &Wilkins, 1983:247–255.
Pitanguy I. The breast. In: Chang W, et al., eds. An Atlas of Reconstruction. Baltimore: Williams & Wilkins, 1984:150.
Pitanguy I. A personal technique for reduction mammaplasty. The International Conference on Plastic Surgery, Beijing, China. 1984; 2:32.
Pitanguy I. Reduction mammaplasty by the personal technique. In: Chang WHJ, et al, eds. The Breast: An Atlas of Reconstruction. Baltimore: Williams & Wilkins, 1984:75–160.
Pitanguy I. Treatment of benign pathologies of the breast. In: de Janeiro R, Belfort P, Pinotti JA, Eskes TKAB, eds. The Proceedings of the XIIth World Congress of Gynecology and Obstetrics, October, 1988:133–138.
Pitanguy I. Principles of reduction mammaplasty. In: Georgiade N, ed. Aesthetic Surgery of the Breast. Philadelphia: W.B. Saunders, 1990:191–213.
Pitanguy I. Reduction mammaplasty: a personal odyssey. In: Goldwin R, ed. Reduction Mammaplasty. Boston: Little Brown, 1990:95–105.
Pitanguy I. Contribution to the surgical treatment of breast deformities. 6th International Congress on Breast Diseases, Boston, June 10–14. The Society for the Study of Breast Diseases, 1990.
Pitanguy I, Radwanski HN. Philosophy and principles in the correction of breast hypertrophy. In: Mang WL, Bull HG, eds. Ästhetische Chirurgie. Alemanha: Einhorn-Presse Verlag, 1996:216–232.
Pitanguy I, Torres E. Histopathological aspects of mammary gland tissue in cases of plastic surgery of breast. Brit Jour Plast Surg 1964; 17(3):297–302.

Abdomen

Pitanguy I. Abdominal lipectomy: an approach to it through an analysis of 300 consecutive cases. Plast Reconstr Surg 1967; 40(4):384–391.
Pitanguy I. Vantaggi dell impiego di contenzione gessata nelle plastiche abdominali. Minerva Chir 1967; 22(10):595–598.
Pitanguy I. Lipectomy abdominoplasty: lipodystrophy of the inner side of the arm. In: Grabb W, Smith J, eds. Plastic Surgery: A Concise Guide to Clinical Practice. 2nd ed. Boston: Little Brown, 1973.
Pitanguy I. Abdominal lipectomy. Clin Plast Surg 1975; 2(3):410.
Pitanguy I, et al. Treatment of abdominal wall eventrations associated with abdominoplasty techniques. Aesth Plast Surg 1984; 8(3):173–179.
Pitanguy I, et al. Abdominoplastik: unsere operativen richlinien. Zentralblatt fur Chirurgir 1988; 113: 765–771.

Body Contour

Pitanguy I. Trochanteric lipodystrophy. Plast Reconstr. Surgery 1964; 34(3):280–286.
Pitanguy I. Dermolipectomies crurales. Ann Chir Plastique 1975; 17(1):40–46.
Pitanguy I. Correction of lipodystrophy of the lateral thoracic aspect and inner side of the arm and elbow dermossenescence. Clin Plast Surg 1975; 2(3):477–483.
Pitanguy I. Dermolipectomy of the abdominal wall, thighs, buttocks, and upper extremity. In: Converse JM, ed. Reconstruction Plastic Surgery. 7. 2nd ed. Philadelphia: W.B. Saunders, , 1977; 3800.
Pitanguy I. Body contour. Am J Cosm Surg 1987; 4(4):283–293.
Pitanguy I. Thigh and buttock lift. In: Lewis JR, ed. The Art of Aesthetic Surgery. 2. Boston: Little Brown, , 1989.
Pitanguy I. Submental liposuction as an ancillary procedure in face-lifting. FACE 1995; 4(1):1–13.
Pitanguy I. Evaluation of body contouring surgery today: a 30-year perspective. Plast Reconstr Surg 2000; 105(4):1499–1514.

Associated Procedures

Pitanguy I. Thigh lift and abdominal lipectomy. In: Goldwyn RM, ed. Unfavorable Results in Plastic Surgery. Boston: Little Brown, 1972:387–398.

Pitanguy I. Team approach to the simultaneous surgical correction of multiple aesthetic problems. 8th International Congress Plastic Reconstruction Surgery, Montreal, Canada, 1983:580–583.

Pitanguy I, Ceravolo M. Our experience with combined procedures in aesthetic plastic surgery. Plast Reconstr Surg 1983; 71(1):56–63.

Pitanguy I, et al. Methodology in combined aesthetic surgeries. Aesth Plast Surg 1978; 2(3):331–340.

4 Remodeling of the Face in Three Dimensions: Soft Tissue vs. Alloplastic Implants

Oscar M. Ramirez
Johns Hopkins University School of Medicine, Baltimore, and Esthétique Internationale, Timonium, Maryland, U.S.A.

Charles R. Volpe
Esthétique Internationale, Timonium, Maryland, U.S.A.

INTRODUCTION

The 21st century has been marked by an intense public awareness of aesthetic surgical procedures. The Internet, broadcast television, and print media have given patients greater exposure to the field of cosmetic surgery. Due to this media exposure, social acceptance of aesthetic surgery is growing. Armed with greater knowledge, more patients are demanding the return to a youthful appearance, utilizing the latest surgical procedures. Nowhere can this be seen more than in the area of facial rejuvenation.

For the clinician, the 21st century marks a period of improved understanding of facial anatomy and the aging process. It also marks a period of government approval of soft-tissue fillers, improved technology, and the description of new operative techniques. With these advances, facial rejuvenation is increasingly approached in a three-dimensional (3-D) manner.

Three-dimensional facial rejuvenation can be accomplished through a variety of techniques. Soft tissue can be manipulated with vascularized fat pad repositioning, fat grafting, and by imbrication techniques. Alloplastic materials can be inserted to augment the skeletal framework and can be utilized as soft-tissue fillers. The increased number of surgical options leads to increased confusion. When should soft-tissue techniques be used? What is the role of alloplastic implants?

By a better understanding of the aging process, the decision to use autogenous materials versus alloplastic implants versus a combination of both becomes clearer. The purpose of this chapter is to outline the authors' approach to 3-D facial remodeling, as part of the rejuvenation process.

UNDERSTANDING THE AGING PROCESS

The aging face is characterized by volumetric changes caused by a reduction of the soft tissues and resorption of bone (1). Soft-tissue changes include deepening of the nasolabial fold and concomitant inferior, lateral, and anterior displacement of the cheek mass (2). With aging, remodeling of the facial skeleton continues with rotation of facial structures downward and inward from the cranial base (3). The volumetric changes affect the central part of the face earlier than the peripheral areas of the face (4).

With this understanding, the concept of the central oval of the face can be explained. The central portion of the face comprises the mimetic and sphincteric muscles allowing facial expressions. The peripheral portion of the face is more static and thus more resistant to the aging process. Thus, the face can be broken down into two distinct aesthetic units: (*i*) the central oval and (*ii*) the peripheral hemicircle (4).

The central oval is composed of the loose, dynamic structures that fall prey to the gravitational forces of nature. Combined with loss of bone volume, it becomes evident that the deflation and gravitational migration of the soft tissues lead to "earlier aging" of the central oval of the face. Characteristic features in the frontal region include visible spasm of the corrugator muscle, deep-set eyes, and the appearance of upper eyelid skin excess. The temporal region becomes hollowed. The lower eyelids demonstrate orbital fat herniation, and in advanced stages, exposure of the lower orbital rim and creation of a "tear trough" deformity. The malar area is characterized by a generalized loss of thickness and ptosis of Bichat's fat pad (BF). Reduction in mandibular volume results in loss of projection of the gonial angles and the chin and produces hollowness around the jowls. Facial expression lines become accentuated due to collagen damage and loss of elastic fibers.

The peripheral hemicircle is susceptible to volumetric change later in life. Significant skin laxity, accumulation of fat in the submental and submandibular regions, platysmal banding, and development of an obtuse cervicomental angle are characteristic.

Due to the individual nature of the aging process, correction can be provided through the use of soft-tissue manipulation and/or alloplastic augmentation.

METHODS OF THREE-DIMENSIONAL AUGMENTATION

Two-dimensional (2-D) face-lifting techniques provide the basic construct upon which 3-D rejuvenation procedures are performed. The 2-D techniques allow rejuvenation through oblique and lateral lifting or through vertical and superolateral lifting. The addition of enhancement in an anterior–posterior (A–P) direction defines the 3-D facial rejuvenation technique. There are four methods available to create 3-D rejuvenation: (i) augmentation of the subcutaneous fatty layers, (ii) imbrication of facial soft tissues, (iii) repositioning of fat pockets as pedicle flaps, and (iv) augmentation of the skeletal framework (Fig. 1).

The authors' approach to 3-D rejuvenation utilizes these methods individually or in combination. Proper diagnosis of the aesthetic deficiencies, whether skeletal or soft tissue, will determine the most effective plan to achieve excellent results. Common sense dictates that restoration of deficient structures with similar tissues will provide the most natural result.

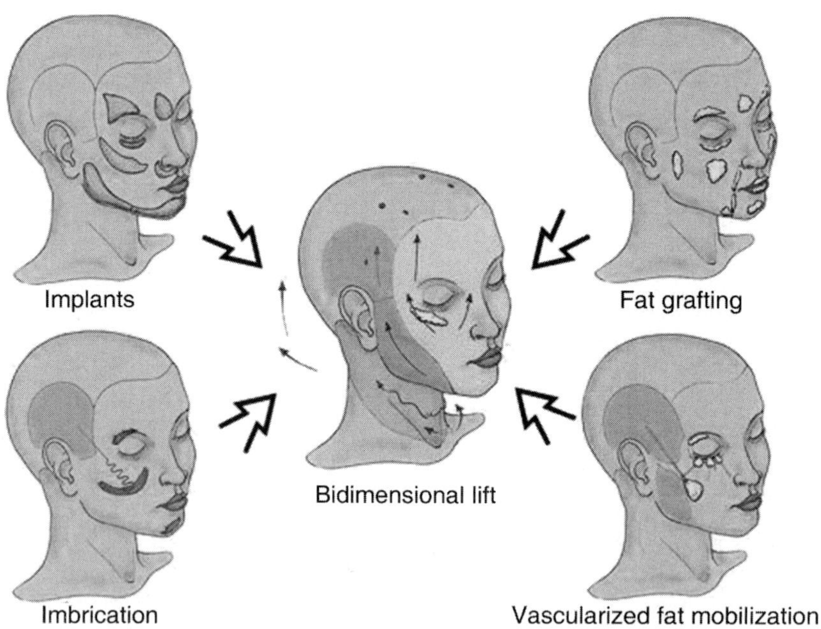

Figure 1 This is a schematic diagram showing the components available for three-dimensional facial rejuvenation. Bidimensional lifting in vertical and lateral planes provides the foundation of the endoscopic face-lift. Weak skeletal support can be corrected with alloplastic implants as shown in the upper left corner of the diagram. Fat grafting, as shown in the upper right corner, is commonly used to enhance areas not corrected by lifting techniques. In addition, fat grafting is used to treat small areas of depression or creases caused by subdermal damage. Imbrication of soft tissues is amenable in the brow, maxillary malar area, and mentum, as shown in the lower left corner. The lower right corner of the diagram shows the areas useful for augmentation by adjacent vascularized fat mobilization. These include upper orbital rim augmentation with the upper eyelid fat pads, the infraorbital rim tear trough area with the lower eyelid fat pads, and cheek augmentation with the Bichat's fat pad. *Source*: From Ref. 5.

PREOPERATIVE ASSESSMENT

Patients are all examined in a well-lit room, in a seated position. An initial assessment is performed, noting current and past medical history, past surgical history, current medications, and allergies. Social and family history is noted. A detailed history of past cosmetic procedures is obtained. A directed physical examination is performed, noting the stigmata of the aging process. Access to patient photographs at earlier stages in their lives is quite helpful in the creation of a surgical plan. Patients are encouraged to provide these if possible. Skeletal models and sample alloplastic implants, and drawings are available in the examination room to assist in the explanation of proposed surgical procedures. A comprehensive collection of preoperative and postoperative patient results is available to the patients for perusal.

PHOTOGRAPHIC DOCUMENTATION

All patients have photographic documentation performed prior to surgery. A full-face (A–P) frontal view, right and left three-quarter (oblique) views, right and left lateral views, and a tilted view are the minimum images acquired. Ancillary images, which include the "expression faces," are acquired based upon the developed surgical plan. The images are printed prior to the operative procedure and are posted in the operating room for intraoperative reference. Similar postoperative photographs are acquired at three months, six months, one year and more, respectively.

SOFT-TISSUE TECHNIQUES

Endoscopic Midface Rejuvenation

Standard face-lift procedures can effectively address the aging process around the jawline and neck. The bidimensional nature of these techniques fails to adequately address the volumetric loss in the midface region. By incorporating the principles of 3-D rejuvenation, more effective treatment of the aging midface can be accomplished. Innovative endoscopic procedures developed by Dr. Oscar Ramirez allows, restoration of midfacial volume without the stigmata of standard techniques (6).

The midface can be approached independently as a midface rejuvenation alone, with inclusion of only the temporal component of the endoscopic forehead lift, or in combination with a full endoscopic forehead rejuvenation. The pure endo-midface procedure is a technique advantageous for younger patients who do not need treatment of the central forehead. The addition of the temporal component allows a more reliable and simpler technique for midface suture anchoring. Patients requiring redistribution of redundant lateral orbital tissues elevated during the vertical lift benefit from the addition of the temporal component of the endoscopic forehead lift. Description of the full endoscopic forehead–midface procedure is beyond the scope of this chapter. However, we will briefly describe the endoscopic midface.

Surgical Technique

The endoscopic midface procedure begins with an incision in the temporal area. This incision is located perpendicular to a tangent drawn from the nasal ala to the lateral canthal tendon and is 2 cm inside the temporal scalp. A 1.8-cm incision is made through the skin and subcutaneous tissue, deep to the superficial temporal fascia.

Dissection is continued by maintaining it above the temporal fascia proper and more inferiorly above the intermediate temporal fascia. The initial dissection can be performed blindly in an inferior direction for approximately 2–3 cm. With the tissues elevated, a Silastic port protector is inserted and the remainder of the dissection is performed under endoscopic control. The temporal vein 2 (sentinel vein) and temporal vein 3 are preserved, in addition to the zygomaticotemporal nerves. The dissection continues in an anterior and inferior direction, remaining above the intermediate fascia. This continues down to the level of the zygomatic arch. The zygomatic arch is entered 2–3 mm above the superior border of the arch. This requires division of the intermediate temporal fascia, thus exposing the periosteum of the zygomatic arch. The authors prefer elevation of the anterior two-thirds of the zygomatic arch periosteum because it enables greater lifting and redistribution of the midface soft tissues. The periosteum of the entire zygomatic arch is elevated when soft tissues lateral to the cheek need to be elevated. Surgeon comfort with the dissection over the zygomatic arch is associated with a significant learning curve. We have found that communication of the midface and temporal dissections is accelerated with preelevation of the zygomatic arch, or at least the superior border of the arch.

The midface dissection at this point continues through an intraoral (upper buccal sulcus) incision. The authors' preferred incision is perpendicular to the alveolar ridge (vertical or oblique) at the level of the first premolar. We find that the vertically or obliquely oriented incision preserves the mucosal integrity at the alveolar ridge, allowing a rapid, watertight closure that is associated with fewer complications. Under direct visualization using a fiberoptic lighted retractor, the initial subperiosteal dissection of the maxilla and malar area is performed. The endoscope is used for the upper malar dissection. The use of the endoscope minimizes trauma to the midface structures caused by excessive traction. It also allows a more precise and cleaner dissection. The endoscope is most useful during periosteal elevation along the lateral half of the zygoma body, its extension underneath the fascia of the masseter muscle, and the anterior two-thirds of the zygomatic arch. A few fibers of the upper (medial) portion of the masseter tendon attached to the fascia can also be elevated from the zygoma. Endoscopic visualization assists in the preservation of the zygomaticofacial nerve.

Dissection continues along the inferior and lateral orbital rim and continues toward the superior border of the zygomatic arch. Skeletonization of the infraorbital nerve is not necessary under most circumstances.

With the initial midface dissection now complete, the endoscope is returned to the temporal area. An assistant elevates the soft tissue of the midface, thus allowing the surgeon to safely connect the temporal and midface dissection pockets under endoscopic control. Gentle elevation during this step protects the frontal branch of the facial nerve from injury. After a wide communication of the temporal and midface pockets is accomplished, the endoscope is reintroduced through the upper buccal sulcus incision.

The inferior orbital rim is dissected further by elevating the inferior arcus marginalis. A 4–0 Polydioxanone suture (PDS) (Ethicon, U.S.A.), introduced endoscopically, is used to imbricate the medial suborbicularis oculi fat (SOOF) to the lateral aspect of the inferior arcus marginalis. It is important to check eye globe mobility at this point with a forced duction test. Improper placement of this imbricating suture can trap or place traction upon the inferior rectus or inferior oblique muscles. Even suture lacing through the fat pad can indirectly affect the pulley system or the inferior rectus muscle. This suture has been designed to efface or obliterate the tear trough deformity.

The lateral aspect of the SOOF is then grasped with a 3–0 PDS suture, providing the first of three volumetric suspension sutures. Both ends of this suture are then passed through the temporal incision, under endoscopic guidance. The suture ends are tagged with a labeled needle driver. The second suspension suture is the cheek imbrication or "modiolus" suture. This suture is placed into the tenuous fascia/fat of the inferior maxillary soft tissue near the upper buccal sulcus incision. Both ends of this suture are then directed through the temporal incision and tagged, as previously described.

Exposure of the BF follows the placement of the third suspension suture. BF is approached through the superomedial wall of the buccal space. The periosteum and buccinator muscle are spread with the use of a blunt dissector. This allows the BF to herniate through maintaining an intact capsular fascia. The fat pad should be carefully dissected free from the wall of the buccal space. The BF should be easily movable for repositioning as a pedicle flap. A 4–0 PDS suture is then woven into the fat pad and the suture ends delivered to the temporal area, similar to the previous suspension sutures. The endoscope should be used to visualize the delivery of the pedicled fat flap over the zygomatic arch.

Each of the suspension sutures is then secured to the temporal fascia proper, in ordered fashion (Fig. 2). The sutures should be placed in the temporal fascia proper, below the level of the temporal incision. The first suture, the BF suspension, should be placed most medially. The inferior malar fascioadipose or "modiolus" suture is placed next, in a more lateral location of the temporal fascia proper. The most lateral suture, the SOOF suture, is the last to be anchored to the temporal fascia proper. This completes the suspension of the midface. Each

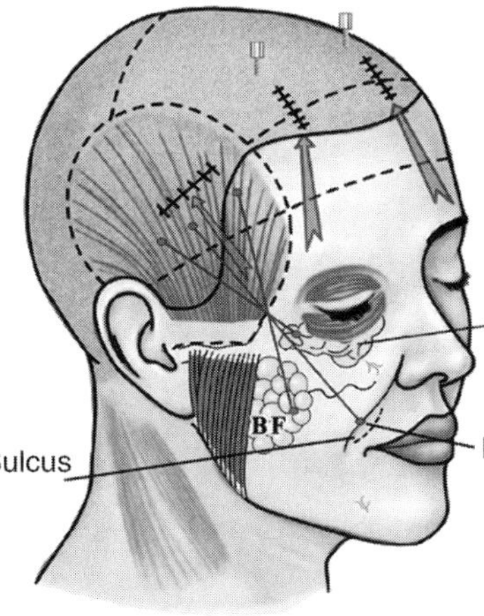

Figure 2 Treatment of the midface is performed with key suspension sutures that provide lifting in a vertical direction. The sutures are placed from the buccal sulcus incision and directed through the temporal pocket created endoscopically. The orientation of the anchoring and fixation of the corresponding sutures into the temporal fascia proper is indicated. The BF suture is woven through the fat pad and directed in a superomedial direction. This adds lateral bulk to the cheek over the zygomatic arch. The modiolus suture is directed in a tangential direction to the nasolabial fold and provides lifting of the lower cheek soft tissues. The SOOF suspension suture is directed most laterally and allows improvement of the tear trough deformity. *Abbreviations*: BF, Bichat's fat pad; SOOF, suborbicularis oculi fat.

suture has a different effect on the aesthetics of the cheek. BF suspension elevates and empties the suprajowl area and gives volume to the cheek. Modiolus suspension elevates the corner of the mouth and imbricates the cheek. The SOOF suspension elevates and gives volume to the cheek.

Butterfly drains are placed bilaterally through separate stab incisions in the temporal scalp. Each drain is carefully directed into the midface and secured to the temporal scalp with a suture. The superficial temporal fascia is then anchored to the temporal fascia proper with two 4–0 PDS sutures, while an assistant provides superomedial traction to the advanced scalp. The intraoral incisions are then closed with interrupted 4–0 chromic catgut sutures (Figs. 3–8).

Bichat's Fat Pad Excision

There is a subset of patients who present for midface rejuvenation, who demonstrate chubby cheeks, significant bulk and pseudoherniation of Bichat's fat pad, and good malar bone support. These patients benefit from excision of Bichat's fat pad rather than suspension. Dissection of the fat pad proceeds as previously outlined. However, care must be taken during resection of the fat pad. Undue traction of the fat pad can result in injury to neurovascular structures and/or Stensen's duct. Meticulous hemostasis should be obtained and can be facilitated by the use of bipolar cautery during Bichat's fat pad excision.

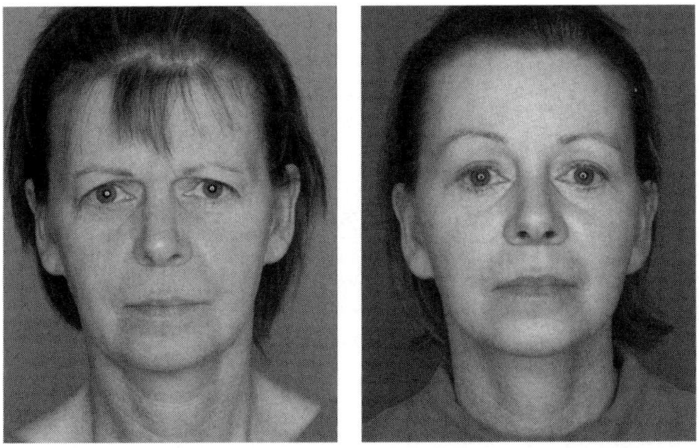

Figure 3 This 50-year-old patient had aging changes significant for her chronological age. She underwent an endoscopic midface-lift in conjunction with an endoscopic forehead lift and a mentopexy Type I (refer to Figs. 19–21). Note the nasolabial folds and the jowling present in the preoperative (*left*) view. Postoperatively (*right*), the patient demonstrates improved midface fullness and symmetry associated with a more youthful appearance.

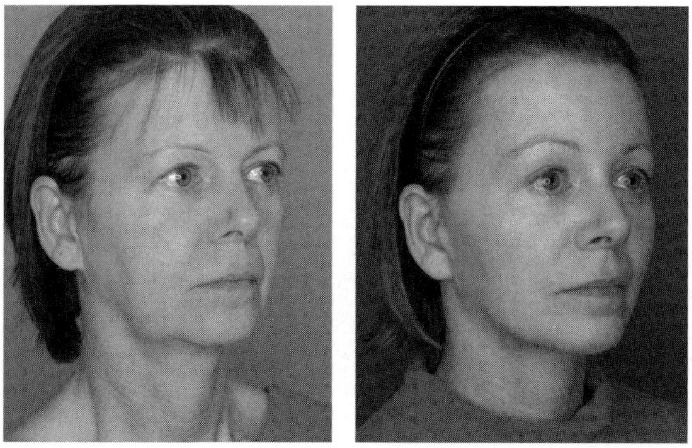

Figure 4 Preoperative (*left*) and postoperative (*right*) three-quarter views of the patient shown in Figure 3. Improvement in midface aesthetic can be clearly seen from the three-quarter view. Support of the cheek mass and transposition of the Bichat's fat pad contribute to the more youthful appearance.

Fat Grafting

Structural fat grafting, as described by Coleman (7), provides an excellent means for treating residual facial asymmetries or contour irregularities. Deep residual creases, such as nasolabial and marionette lines, can also be effectively treated. The fat grafts are typically harvested from the lower abdomen toward the end of the midface procedure. Grafts can be harvested from the hips, medial thighs, or posteromedial knee region in patients with a paucity of anterior abdominal fat.

Postoperative Care

The patients are monitored for 23 hours and discharged home under the care of a well-informed relative or practical nurse. The butterfly drains are attached to vacuum tubes and changed periodically during the next 48 hours. We find that evacuation of this fluid minimizes the amount of facial edema, postoperatively. Drain output of 10–20 mL should be expected, on average. Drain removal occurs typically on the second postoperative day. Antibiotics, started prior to surgery, are continued for five days, postoperatively. Steroids are not routinely given. Supportive taping of the midface begins at the end of the operative procedure and continues for approximately 7 to 10 days.

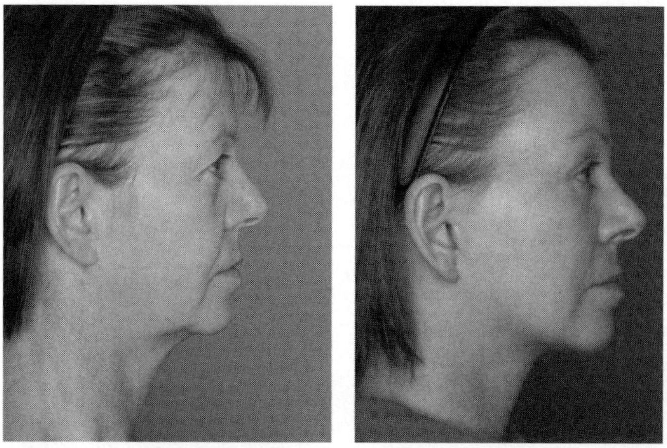

Figure 5 Preoperative (*left*) and postoperative (*right*) lateral views of the patient in Figures 3 and 4. Midface rejuvenation provides significant improvement of the lower eyelid-to-cheek transition. In addition, the degree of jowling is reduced and softening of the nasolabial fold results.

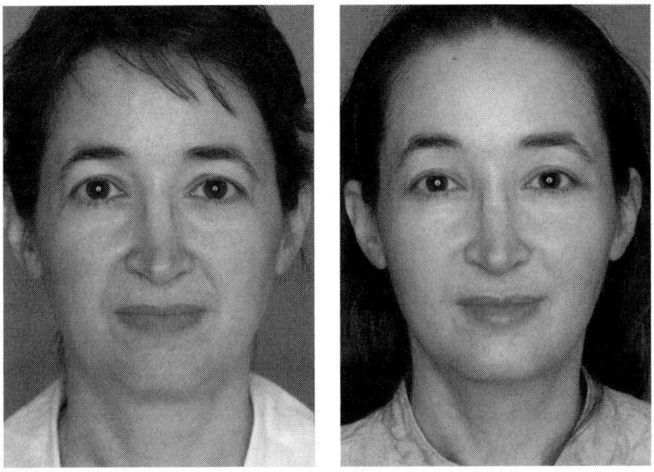

Figure 6 This is a 46-year-old patient who underwent an endoscopic midface procedure in conjunction with an endoscopic forehead lift and mentopexy Type II (refer to Figs. 22–24). Preoperative (*left*) and postoperative (*right*) frontal views are shown, respectively. Note the improved cheek mass position and softening of the nasolabial folds.

Complications

Complications related to the endoscopic midface and endoscopic temporomidface procedures include nerve injury, hematoma, infection, and alopecia. Nerve injury, perhaps the most devastating complication, is typically seen with excessive traction during endoscopic manipulation. In an effort to decrease traction-related nerve injury, we prefer to use a 4-mm endoscope and a blunt Cobra-tip sleeve. Retraction is avoided when possible, and slender retractors are implemented when necessary. Miniaturized instruments for dissection and manipulation have also been employed. With implementation of these steps, neuropraxia of the frontal branch of the facial nerve occurred in 0.4% of patients. Neuropraxia of the zygomaticus branch of the facial nerve and the infraorbital nerve occurred in 0.2% and 0.4% of patients, respectively (4). No permanent injury to motor nerves has been observed to date.

Hematoma and infection can be minimized with meticulous operative technique and adequate irrigation of the subperiosteal pockets with antibiotic solution prior to closure. Hematoma has been seen in a single patient, on postoperative day 4. This late presentation occurred secondary to an acute hypertensive episode. The hematoma was drained and the patient recovered uneventfully. Infection has been seen in one patient undergoing an endoscopic midface procedure. The patient complained of severe pain in the cheek, 10 days postoperatively. Fluctuance of the cheek mound and tenderness was noted. Incision and drainage of the collection resulted in resolution of the infection without further sequelae.

Alopecia is rarely seen following the endoscopic midface procedure. Adequate infiltration of local anesthetic, preoperatively, and judicious use of electrocautery can prevent unnecessary alopecia.

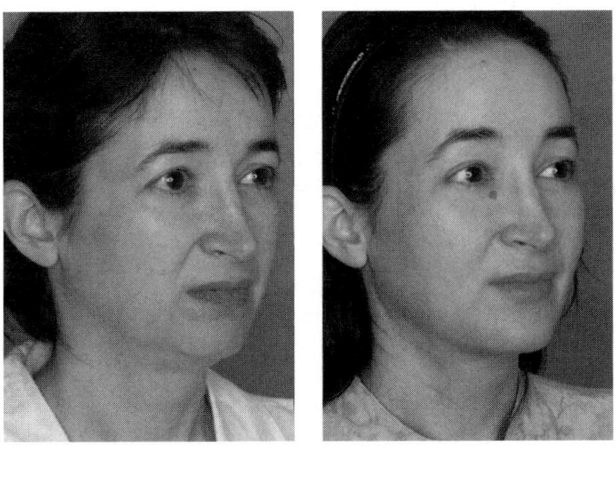

Figure 7 Preoperative (*left*) and postoperative (*right*) three-quarter views of the patient shown in Figure 6. Fullness of the lateral cheek mass in the postoperative view clearly defines a more youthful appearance.

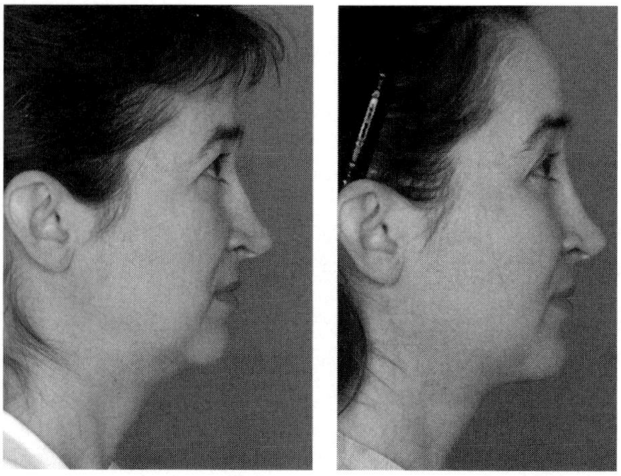

Figure 8 Preoperative (*left*) and postoperative (*right*) lateral views of the same patient. Note the smooth transition from the lower eyelid to cheek in the postoperative view.

ALLOPLASTIC IMPLANTS

Introduction

Facial rejuvenation procedures are increasing, involving the use of implantable biomaterials. The armamentarium of alloplastic implants available to the aesthetic and reconstructive surgeon is constantly changing. With the silicone breast implant crisis of the 1990s as a reminder, the use of alloplastic implants in facial rejuvenation should be judicious, and such implants should be placed with a clear understanding of their biocompatibility and morbidity. An ideal implant would be truly biocompatible and free of morbidity.

Although an implant of this nature fails to yet exist, modern implants that show a high degree of biocompatibility and demonstrate minimal morbidity when properly introduced have been developed.

Soft-Tissue Response to Augmentation

The ability to adequately correct contour deficiencies during facial rejuvenation procedures depends on a variety of factors, including, but not limited to, loss of skeletal volume, laxity of the connective tissue support, and gravitational migration of the soft tissues. Utilizing cephalometric analysis, attempts have been made to predict the soft-tissue response to craniofacial skeletal manipulation (osteotomy) (8,9). When considering the variables involved in creating aesthetic contour deformities, accurate prediction of the soft-tissue response to augmentation becomes less clear. To date, clinical studies demonstrating the predictable soft-tissue response to alloplastic augmentation fail to exist. Successful correction of facial contour deficiencies requires part artistic aptitude, part sound clinical skill, and the judicious use of implant sizers. The adage of "measure twice, cut once" truly applies to the use of alloplastic implants in facial rejuvenation surgery.

Choice of Alloplastic Implant Material

A cursory look through any aesthetic or reconstructive surgery journal will demonstrate the variety of alloplastic implants on the market. Keeping with the premise that an ideal alloplastic implant should be biocompatible and result in low patient morbidity, the choices narrow. Rubber polysiloxane (silicone) and high-density porous polyethylene implants are, currently, the most common alloplastic materials available for facial augmentation procedures.

Solid silicone implants are manufactured in a wide variety of shapes and sizes. The implants are soft and pliable and can be inserted with ease. The smooth surface of silicone implants does not permit vascular or soft-tissue ingrowth. Fibrous tissue encapsulation is characteristic of solid silicone implants. Morbidity related to silicone implants include infection, extrusion, and displacement, as well as bone erosion by the implants (10). The process of encapsulation makes removal of silicone implants technically less challenging when necessary.

High-density porous polyethylene implants such as Medpor (Porex Surgical, Newnan, Georgia, U.S.A.) are also manufactured in a variety of shapes and sizes. In contrast to silicone, the porous nature of these implants allows ingrowth of both soft tissue and bone (11). The morbidity related to porous polyethylene implants includes infection, extrusion, and seroma formation. The incorporation of the polyethylene implant into native tissue accounts for a significantly lower risk of infection and extrusion compared to silicone implants (12). However, morbidity can be significantly increased when removal of porous polyethylene implants is necessary. Bone and fibrous tissue ingrowth can make implant removal a formidable task. Patients must be informed of these characteristics when considering alloplastic facial augmentation with porous polyethylene implants.

Malar Implants

Midface rejuvenation can be accomplished with alloplastic implants in select patients. Although our bias tends toward soft-tissue augmentation of the cheek area, occasionally, patients request cheek rejuvenation without the desire for a full endoscopic procedure. Alloplastic implants provide an expedient way to achieve improved malar aesthetics. Several high-density porous polyethylene and solid silicone implants are available for malar augmentation. We prefer to use high-density porous polyethylene implants to provide subtle contouring of the midface. Medpor RZ Malar Shapes implants are available in 3- and 5-mm sizes. The implants are manufactured individually and specifically for right- or left-side implantation. The RZ malar implants are designed to provide the greatest projection central to the malar prominence and then taper toward the zygomatic wing. This specific shape creates a delicate malar augmentation in an anterior projection. Perceived facial width is not increased with these implants. The implants are manufactured with a notched medial edge so that the implant can be safely placed around the infraorbital nerve and foramen. We prefer to place the implants through a standard gingival buccal sulcus incision, described previously in the section on "Endoscopic midface Rejuvenation." Heavy absorbable sutures such as 3–0 PDS or rigid fixation with titanium screws can stabilize the implant in the desired position.

Mandibular Matrix System

Size and shape of the mandible affects the harmonious relationship of the skeletal support and the soft-tissue envelope that defines a beautiful face. The mandible is the framework of the lower face. Deficiencies in mandibular volume and shape can negatively affect the aesthetics of the mouth, chin, and neck. The mandibular matrix system was developed to address the absence of an inadequate mandibular contour (13). The mandibular matrix system allows a method of skeletal support restoration that can be applied to the entire mandible.

The system is composed of a series of implants made from porous polyethylene. The excellent biocompatibility characteristics make porous polyethylene the authors' choice for alloplastic augmentation of the mandibular framework. The implants allow for rapid vascularization and tissue ingrowth. The rapid integration of the implant material makes porous polyethylene the ideal alloplast for a mobile and dynamic structure such as the mandible. The mandibular matrix system can be fashioned to mimic the normal contour of the jawline. The multiple components of the implant system allow augmentation of the entire mandible or individual segments that may be deficient.

The implants have been designed to provide "tridimensional" restoration of the mandible. The implants wrap around the inferior border of the mandible. Due to this shape, the implants are self-stabilizing and require minimal or no screw fixation. This is a significant advantage as compared to 2-D onlay implants. In addition, the component system allows the restoration of the entire mandibular contour through minimal access incisions. The system is composed of a two-piece extended wraparound chin implant and gonial angle implants specifically designed for the right and left mandibular angles, respectively. A prejowl implant can replace the geniomandibular component or can be included as an onlay in this system when necessary.

The Implant System

Extended Wraparound Chin Implant

These implants are available as square or round implants, as viewed anteriorly. The implants are available in three sizes: small, medium, and large. These sizes correspond to 3, 5, and 7 mm of anterior projection, respectively. Each implant comprises right and left sides that are joined in the center by an alignment tab. The alignment tab is designed to allow stabilization of the two halves of the implant. Use of the alignment tab becomes optional when proper alignment of the implant along the inferior mandibular border is jeopardized.

Mandibular Angle Implant

These implants are designed to wrap around the inferior and posterior borders of the mandibular or gonial angle. The implants are specifically manufactured in right and left sides and are available in small, medium, and large sizes. These sizes correspond to 3, 7, and 11 mm of lateral projection, respectively. The greatest projection of the implant is at the level of the new gonial angle.

Adjunctive Implants: Prejowl and Button Chin Implants

Prejowl Implant

The prejowl implant is designed for patients who demonstrate a significant geniomandibular groove but do not require chin augmentation. The implant is supplied in two parts, divided medially. The implant has a 4-mm maximal projection that corresponds with the level of the prejowl depression.

Button Chin Implant

The button chin implant is a small tridimensional implant designed for patients who require improved anterior projection of the chin but do not require lateral augmentation along the mandible. The implant is available in 4 mm thickness. The implant is designed to comfortably wrap around the symphysis of the mandible. The wraparound feature provides stability to the implant, making rotation or migration of the implant virtually impossible.

Indications for Use

The authors have used the mandibular matrix system implants in patients with a congenital small mandible, edentulous patients, and patients seeking aesthetic improvement of the jawline. With total or partial loss of dentition, mandibular volume is severely affected. There is significant bony resorption of the mandibular body characterized by loss of height. Loss of chin projection is also characteristic. The generalized loss of bony support leads to skin laxity and excess around the jawline, the presence of jowls, lower lip redundancy, and chin ptosis. Failure to address the loss of structural support during rejuvenation of the soft tissue typically results in a poor aesthetic outcome. The mandibular matrix system provides an excellent construct to redefine the jawline, especially when combined with standard cervicoplasty procedures.

Surgical Technique

The surgical technique employed with the insertion of the mandibular matrix system has been refined since the early description in 2000. General anesthesia is recommended for all cases. When combined with adjunctive aesthetic procedures, the matrix system should be placed as early as possible. Access incisions should be closed immediately, in order to prevent possible contamination. Retromolar and lower buccal sulcus incisions can be used for the insertion of the mandibular angle implants and extended chin implants, respectively. The authors, however, now place both the mandibular angle and extended chin implants through a 3-cm submental incision and with the assistance of the 4-mm endoscope. The mandibular angle implants are secured with a 2–0 PDS suture, and the extended chin implants are secured with small titanium self-drilling or self-tapping screws, in bicortical fashion.

Careful planning is necessary for the placement of the submental incision. Augmentation of the bony symphysis will advance the soft-tissue envelope. This tends to rotate the submental incision anteriorly. Therefore, we typically place the incision 1 cm posterior to the submental crease. By doing this, the incision remains hidden in the submental area.

The dissection is carried down through the subcutaneous adipose tissue to the level of the platysma. A thick subcutaneous dissection is then performed 2 cm anterior and 2 cm posterior to the incision. The platysma, mentalis muscle, and periosteum are then divided in the midline, perpendicular to the direction of the submental skin incision. A subperiosteal dissection is then performed in an anterior direction, to the level of the mentolabial fold. This can be performed under direct visualization, with the aid of a lighted Aufricht retractor. Care must be taken to avoid perforation of the oral mucosa.

The dissection continues laterally to expose the entire anterior and inferior surface of the mandible. This dissection is facilitated with the use of a No. 4 Ramirez elevator (Snowden-Pencer, U.S.A.). The mental nerves must be identified and carefully dissected free from the surrounding structures, but skeletonization of the nerves should be avoided. Nerve injury can be prevented by early identification of the structures and avoidance of excessive retraction. The lateral dissection proceeds to the level of the anterior border of the masseter muscle. This can be accomplished with the assistance of the 4-mm endoscope or small fiberoptic lighted retractor. At this point, dissection is complete for the insertion of the extended chin implant Silastic sizers.

Insertion of the mandibular angle implants requires careful dissection of the pterygomasseteric sling. The 4-mm endoscope is inserted and a subperiosteal dissection continues with an angle periosteal retractor (Snowden-Pencer, U.S.A.). The pterygomaxillary sling is elevated in continuity (Fig. 9). Under direct visualization, the inferior aspect of the mandibular angle is freed from the tendinous and periosteal attachments. The posterior border of the ascending ramus is cleared in a similar fashion. The bony surface of the mandibular angle is then exposed sufficiently in anterior, inferior, and posterior directions to allow the insertion of Silastic mandibular angle implant sizers.

With the dissection complete, the cavity is irrigated with antibiotic solution followed by packing with neurosurgical pledgets soaked in diluted Betadine and epinephrine solution (1:30,000). The pledgets are left for several minutes to provide hemostasis and improve endoscopic visualization during implant placement.

As stated previously, oral incisions can be used for the placement of the implant system. However, the authors feel that this approach may increase the incidence of bacterial seeding of the implant and development of early postoperative infection.

Comfort with the endoscopic approach and access to the appropriate instrumentation should act as a guide to the method of implant introduction.

The extended chin and mandibular angle implants have been developed with corresponding Silastic sizers. Each sizer has a similar projection, length, and depth at the groove of the implant. The mandibular implant sizers are introduced followed by the extended chin implant sizers. The endoscope is then introduced to assess the fit of the sizers and the adequacy of the soft-tissue dissection. The external contour of the jawline is then assessed. The appropriate-sized implants are chosen based upon fit and desired aesthetic contour. Calipers are then used to measure the distance of the mental nerves from the midline and the lower border of the mandible. These measurements are recorded and transferred to the chosen extended chin implant. Grooves in the extended chin implant can then be carved with the use of a 10° scalpel and a cutting board. Adequate space (2–3 mm) around the mental nerve foramina should be created. Further carving of the extended chin and mandibular angle implants can be performed with a scalpel and/or a high-speed burr. All carving should be

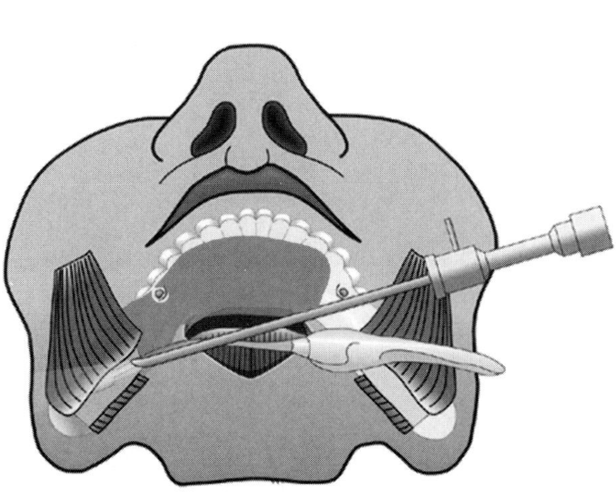

Figure 9 The endoscopic dissection of the pterygomasseteric sling. Note the dark gray area highlighted on the mandible. This represents the area of subperiosteal dissection required for placement of the mandibular matrix system.

done on a back table away from the patient. The prepared implants are then washed of debris and soaked in antibiotic solution.

The sizers are removed and the endoscope is inserted to assure that hemostasis has been achieved. A smooth, sterile plastic sleeve is then rolled into a conical shape and inserted into the incision. This sleeve isolates the implant from the skin surface and creates a smooth, protected surface for the rough porous polyethylene to slide against. Without the sleeve, insertion of the implant can be a humbling experience. The mandibular implants are then directed to the proper anatomic location under endoscopic guidance or with a small fiberoptic-lighted retractor. The implants can be manipulated with the assistance of two periosteal elevators.

The mandibular angle implant is then fixed into position with either a small titanium screw or a 2–0 PDS (Ethicon, U.S.A.) suture passed through a predrilled bicortical hole through the body of the mandible. The wraparound design of the mandibular angle implant prevents rocking of the implant when properly placed and allows fixation of the implant along its anterior border. If screw fixation is chosen, trajectory of the infra-alveolar (mental) nerve must be noted prior to drilling.

With the angle implants secured, the extended chin implants are inserted in a similar fashion. Use of the smooth plastic sleeve during implant insertion cannot be overstressed. Smooth insertion with minimal retraction will reduce the incidence of injury to the mental nerves. The extended chin implant is then positioned along the inferior border of the mandible. The location of the mental nerve is checked prior to screw fixation of the implant. Each side of the chin implant is fixed with a single small titanium screw in bicortical fashion, after predrilling. The lateral aspect of the extended chin implant should overlap the anterior border of the mandibular angle implant when attempting to achieve a wide profile. The lateral wings of the extended chin implant can be trimmed (no overlap with the angle implant) to maintain a narrow profile (Fig. 10).

Should the use of prejowl implants or a button chin implant be indicated, the implants can be placed through the same submental exposure. Fixation can be achieved with small titanium screws in either a unicortical or bicortical fashion. Aesthetic outcome will dictate the role these alternative implants play.

Prior to closure, the surgical cavity is irrigated with antibiotic solution. The platysma is sutured in the midline with interrupt sutures. If other aesthetic procedures are to be performed at the level of the neck, the skin incision is covered with a bio-occlusive dressing. This prevents tissue desiccation prior to skin closure. Skin closure, when appropriate, is performed with 5–0 or 6–0 Prolene (Ethicon, U.S.A.) interrupted sutures. A bio-occlusive dressing is

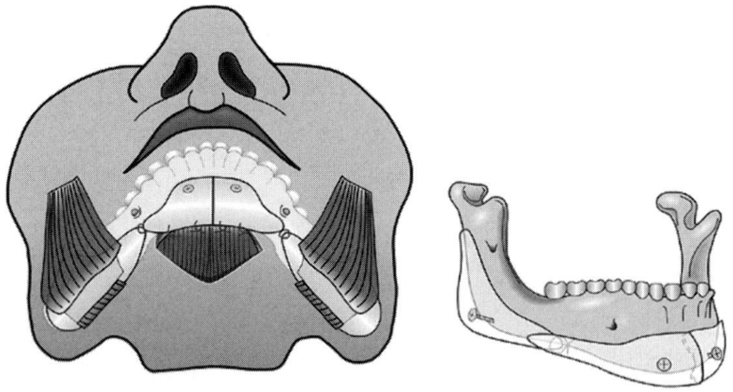

Figure 10 Final placement of the entire mandibular matrix system. The gonial angle implants are positioned along the mandible beneath the pterygomasseteric sling. Note that the implants are secured with titanium screws. The authors secure the chin implants with titanium screws as depicted. The lateral wings of the chin implant should overlap the gonial angle implants as shown to the right. This maintains a smooth contour to the augmented mandible. Although screw fixation of the gonial angle implants can be used, the authors prefer to secure the angle implants with a single 2–0 PDS suture placed through a drill hole in the inferior portion of the mandible. Significant support provided by the pterygomasseteric sling makes suture fixation of the gonial implants possible. *Abbreviation*: PDS, Polydioxanone (Ethicon, U.S.A.).

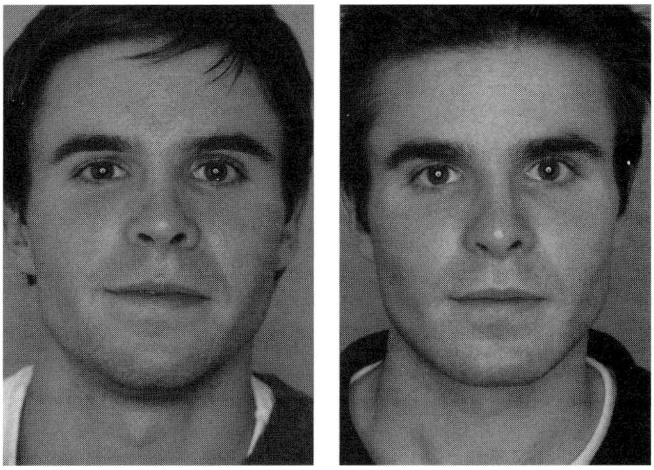

Figure 11 Anterior–posterior preoperative (*left*) and postoperative (*right*) views of a 20-year-old patient who underwent placement of the mandibular matrix system. The patient's preoperative concerns centered around the relative mandibular asymmetry and the narrow, pointed chin. Improved definition of the mandibular angles and balanced chin width are shown in the postoperative view.

applied over the incision after closure. A tight face-lift dressing is applied at the end of all procedures to reduce swelling and dead-space fluid accumulation (Figs. 11–16).

Postoperative Care

Oral antibiotics are given for 7 to 10 days. If oral incisions are used, antibiotics are continued until the incisions have healed. Patients are placed on a full liquid diet for one week. Diet is advanced to soft diet for one to two weeks before advancing to a regular diet. A supportive neck/chin strap is worn for 14 days.

Complications

The mandibular matrix implant system provides an excellent method for improving the aesthetic contour of the jawline. Complications related to the procedure include early and late infection, displacement of the implants, and patient dissatisfaction.

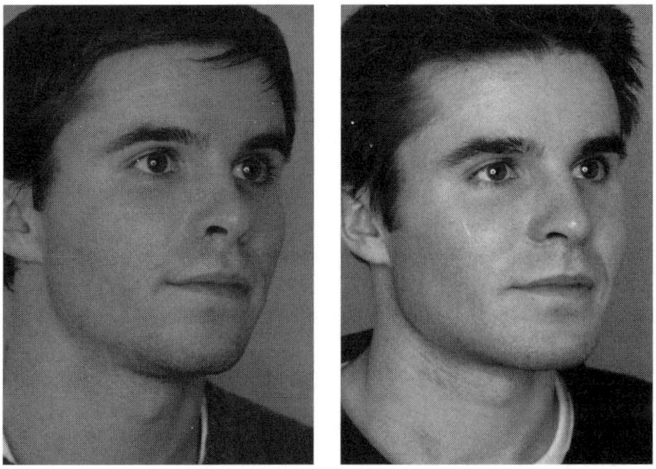

Figure 12 Three-quarter views of the patient in Figure 11. Preoperative (*left*) and postoperative (*right*) views are shown. The mandibular matrix system improves the definition of the entire mandible. Aesthetic balance of the mandible is achieved postoperatively with greater definition of the mandibular angle and chin width.

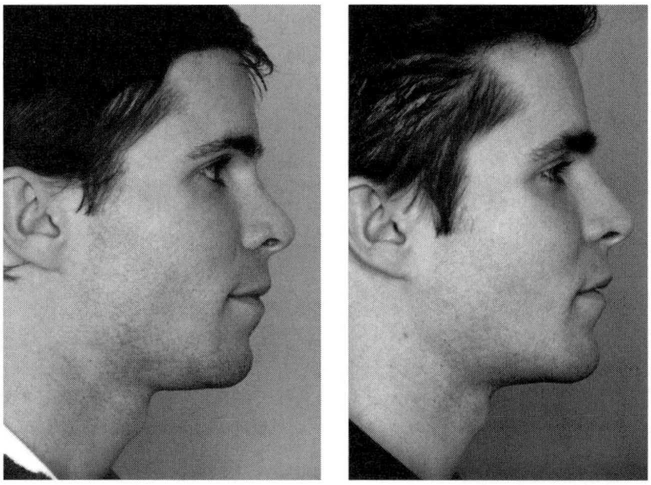

Figure 13 Lateral views of the patient in Figures 11 and 12—preoperative (*left*) and postoperative (*right*). Note the improvement of chin projection and shape with the extended wraparound chin implant of the mandibular matrix system.

Early infection can be treated with prompt recognition, irrigation and drainage, and the administration of antibiotics. To date, all infections in the authors' practice have been managed with conservative treatment, without the development of late infection.

Displacement of the implants typically occurs early in the postoperative course. Early reoperation is required to correct the position of the implant. Given the rapid fibrovascular ingrowth into porous polyethylene, implant displacement outside of the early postoperative setting is unlikely to be seen.

Patient dissatisfaction, though not typically considered a postoperative complication, deserves special mention. In the authors' practice, there is a subset of patients who present with adequate-to-borderline mandibular/chin size and projection, but desire enhancement of the mandibular contour. These patients have very critical aesthetic perceptions and are looking for aesthetic perfection in the surgical result. They expect immediate results and often

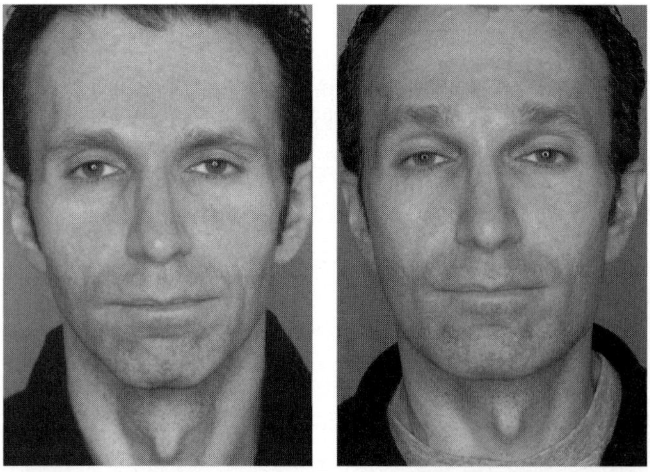

Figure 14 This 42-year-old patient demonstrates relative asymmetry of the upper and lower face. Preoperative anterior–posterior (A–P) view (*left*) shows a sharp, pointed chin and poor projection of the mandibular angles. Postoperative A–P view (*right*) after placement of the mandibular matrix system. Note the improved balance of the upper and lower face. The wraparound chin implant improves lower facial shape and the increased biangular distance provided by the gonial angle implants improves the overall mandibular width.

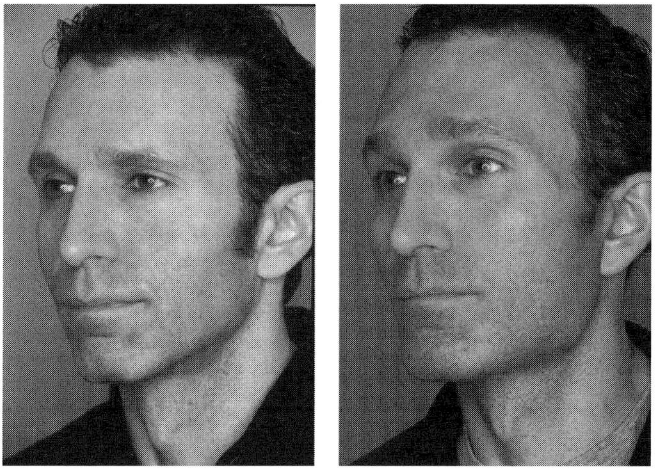

Figure 15 Three-quarter views of the patient in Figure 14. The preoperative view (*left*) shows the asymmetry of the broad upper face and narrow lower face. Postoperatively (*right*), improved definition of the mandibular angle and projection of the chin create a more balanced aesthetic result. Harmony between the upper and lower face has been achieved.

become distraught over their appearance in the early postoperative phase. We have coined the phrase: "The Dorian Gray Phenomenon" to describe this process. The patients may request early removal of the implant system if the results do not meet their expectations. These patients, when recognized preoperatively, are counseled to expect up to 12 weeks of recovery before the final aesthetic results are evident. If still dissatisfied with the results, further procedures can be discussed to augment or reduce the size of the implant system. Complete removal of the implants should be avoided. These patients must be aware that skeletal-to-soft-tissue disproportion may become accentuated by complete removal of the implant system.

THE COMBINED APPROACH (SOFT TISSUE WITH OR WITHOUT IMPLANTS)

Mentopexy

The aging chin is a complex entity that frequently is not properly addressed during facial rejuvenation procedures. Gonzales-Ulloa coined the term "witch's chin" deformity to describe the characteristic sagging soft tissues of the aging chin (14). The witch's chin deformity more properly consists of ptosis of the premental soft tissues, a prominent submental crease, and often a loss of bony projection.

Chin pad ptosis can occur as a normal process of aging and as an iatrogenic process. Zide points out that the ptotic chin can result from gravitational migration of the soft tissues

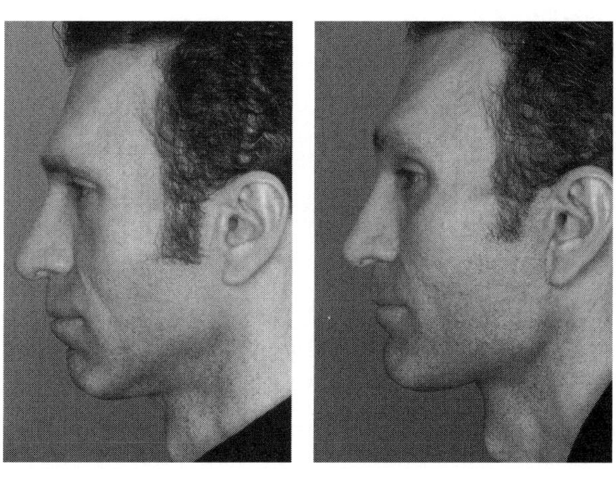

Figure 16 Lateral views of the patient in Figures 14 and 15—preoperative (*left*) and postoperative (*right*). Note the improved projection of the chin and definition of the mandibular angle.

alone and can present as a relative ptosis due to a deficient soft-tissue configuration behind the submental fold (15). Lesavoy et al. state that three primary situations give rise to the deformity: (*i*) loss of bony projection and mentalis muscle origination concomitant with gravitational elastosis of overlying soft tissues, especially in edentulous patients; (*ii*) imbalance of the soft tissue–to–bony projection relationship as well as loss of mentalis muscle origination that occurs after osseous reduction of the mandible; and (*iii*) loss of mentalis muscle origination, bone resorption, and capsular contracture that occurs with removal of (Silastic) prosthetic chin implants, particularly those placed in a subperiosteal position, especially those of longstanding duration (16).

In an effort to address the complex pathophysiology of the witch's chin deformity, the authors present a multivariate approach toward correction of the ptotic chin. Soft-tissue manipulation and the use of alloplastic implants play a role in the treatment of the ptotic chin. A subperiosteal dissection performed through a submental incision is used for each of the procedures described.

Mentopexy—Type I

The Type I mentopexy procedure involves simple elevation of the ptotic soft-tissue envelope with a 3–0 PDS suspension suture. This technique is ideally suited for patients who demonstrate ptosis of the soft-tissue mass of the chin without loss of skeletal support (Fig. 17).

Mentopexy—Type II

The Type II mentopexy procedure provides elevation of the soft-tissue envelope and imbrication of redundant soft-tissue mass, with a 3–0 PDS suture placed in a purse-string fashion. This technique, similar to the Type I procedure, is suited for patients showing ptosis of the soft-tissue chin without diminution of skeletal support. The purse-string technique allows reefing of redundant tissue laterally. The purse-string can also be used to create or augment an existing midline dimple (Fig. 18).

Mentopexy—Type III

Mentopexy can be performed in conjunction with alloplastic augmentation of the chin. We classify this procedure as a Type III mentopexy. The primary indication for this technique is significant diminution of skeletal support in the symphyseal region of the mandible in combination with severe soft-tissue ptosis of the chin (witch's chin). Diminution of the skeletal support commonly is seen in edentulous patients and patients with a history of a longstanding Silastic chin implant placed in a subperiosteal plane. This complex of bony and soft-tissue involvement must be recognized preoperatively. Unless each component is adequately

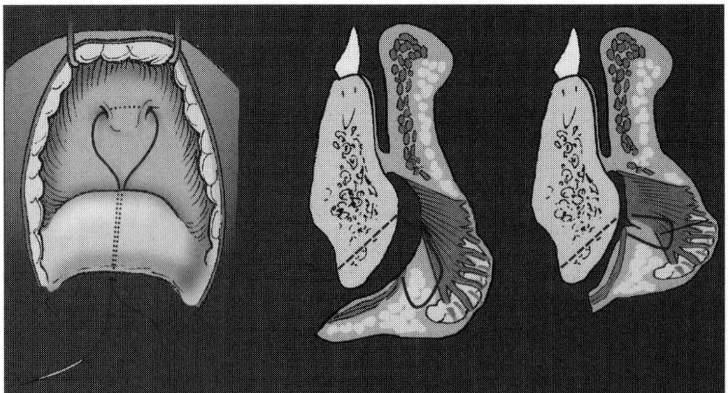

Figure 17 Mentopexy Type I. The left image depicts the view seen from inferior to superior. The suture is placed in the chin soft tissue at the inferior aspect of the mentalis muscle. The middle and right-side images show the effect provided by suture fixation. The chin soft tissue is elevated in a superior and anterior direction. The 3–0 PDS suture is passed through a midline hole drilled through the inferior border of the mandible and is secured to the posterior aspect of the mandible.

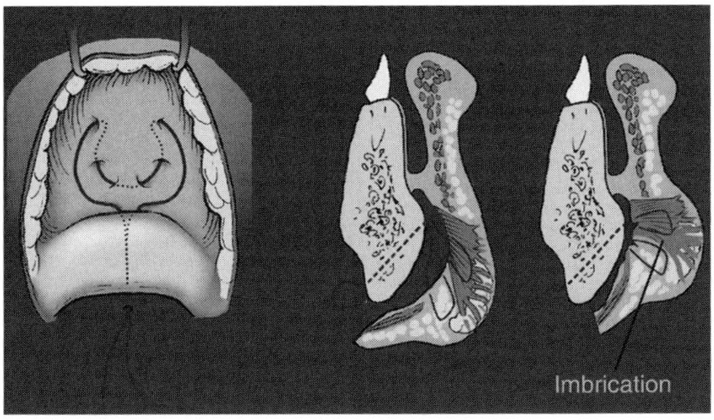

Figure 18 Mentopexy Type II. The purse-string 3–0 PDS suture provides elevation and imbrication of the chin soft tissue. Fixation follows as described in Figure 17.

addressed, postoperative aesthetic results will be significantly compromised. Augmentation of the skeletal support and repositioning of the soft-tissue envelope are necessary to achieve a balanced aesthetic outcome.

The chin implant is secured with small titanium screws in a bicortical fashion. The preferred suture technique (Type I or Type II) used during the mentopexy procedure is fixed to the porous polyethylene implant at the appropriate level to achieve the desired aesthetic result.

Mentopexy—Type IV

The Type IV mentopexy procedure involves redraping of the soft-tissue mass of the chin. The periosteum is carefully scored in a cephalad direction at several points lateral from midline. This scoring technique allows the soft tissue to be redraped along the mandibular border. This technique is preferred for patients demonstrating increased skeletal projection of the mandible, who do not want reduction genioplasty. This technique, combined with standard cervicoplasty procedures, can provide lasting aesthetic results.

Surgical Technique

The mentopexy procedure begins with a 3-cm submental incision, placed one finger's breadth posterior to the native submental crease. The skin and subcutaneous tissue are dissected down to the level of the platysma. A skin/subcutaneous tissue flap is then generated, 2 cm in both the anterior and posterior direction. The platysma is then incised in the midline up to the level of the inferior border of the mandible. The periosteum is divided, in a similar fashion, allowing the remainder of the procedure to be performed in a subperiosteal plane. A blunt-tip periosteal elevator is then used to elevate the periosteum of the mandible in an anterior and lateral direction. Anterior dissection proceeds to the level of the oral mucosa. Perforation of the oral mucosa is to be avoided. The periosteal dissection proceeds laterally to the anterior border of the masseter tendon. Care must be taken when dissecting around the mental nerve foramena. We do not skeletonize the mental nerves, in an effort to prevent traction-related neuropraxia.

The Type I and Type II mentopexy procedures utilize suspension of the ptotic soft-tissue structures. Suspension is performed with placement of the 3–0 PDS suture at the level of the lowermost aspect of the mentalis muscle/periosteum. A bicortical drill hole is then created in the midline of the mandibular symphysis. The drill hole should be directed in a caudal fashion as shown in Figs. 17 and 18. The suture is then directed through the bone and tied along the posterior border of the mandible. Evaluation of the proper chin position is noted prior to skin closure.

The Type III mentopexy procedure follows in a similar fashion. Several caveats should be noted with this technique. Location of the mental nerves should be noted prior to chin augmentation. We routinely measure the distance of each mental nerve from the midline as well as the inferior border of the mandible with the use of calipers. These measurements are then transferred to the chin implant. Any overlap of the implant is removed, leaving a 2- to 3-mm gap around the mental nerve foramena. The implants are secured to the bone with small titanium screws placed in a bicortical fashion. The suspension suture is then driven through

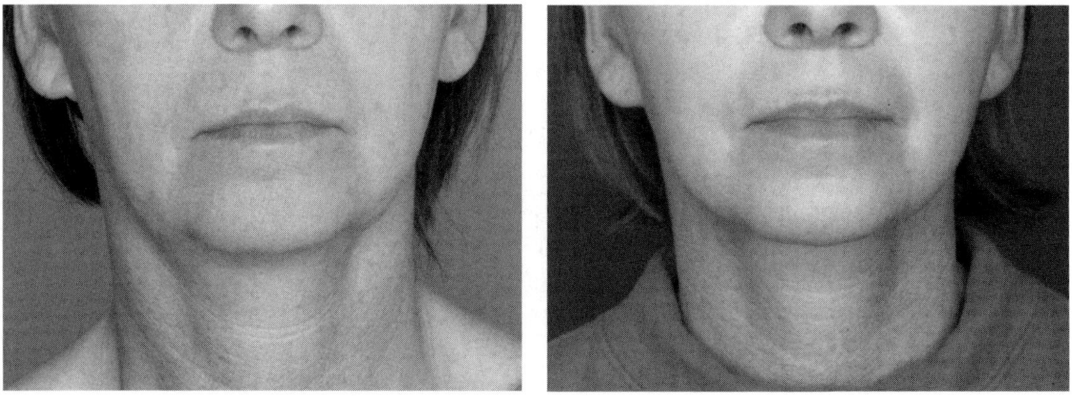

Figure 19 Preoperative (*left*) and postoperative (*right*) views following a mentopexy Type I procedure as seen from the anterior–posterior projection.

the porous polyethylene implant at the desired level. It is not necessary to place the suture through the mandible, as described for the Type I and II technique.

The Type IV mentopexy technique, being a redraping technique, does not require suture fixation. Care must be taken during periosteal scoring to prevent injury to the underlying mentalis musculature. Scoring can be performed with a scalpel or electrocautery placed on a low setting. Complete mobilization of the periosteum to the level of the anterior masseter tendon is crucial for the success of this technique.

When the proper aesthetic result is achieved, the dissection pocket is irrigated with antibiotic solution. The platysma is approximated in the midline with interrupted sutures. The skin edges are approximated with 5–0 or 6–0 Prolene sutures. Tape is then applied to the chin for support. If adjunctive aesthetic procedures are to be performed in the neck, the submental incision is covered with a protective bio-occlusive dressing to prevent desiccation. The incision is then closed at the completion of the case (Figs. 19–24).

Postoperative Care

A bio-occlusive dressing is placed on the submental incision for two to three days. Supportive taping of the chin begins in the operating room and continues for seven days, postoperatively. The sutures are removed on postoperative day 3 to day 5 to prevent crosshatching.

Complications

Neuropraxia of the mental nerves is the most commonly encountered complication of this procedure. Careful identification of the mental nerves early in the course of dissection and gentle

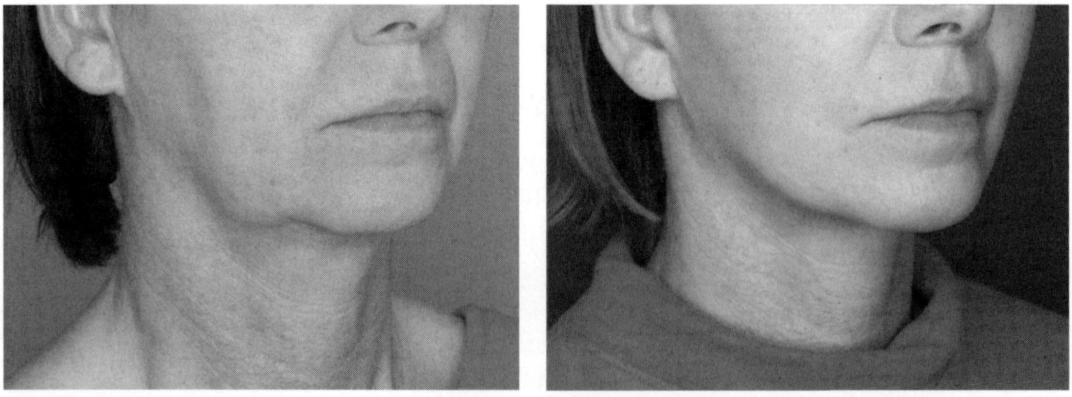

Figure 20 Three-quarter views of the patient in Figure 19. Preoperative (*left*) and postoperative (*right*) views.

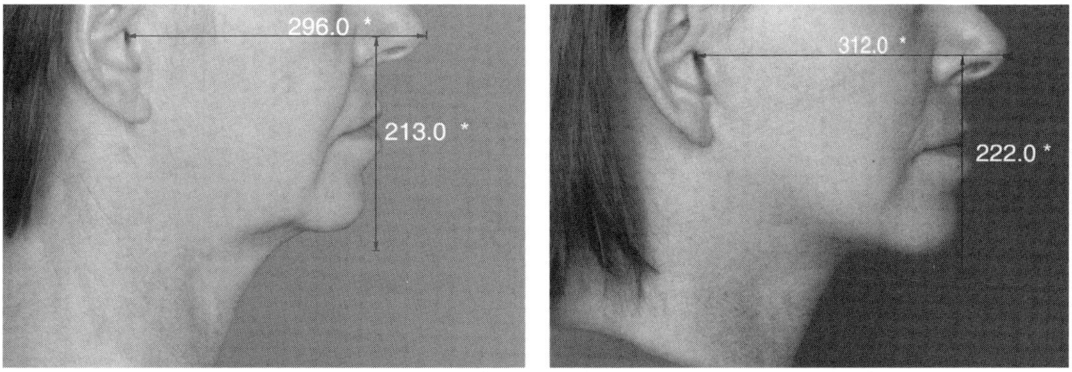

Figure 21 Lateral views of the patient in Figures 19 and 20. Note the chin pad ptosis and poor anterior projection of the chin in the preoperative view (*left*). Postoperatively (*right*), the reference lines demonstrate the improved anterior projection of the chin following the Type I mentopexy.

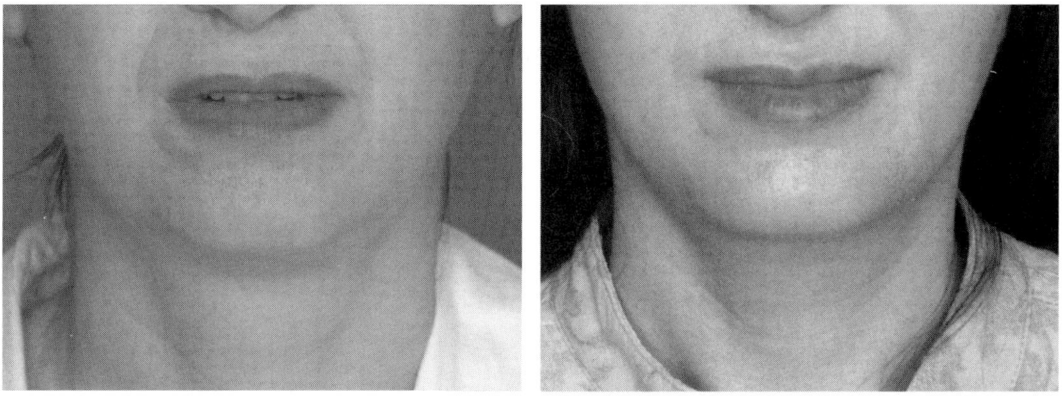

Figure 22 Anterior–posterior views of a Type II mentopexy patient. Preoperative (*left*) view and postoperative (*right*) result are shown.

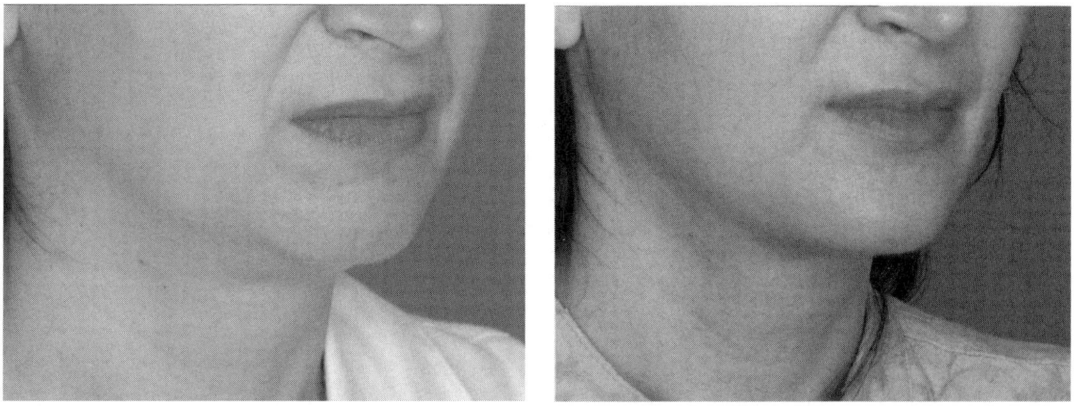

Figure 23 Three-quarter views of the patient in Figure 22. Preoperative (*left*) and postoperative (*right*) images are shown. The Type II mentopexy was performed to address the mild clefting in the chin soft tissue seen in the preoperative view. The purse-string suture of the Type II mentopexy obliterated the soft-tissue cleft and provided improved chin aesthetics.

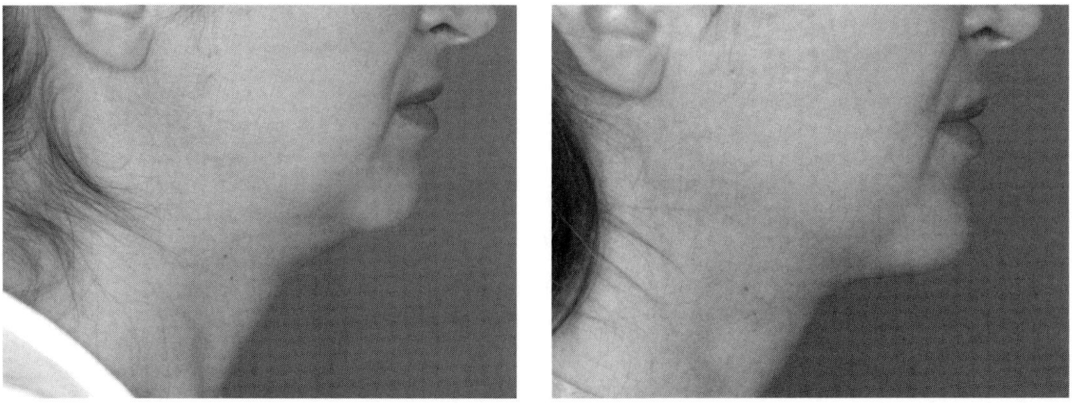

Figure 24 Lateral views of the patient in Figures 22 and 23. Ptosis of the chin in the preoperative (*left*) view is corrected with the mentopexy procedure as shown with the postoperative result (*right*).

retraction cannot be overstressed. Implants placed should not impinge upon the mental nerves. Leaving a 2- to 3-mm space around the foramena should always be observed. Most cases of neuropraxia resolve within several weeks. Permanent nerve injury has not been observed in the authors' practice.

SUMMARY

Being cognizant of the face's 3-D structure, it becomes evident that facial rejuvenation should be performed with "tridimensionality." The senior author has developed revolutionary techniques to accomplish this goal. This approach to facial rejuvenation is founded upon a clear understanding of the facial aging process. Both gravitational migration of soft-tissue structures and loss of skeletal support play significant roles in the aging face. We have shown that repositioning the soft-tissue envelope in a subperiosteal plane can significantly improve facial aesthetics.

The authors firmly believe that autogenous tissue should be used in the sculpting process whenever possible. The endoscopic midface procedure derives its success from the ability to reposition these autogenous tissues. The endoscopic midface procedure demonstrates that significant soft-tissue remodeling can be accomplished without the need for alloplastic implants.

Alloplastic materials have a contributory role, as well. Although no implant material is perfectly biocompatible, alloplasts, such as porous polyethylene, have been shown to be safe and effective for correction of skeletal deficiencies. The mandibular matrix system described in this chapter is ideally suited for correction of aesthetic contour deficiencies around the jawline. The segmental design of the implant system offers surgeons the flexibility of minimal access incisions and the versatility to correct partial or complete contour deficiencies.

There are occasions where a combined use of native soft tissue and alloplastic implants is indicated. We present a novel approach to the treatment of the ptotic chin. The witch's chin deformity has long been a misunderstood and mistreated entity. Using a combined approach, we have demonstrated that both soft-tissue manipulation and bony augmentation with implants can play a role in the treatment of the ptotic chin.

REFERENCES

1. Delmar H. Anatomy of the superficial parts of the face and neck. Ann Chir Plast Esthet 1994; 39(5):527–555 (in French).
2. Yousif NJ et al. The nasolabial fold: a photogrammetric analysis. Plast Reconstr Surg 1994; 93:70.
3. Pessa JE. An algorithm of facial aging: verification of Lambro's theory by three-dimensional stereolithography, with reference to the pathogenesis of midfacial aging, scleral show, and the lateral suborbital trough deformity. Plast Reconstr Surg 2000; 106:479.

4. Ramirez OM. The central oval of the face: tridimensional endoscopic rejuvenation. Facial Plast Surg 2000; 16(3):283–298.
5. Ramirez OM. Full face rejuvenation in three dimensions: a "face-lifting" for the new millennium. Aesth Plast Surg 2001; 25:152–164.
6. Ramirez OM. Three-dimensional endoscopic midface enhancement: a personal quest for the ideal cheek rejuvenation. Plast Reconstr Surg 2002; 109(1):329–340.
7. Coleman SR. Structural fat grafts the ideal filler. Clin Plast Surg 2001; 28(1):111–119.
8. Hershey HG, Smith LH. Soft-tissue profile change associated with surgical correction of the prognathic mandible. Am J Orthod 1974; 65:483.
9. Hohl TH et al. Craniofacial osteotomies: a photocephalometric technique for the prediction and evaluation of tissue changes. Angle Orthod 1978; 48:114.
10. Friedland JA, Coccaro PJ, Converse JM. Retrospective cephalometric analysis of mandibular bone absorption under silicone rubber chin implants. Plast Reconstr Surg 1976; 57:144.
11. Wellisz T, Kanel G, Anooshian RV. Characteristics of the tissue response to Medpor porous polyethylene implants in the human facial skeleton: the long term effects of biomedical implants. J Long Term Eff Med Implants 1993; 3:223.
12. Rubin JP, Yaremchuk MJ. Complications and toxicities of implantable biomaterials used in facial reconstructive and aesthetic surgery: a comprehensive review of the literature. Plast Reconstr Surg 1997; 100(5):1336–1353.
13. Ramirez OM. Mandibular matrix implant system: a method to restore skeletal support to the lower face. Plast Reconstr Surg 2000; 106(1):176–189.
14. Gonzales-Ulloa M. Ptosis of the chin: the witch's chin. Plast Reconstr Surg 1972; 50:54.
15. Zide BM. The mentalis muscle: an essential component of chin and lip position. Plast Reconstr Surg 2000; 105(3):1213–1215.
16. Lesavoy MA, Creasman C, Schwartz RJ. A technique for correcting witch's chin deformity. Plast Reconstr Surg 1996; 97(4):842–846.

5 Reshaping of the Periorbital Region

Frank Trepsat
Clinique de Genolier, Geneva, Switzerland

INTRODUCTION

Since the early days of aesthetic facial surgery, improving the eyelid region has been an important part of the technical developments in the treatment of this telltale area of aging. One of the crucial points in facial rejuvenation is the restoration of a youthful, natural, rested look. Indeed, when you look at someone, you actually do not look at the eyelids, but you do see them, and the first impression that you get is based on what you have seen. On the contrary, you never look at the neck unless someone with an unusual appearance makes you wonder if that person could have had a face-lift.

As far as the upper eyelid region is concerned, most patients arrive saying, "Doctor, I have too much skin on my upper eyelids. Please get rid of it for me!" The various surgical techniques that have been developed enable the removal of this excess skin by methods of varying sophistication. Certain authors have focused on the level of the incision or the amount of skin to be removed, while others have described techniques refining the location and extent of the palpebral fold (1). But removing some tissue from the eyelids or recreating a fold does not restore youth; it just, in many cases, changes the face into a different one that has never before existed. If you want to look like you did some years ago, you have to consider what has changed; when you do that, you realize that the problem is not a skin excess but a lack of tissue fullness.

When the first frontal coronal lifts were performed (2–5), interest was focused more on how much the scalp should be tightened and where to tighten it than on analyzing the characteristics of youth. With the more subtle and refined endoscopic frontal lifts, authors (6–8) became more interested in trying to keep as natural a look as possible but, at that time, had in mind only the movements of the eyebrows and the eyelids in a two-plane geometrical space. Aging in the frontal area is a change of shape; just consider the shape of the frontal area of a child and his grandmother: the child has a soft, rounded forehead and the grandmother has a centrally depressed frontal bone, depressed temporal fossa, and the corrugator muscles showing through a thinned subscalp layer. Endoscopic experts improved our knowledge of functional anatomy (9,10) and interest turned to understanding the processes that produce an aged look.

In the lower eyelid region the request is similar: "Please get rid of these bags under my eyes and pull my skin like this," and patients invariably pull the skin of their lower eyelids upward. All the classical techniques described up to now tell us how to remove the excess skin and how to tighten it from above or laterally without obtaining an ectropion, and how to remove the excess fat bulging through the skin. But everybody thinks in terms of gravity pulling the lateral canthus and the lower eyelids from below. Authors described ingenious techniques to tighten the lateral canthus, which, in most cases, has not changed at all: it is just the deflation of the whole area, which aspirates from below the lower eyelids and pulls downward the lateral tendon. Indeed, the loss of the supporting pillar that represents the malar fat pad pulls downward the nonsupported lower eyelid. Just think of the appearance of someone with Franceschetti syndrome: the problem comes from below and not from above.

The papers by Loeb (11) developed later in his article by Hamra (12) are landmarks because they allowed us to realize that preserving fat is important. To preserve first is a good idea, to replace the lost fat is the next step. The description of the first midface-lift by Tessier (13) was a historic landmark in that he considered the middle third of the face as a unit, including the lower eyelid region, but did not focus on the importance of the palpebromalar junction.

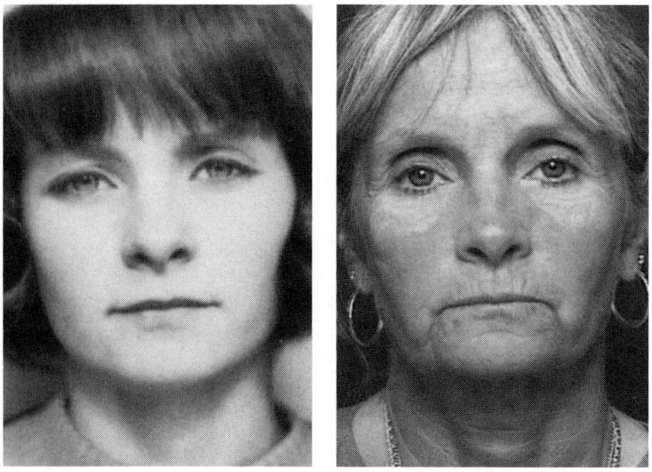

Figure 1 Periorbital aging is mostly due to fat atrophy.

Laser resurfacing was for a while very much in fashion and seemed very promising, but in the long run many plastic surgeons stopped using it because of its tendency to bleach the skin and also because of the risks of ectropion because it shrinks the skin, which then contracts and pulls down.

Fat grafts have been performed for a very long time, but take was unpredictable and resorption was frequent. It had the reputation of unpredictability although some plastic surgeons used small fat grafts on a regular basis with confidence.

The very detailed and precise description of micro–fat grafting (lipostructure) by Coleman (14) marked for us the start of a new era because it gave us the possibility of restoring reliably many of the characteristics of youth. He described in 1994 (15) the way he treats the periorbital region, as did Fagien in the upper eyelid (16), and Lambros in the midface (17) with micro–fat grafts. Erol improves the midface with a tissue cocktail (18).

For a long time, other successful ways of restoring a youthful facial shape were developed successfully with the use of implants or prostheses: Flowers described the polar bear syndrome due to an alteration of the shape of the malar bone and its correction by silicone prosthesis, and published many papers on the palpebral region. Terino (19) focused his interest and expertise on developing prostheses to improve the chin area, the malar zone, and the jawline, and he has vast experience in this field. Ramirez (20) includes in his facial rejuvenation program the insertion of a prosthesis to improve the angle of the mandible and the jawline. But fear of infection and of detection of the implants kept many of us away from these techniques, although they were very successful in the hands of experts.

The analysis of the aging process of each patient may be different, but there are constant findings that may be shown during the first consultation with a prospective patient. Ask the patient to bring along a full-face view taken a long time ago, or that is pleasing. This picture is then scanned and compared on the screen with the same view taken the day of the consultation.

When comparing two pictures of the same patient taken 30 years apart, you will notice in Figure 1 the upper eyelids have a sunken appearance, and there is a tear trough deformity in the lower eyelids.

ABOVE THE INTERCANTHAL LINE

A downward slant of the tail of the eyebrow due to a loss of skin elasticity in the temporal region and also due to a loss of volume of the entire frontal region is caused by modifications in the shape of the calvarium as well as a decrease in the thickness of the soft-tissue layers. As a result, it seems that there is too much skin in the lateral part of the upper eyelid and the patient has a hooded appearance. Some patients try to get rid of this excess skin lying on their eyelashes by elevating their eyebrows, thereby accentuating their aged look (Fig. 2).

This impression of excess skin is enhanced even more by a significant fat resorption occurring mostly in the lateral compartment of the upper eyelid and eyebrow fat in the fatty

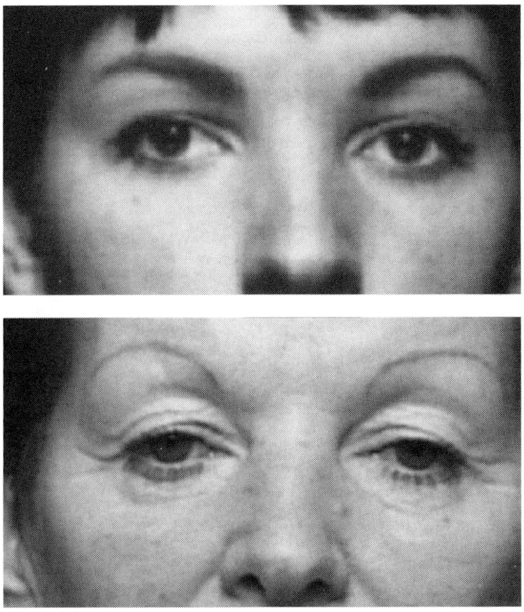

Figure 2 In some cases, apparent skin excess leads to frontal hyperactivity.

layer of Charpy or retro orbicularis orbital fat (ROOF). The inner upper eyelid fat compartment, which resembles more the type of fat encountered inside the extraocular cone, is less prone to reabsorbtion and is therefore more visible after resorption of the lateral compartment; so the upper eyelid skin, deflated in its lateral two-thirds, is also deprived of the vascularization induced by the presence of youthful fat. As a result, it is less elastic, more wrinkled, and is pushed downward by the weight of the eyebrow. As the inner fat compartment resists the aging process better, we see quite frequently hollowness in the region of the pulley of the grand oblique muscle that separates the two fat compartments in the upper eyelid.

As the skin loses its elasticity, the fibrous attachments between the tarsus and the skin tend to loosen and wrinkles may be seen in this usually smooth region; as a result, great care is necessary in searching for a slight senile ptosis that could impair the operation.

The glabella is also involved in the aging process: the calvarium shape changes and so does the upper orbital rim. There is a thinning of the central part of the glabella fat layer revealing the hypertonic and hypertrophied corrugator muscles; this gives an angry, unhappy look with a lowering of the head of the eyebrows and deep vertical wrinkling between the eyebrows.

BELOW THE INTERCANTHAL LINE

The slight downward migration of the lateral part of the lower eyelid is due to a loss of its support by the malar fat pad. This loss of a supporting pillar is a major element in the aging of the lower eyelid and must be dealt with, if rejuvenation of the patient's face, and not only the eyelids, is what is really wanted. The face should be considered as a whole, not made of separate bits and parts that can be repaired without any relationship with the others (frontal region and eyebrows for the upper eyelid and malar area for the lower eyelid region).

This loss of support is due to a loss of thickness in the suborbicularis orbital fat pad (SOOF) (21) between the orbital retaining ligament (ORL) and the zygomaticocutaneus ligament (ZCL) described by Mendelson et al. (22), as well as a loss of volume in the malar fat pad in front and behind the orbicularis oculi muscle, and the downward migration of the rest of this malar fat pad. These two events produce a tear-trough deformity that circles the aging lower eyelid.

As, simultaneously, the orbicularis oculi muscle loses some of its tone and the septum orbital weakens, they give way to a protrusion of the three fat bags in the lower eyelid, which lie on the distended ORL.

Thus, descending from the ciliary margin, you will notice: the aging, thin inelastic skin covering the lower tarsus, the bulge of the protruding intraorbital fat, and then, the furrow

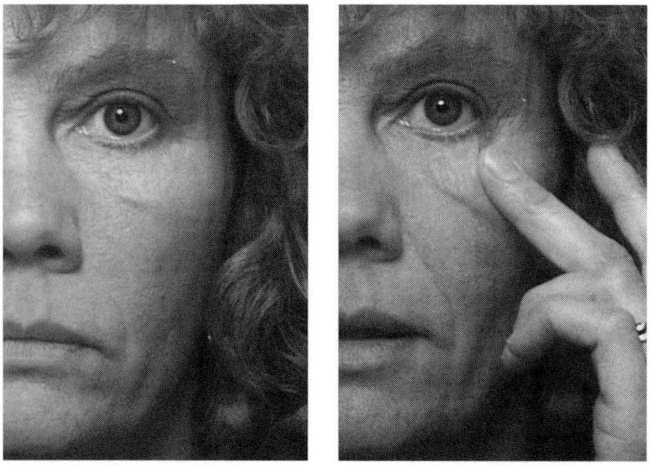

Figure 3 Skin attachment of zygomatico-cutaneus ligament.

due to the cutaneous insertions of the orbicularis retaining ligament (tear-trough deformity) and, further down, the insertion of the zygomaticocutaneous ligaments, marking the palpebromalar fold and its frequent edema. These anatomical data have been very well described by Mendelson and coworkers (Fig. 3) (22,23) after the description of a facial system by Pessa (24) and explains the black eye inferior limit. Between these two ligaments there is atrophy of the fibrous fat lying close to the malar bone in the of the prezygomatic space behind the orbicularis muscle. Descending still further, there is bulging fat retained just above the nasolabial fold caused by a third retaining ligament (25).

PROPOSED SOLUTIONS

Patient Markings

Markings are made in the room before any preop medication.

The patient is in a sitting position and we make use of the comparison between the pictures taken at the first visit and the old scanned pictures. Great precision is necessary when evaluating the volume dissymmetries and making the patient aware of them. Sometimes, it is very useful to use a mirror to fully understand what the patient actually sees when looking in a mirror and what the patient wants; I usually mark in red the areas that need reduction, and in black the ones to increase. At this stage, I never try to mark the eventual excess skin in the upper eyelids because, after the frontal lift and lipostructure, the need for skin resection will be completely different or nonexistent.

In the upper eyelids and eyebrow region I mark a first line, which is just above the upper eyelid crease, and a second upper line that is 0.5 mm above the eyebrow and that goes laterally upward 10 mm above the tail of the eyebrow: this is the area in which we want to recreate a pleasant, young upward shape (Fig. 4).

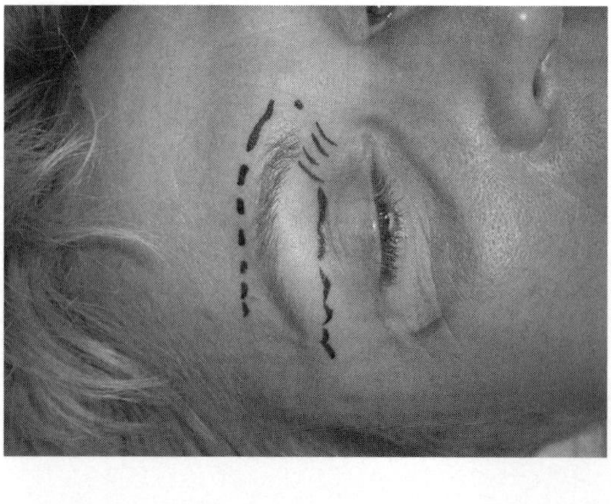

Figure 4 Area in which fat should be grafted above the intercanthal line.

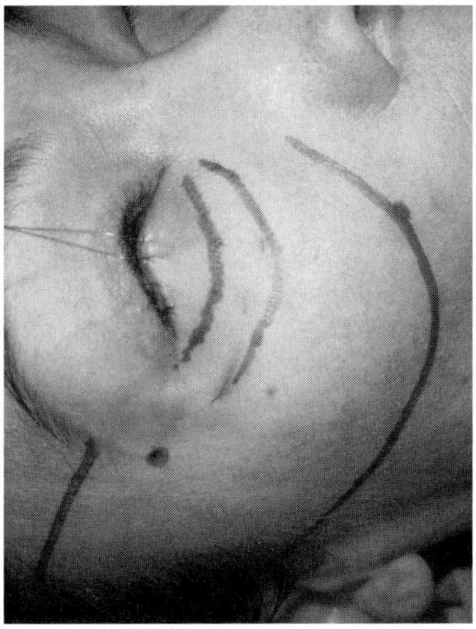

Figure 5 Area in which fat should be grafted below the intercanthal line.

In the lower eyelid region, I first delineate the exact spot at which you can see the change of fat thickness at the transition zone to the malar fat pad. I then draw a line following the lower limit of the tarsus to the lateral canthus parallel to the orbital rim; between these two lines, fat will be grafted deep to the orbicularis oculi muscle just in front of the orbital rim and just above the ORL in order to correct the hollowed area of the tear-trough deformity (Fig. 5).

Then, depending on the degree of skeletonization of the malar region, the area to be reshaped is delineated in continuity, moving toward the canine fossa. This region is the one situated between the ORL and the ZCL.

Fat Harvest

Fat harvest is done at the beginning of the operation with the patient in a prone or supine position. If the patient is very thin, we only inject a small amount of local anesthesia at the site of the stab incision made for the insertion of the suction cannula. Nothing is injected into the region we intend to take fat from, because it does not usually bleed, and, furthermore, this could lead to a false evaluation of the volume obtained. For the lower palpebral region, I find that the inner part of the knee has the most suitable fat quality: it is less fibrous and suppler in nature, and the tissue particles obtained are smaller. In this location, and for the lower eyelid, I suction fat tissue with a multiholed cannula (Fig. 6). Each hole is 1 mm in diameter, and I immediately calibrate the fatty tissue particles that I will graft. It is quicker than with a small cannula with one hole, and the size of each particle will correspond to the diameter of the thin cannula that I will use for fat grafting to this special destination. As in all fat-obtaining processes, the most important thing is to avoid damaging the adipocytes. Before adapting the cannula to the syringe, pull the plunger 1 cm so you will have 1 cc of air between the plunger and the fat. When you

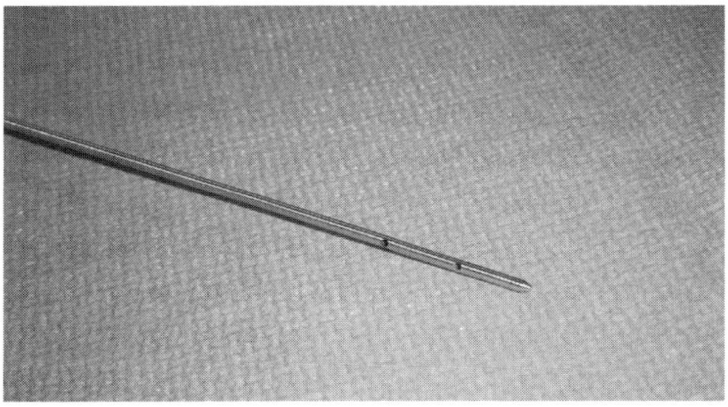

Figure 6 Multiholed cannula used for harvesting fat.

pull the plunger, you will not apply one bar of depression, which would kill the fat cells by vaporization. The expansion of the air will act like a shock absorber; when you aspirate fat do not pull the plunger more than 2 cm away from the fat coming in to prevent damage to the fat.

Once you have 10 cc of fine fat, which will be dedicated to the lower eyelid region, you may take another harvesting cannula to get fat for less-demanding areas. This cannula is also multiholed, but because this fat will be grafted with a 1.5-mm cannula, the holes are 1.5 mm. The remaining fat harvesting is done in the usual locations in which the fat is resistant to diet: inner part of the thighs, saddlebags, love handles, abdomen, buttocks, and the back, if the patient is very thin.

You should plan to gather an amount that is double what you intend to graft, not because of reabsorption, which is actually rare, but because after centrifugation, the usable amount is usually half of the harvest. The other half is blood, oil, and cells damaged by the traumatic aspiration.

The 10-cc syringes full of fat are then put into a centrifuge for three minutes at 3000 revolutions per minute. The fat specially harvested for the lower eyelids should be marked in order not to be mixed with the other syringes. This allows the useful part (the intact fat particles) to be separated from the useless parts: the oil that is produced by the damaged cells and blood. From experience we know that in overweight patients, the quality of the fat particle survival is not very good because their large cells are filled with lipids and, on the contrary, in very thin patients, the proportion of usable cells for the same volume of fat tissue is higher.

Frontal Lift

This should be done prior to any fat grafting because the remodeling to be done can only be appreciated after proper repositioning of the facial structures.

In almost every case, we perform a frontal or temporal face-lift through one lateral incision and two paramedian ones with the use of the endoscope, if we want to weaken the corrugator and procerus muscles.

Naturally, all the retaining structures and especially the upper orbital rim periosteum should be released to allow upward movement of the tail of the eyebrow.

The fixation of the upward mobilization is secured either by a resorbable screw inserted into the calvarium or by resorbable stitches to the temporal aponeurosis if the anterior extent of the muscle allows it. If necessary, we would perform a classical pretracheal lary incision in order to reduce the height of the frontal area.

Fat Grafting Above the Intercanthal Line

Before proceeding to the fat grafting, we may have to remove the most nasal compartment of upper eyelid fat, which most of the time shows more because it does not decrease, unlike the middle fatty compartment, in the vicinity of the pulley of the oblique muscle.

Cannulas

The cannulas used in the upper eyelid and eyebrow region are malleable, rather pointed at the end, but, of course, not as sharp as a needle, and their diameter is 1 mm (Fig. 7). They are malleable so that they can be bent in order to follow the orbital curvature of any patient. They are sharper than the usual cannulas so as to be very easy to insert into the exact location where very small particles of fatty tissue are to be grafted, and their diameter is the same as the holes of the harvesting cannulas to avoid trauma to the fragile fatty tissue. The syringes are 1-cc syringes with Luer lock adapters. A new syringe must be used for each cc grafted. The plunger of a new syringe glides very easily and, as a result, when applying gentle pressure with the base of your thumb you will be able to be precise enough to graft particles of fat of one hundredth of 1 cc. In doing so, each grafted particle of fat will "take," and there is no risk of creating visible lumps.

The entrance sites are situated at the inner portion of the eyebrows, on each side of the glabella, and the grafting will be done in one oblique and upward direction, without criss-crossing.

You should think of the task as reshaping an anatomical region rather than an anatomical structure. This is because that which has shrunk away is the entire periorbital region

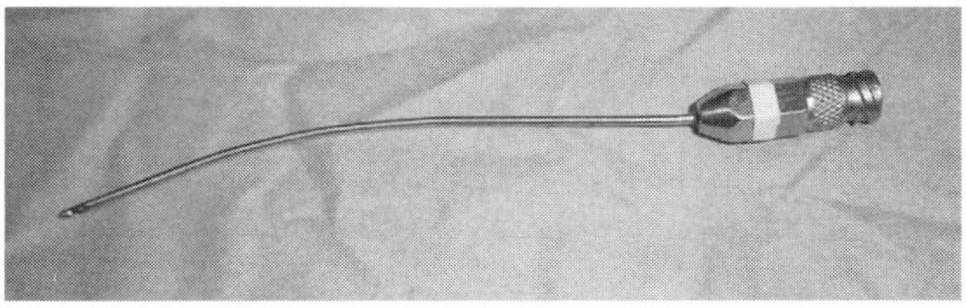

Figure 7 Cannula used for fat grafting in the upper eyelid region and in the malar area.

and not just the part of the eyelid fat that is above the fold. The area to be reshaped therefore extends from the eyelid fold to at least 1 cm above the eyebrow, going upward to the lateral part of it. In the lower part of the frontal area, the fat should be deposited in all the layers from the bone, or from the galea if a frontal lift has been performed, to just underneath the scalp, taking care to deposit the very small particles of fatty tissue evenly. In the upper eyelid, between the fold and the eyebrow, no fat should be grafted between the muscle and the skin because it is not a normal location for fat and any irregularity would show. The fat grafting is done very gently when pulling away the cannula by applying a very light pressure with the base of your thumb on the plunger. In this way, you are very precise in depositing a very regular layer of tiny particles of viable fat tissue. This fat grafting should not be done in the previously undermined plane of the frontal lift where it would not "take" because of the lack of recipient vascularized tissue, but in the scalp, over the galea aponeurosis (Figs. 8 and 9).

Once you have completed the restoration of the shape of the eyelid and eyebrow region, you may consider an upper eyelid skin resection and make an evaluation of the eventual amount of skin to be resected. This is done by pinching the upper eyelid skin with forceps, or by assessing the amount of excess skin as is done when performing an abdominoplasty (26). We always remove more skin in the lateral part of the eyelid; only skin is resected, with the muscle left intact for volumetric reasons, and also because we want to create a fuller eyelid, not a hollowed-out eyelid. Furthermore, because we have just grafted fat underneath the muscle, every particle should be left intact. Fat resection in the inner part of the eyelid can be done in a conservative manner if it is absolutely necessary, and it can be done through the conjunctiva as described by Januszkiewicz and Nahai (27). Excess fat in the lateral compartment should not be resected but can be translocated upward to the orbital rim.

Laser skin treatment can be done at the end of the procedure, and this does not at all impair the take of the fatty tissue.

Fat Grafting Below the Intercanthal Line

Patients with Baggy Eyelids and Tear-Trough Deformity

In this situation, we always begin by treating the fat herniation first. I value the fat sliding procedure described by Hamra (12), but I think that if I did it, it would not be possible to

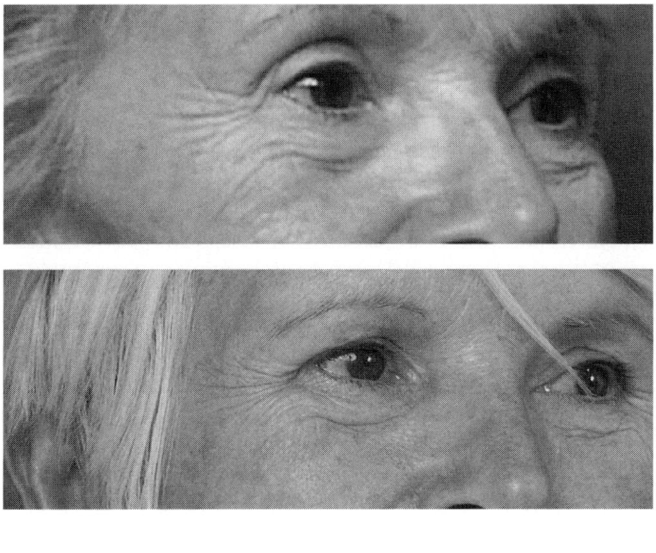

Figure 8 Lower eyelid transconjunctival blepharoplasty and periorbital fat grafting to correct sunken upper eyelid.

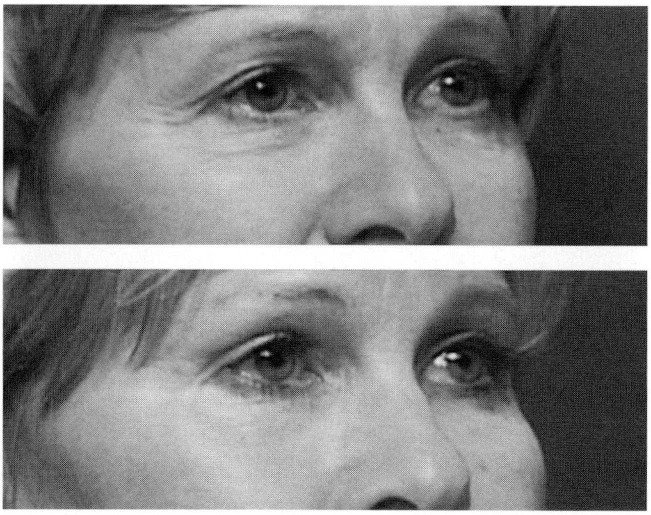

Figure 9 Temporal lift, fat grafting of the upper eyelid region, lower blepharoplasty, and micro-fat grafting of lower eyelids and malar area.

perform the lipostructure without disturbing the newly translocated fat, and I also think that usually, in order to reshape the lower eyelid and malar region, more fat than the quantity that can be transposed is necessary.

For these reasons, before fat grafting, I always perform a transconjunctival standard blepharoplasty, resecting the excess fat flush with the orbital rim. It is below this level that we will improve the thickness of the SOOF with micro–fat grafting. We never make subcutaneous or submuscular eyelid dissection, first because there is no need for skin resection in most cases, and second, after such undermining it would not be possible to perform fat grafting. If, after the completion of the operation there is still notable excess skin, a very conservative skin pinch resection or a light laser resurfacing can be performed. But in fact, there is a genuine upward pushing up action due to the restoration of the malar pillar, which reduces the apparent excess of skin. The delicate and sophisticated techniques of canthopexies (28,29) are, in my opinion, less necessary than once thought, unless the patient wants a very different slant to the palpebral fissure.

The main purpose of fat grafting is to correct the tear-trough deformity and to move the transition zone between the eyelid and the malar area upward. Our goal is also to restore the youthful projection of the malar eminence, in subtle continuity with a shorter lower eyelid.

If a face-lift is to be done, we usually begin by doing the lipostructure, including the lower eyelid, and then we perform the face-lift on an already-reshaped face.

Because we started using lipostructure for the midface region, we have abandoned the midface-lifting we used to do because in our experience, it did not sufficiently improve the key transition zone between the malar eminence and the lower eyelid. Even the more sophisticated midface rejuvenation techniques with sculptural effects (30,31) use fat grafting or dermo–fat graft to improve this area.

The cannula used to graft fat in the lower eyelid is finer than for the upper eyelid: it is 19 gauge in diameter (Fig. 10), and the syringe is 1 cc. The fat comes from the inner part of the knee, harvested with a multiperforated cannula. The holes of this multiperforated cannula are of the same diameter as the 19-gauge cannula that will be used to deposit fat (Fig. 11), so there will not be any pressure trauma when pushing the fat through the very small cannula used for the lower eyelid region. The volume usually harvested for this region is 4 cc, which after centrifugation will give 2 cc of pure fat that will be used exclusively for correcting the tear

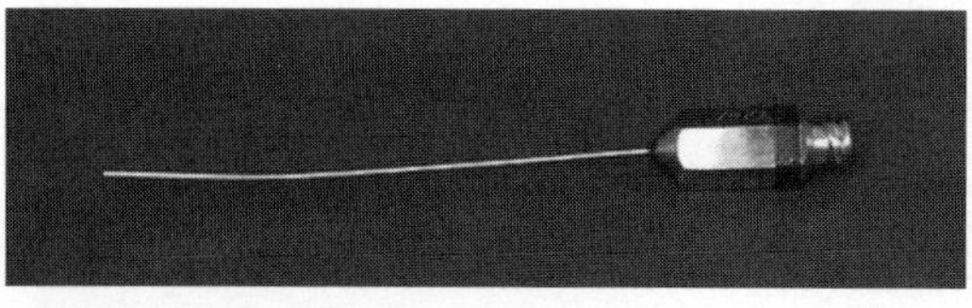

Figure 10 Fine cannula used for lower eyelids.

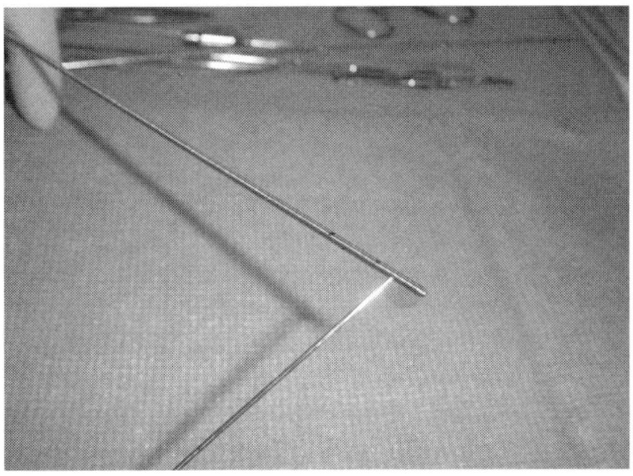

Figure 11 Diameters of holes and grafting cannulas are the same.

trough. For the malar eminence, which is always improved at the same time in order to get a nice natural curvature of the midface, we use fat from the saddlebags or the abdomen, which can be harvested with bigger cannulas.

First, I treat the inner part of the tear-trough deformity: the entrance site of the cannula is at the axis of the deformity. After pretunneling, I graft 0.1 or 0.2 cc of fine fat evenly, deep into the orbicularis oculi muscle, and you actually see that there is no more tear trough. Never overcorrect, because if you perform the operation properly, everything will take and overcorrecting would end up with a bulge.

I then correct the subtarsus part of the lower eyelid: I no longer graft fat into the subcutaneous layer because it is an area in which the least irregularity would show and there has never been much fat there. Fat resorption occurs mainly in the suborbicularis layer so the graft is always done underneath the orbicularis oculi muscle (Fig. 12).

I pretunnel the zone between the tarsus and the transition zone in order to prepare the recipient zone in which I will, very gently and as evenly as possible, deposit tiny particles of fat. The 1-mm stab incision is situated in the region of the crow's feet and, with the cannula disconnected from the syringe, I do 20 to 30 passes underneath the orbicularis, in the SOOF, to prepare the lipostructure. I usually do only two incisions, and I do not crisscross from another entrance site. I do not graft from an entrance site situated below the eyelid, and I do not go upward because I have had bad experiences doing so, creating baggy eyelids by grafting behind the septum orbitale. One stab incision is in the crow's feet and another is in the upper part of the sideburn.

I then take the 1-cc syringe with a content of 0.4 cc of fat harvested from the inner part of the knee and deposit this fat, as regularly as possible, from the lateral incision to the inner part of the eyelid, and from the lower border of the tarsus to the lower end of the tear trough. You can actually see the hollowness of this region disappear. If a hematoma develops, do not panic, just stop the lipostructure, apply gentle pressure, and return to this area at the end of the procedure.

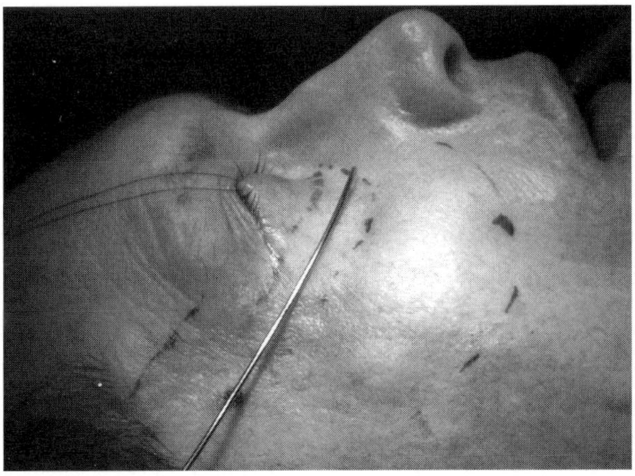

Figure 12 Fat grafting in the lower eyelids should be done underneath the orbicularis and from a lateral approach.

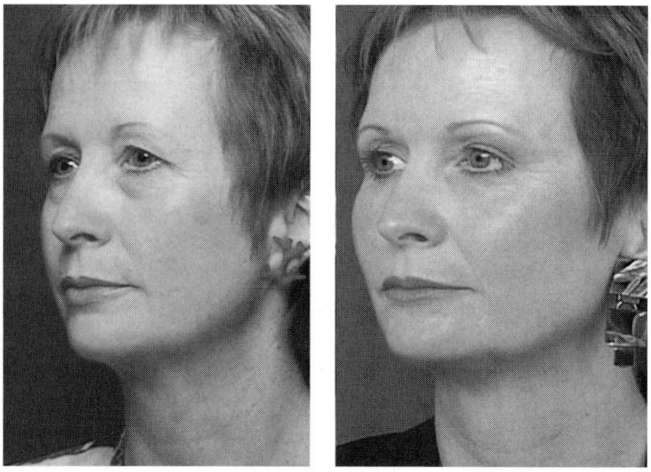

Figure 13 Periorbital fat grafting combined with upper and lower blepharoplasties.

If, at the end of the lipostructure (combined or not with conjunctival baggy eyelid treatment), you think that there is excess skin, it can be treated by means of a pinch excision just below the eyelashes. A standard blepharoplasty with submuscular undermining should not be performed under any circumstances, because the fat graft would not survive in a dissected plane. On the contrary, a peeling or a laser resurfacing can be done at the same operative session.

Having done the correction of this region, you must continue the lipostructure in continuity to the mid- and lower-malar region in order to rejuvenate the whole midface. Through the same crow's feet stab incision and, still obliquely, without crisscrossing your paths, you will graft a total amount of 6–15 cc of fat into all the layers, from the bone to under the surface of the skin below the lower limit of the orbicularis (Figs. 13–15).

Patients Without Baggy Eyelids but with Tear-Trough Deformity

In this situation the goal is to restore a normal thickness of fat in front of the squelettonized orbital rim, which shows through the skin and could be mistaken for a fat protrusion (Fig. 16). This is really due to a downward migration of the malar fat pad, but also to a selective, genetically programmed fat resorption as can be seen in other parts of the body. It is also interesting to observe that this fat thinning occurs almost exactly behind the surface of the orbicularis oculi muscle, as if its repeated contractions could, in the long term, lead to fat resorption.

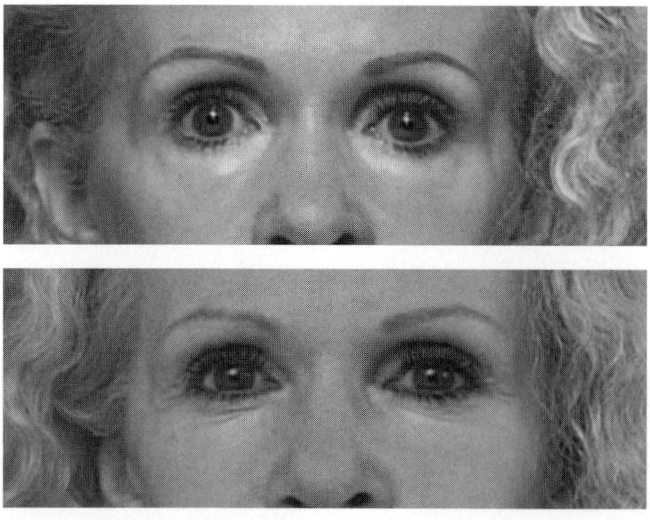

Figure 14 Periorbital fat grafting combined with face-lift and lower blepharoplasties.

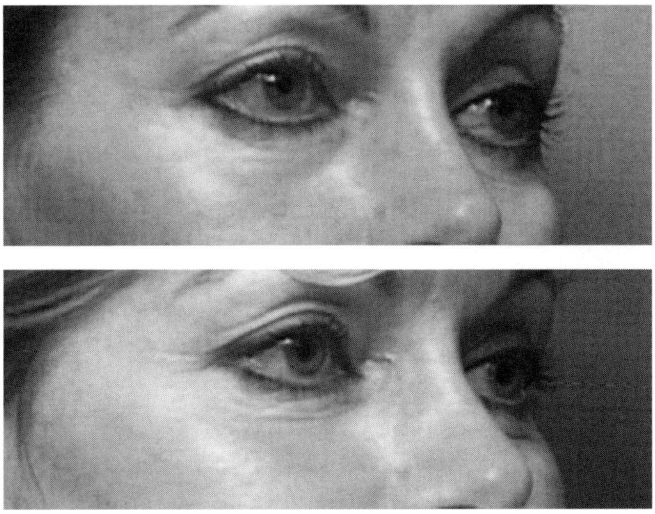

Figure 15 Lower blepharoplasty with fat grafting below the intercanthal line.

The procedure is exactly the same but without the conjunctival approach. Begin by gently grafting fat in the long axis of the inner part of the tear trough, after pretunneling, and then correct the orbital skeletonization through a lateral incision situated in the crow's feet (Fig. 17).

Unfavorable Results and Secondary Corrections

Above the Intercanthal Line

In the upper eyelids and eyebrows, it has occasionally been necessary to make secondary corrections, because in my early days I was a little inhibited and did not graft enough fat. You should graft at least 2.5 cc in order to obtain an improvement. To avoid skin irregularities, graft between the bone and the muscle, not just below the skin. Grafting only between the eyebrow and the upper eyelid crease did not give a pleasant and youthful shape to the area.

Below the Intercanthal Line

When I began performing periorbital lipostructure, I inadvertently grafted fat inside the septum. This resulted in increased puffiness in the lower eyelid, very different from the result

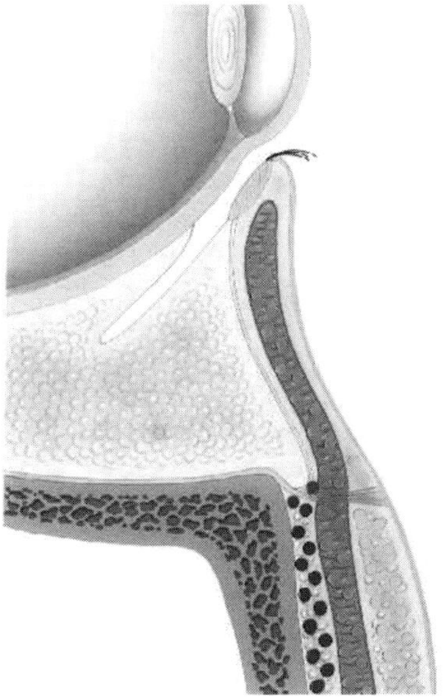

Figure 16 Fat should be grafted underneath the orbicularis.

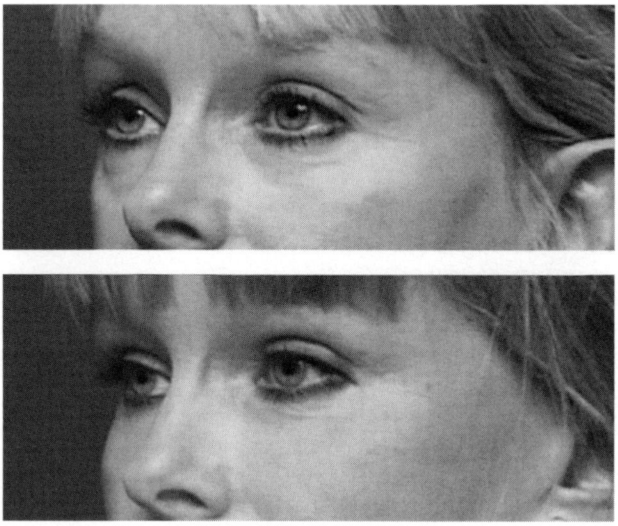

Figure 17 Periorbital rejuvenation by fat grafting alone.

expected by both patient and surgeon. At that time I used to make my stab incision and graft from below the orbit. The movement of the cannula was thus upward. My mistake was to enter the septum and to graft fat inside the lower eyelid bags.

Treatment was very simple: through a transconjunctival incision I found the grafted fat, a little redder than usual, and resected the excess.

In order to avoid this I decided to graft fat in front of the orbicularis to avoid entering the septum orbital, and do it from a lateral stab incision in the canthal region. In most cases, it was very encouraging, provided that care was taken to distribute the grafted fat particles very evenly, because the problem that resulted from going in from below did not occur anymore.

But in many cases, the patients complained of lumps. Sometimes the lumps were almost invisible, but sometimes really conspicuous underneath the skin, mostly visible on tangential views, disturbing for both patient and surgeon. I treated them with diluted injections of steroids and, in some cases, by a direct excision through the skin.

On one occasion, a patient developed a subcutaneous infection that I treated by conservative debridement, without sequelae, and the patient was ultimately satisfied.

Because I started spreading the fat particles underneath the orbicularis oculi muscle, with the aim of filling this region in continuity with the malar region and with the canine fossa below, the only imperfections that I have been faced with are as follows:

1. A slight edema at the inferior limit of the orbicularis oculi muscle (malar mound) like that sometimes observed after standard blepharoplasties. These edemas are difficult to treat, as we all know.
2. An incomplete survival of the grafts, mostly in patients over 60 years of age, leading to a repeat lipostructure, under local anesthetic in most cases.

Under pressure, fat embolisms leading to visual impairment have been reported after fat injection. I do not think that the risk is as great when you gently graft the fat when pulling back a blunt cannula. Extra care is nevertheless necessary in the glabella region and in the vicinity of the angular vein.

CONCLUSION

Since I began performing lipostructure in 1998, all my blepharoplasty patients have had a combination of fat grafting and surgery. I will continue doing my best to improve the results and, because I have had a long-term follow-up, I am confident about the long-term results.

REFERENCES

1. Flowers RS. The art of eyelid and orbital aesthetics: multiracial surgical considerations. Clin Plast Surg 1987; 14:703.
2. Vinas JC, Cavaglia C, Cortinas JL. Forehead rhytidoplasty and brow lifting. Plast Reconstr Surg 1976; 57:445.
3. Tessier P. Ridectomie frontale—lifting frontal. Gaz Med France 1968; 75:5565.
4. Marchac D. Le lifting frontal. Ann Chir Plast Esthet 1982; 27:121.
5. Trepsat F. Le choix des incisions et des myoplasties dans les liftings. Ann Chir Plast Esthet 1989; 34:9.
6. Gore GB, Vasconez LO, Graham HD. Endoscopic brow lift. Clin Plast Surg 1995; 22(4):619–631.
7. Isse NG. Endoscopic facial rejuvenation. Clin Plast Surg 1997; 24:213.
8. Trepsat F, Delmar H. L'apport de la vidéo endoscopie dans la chirurgie de rajeunissement de la face. Ann Chir Plast Esthet 1994; 39(5):647–665.
9. Ramirez OM, Maillard GF, Musolas A. The extended subperiosteal face lift: a definitive soft tissue remodeling for facial rejuvenation. Plast Reconst Surg 1991; 88:227.
10. Byrd HS, Burt JD. Achieving aesthetic balance in the brow, eyelids, and midface. Plast Reconstr Surg 2002; 110(3):926–933.
11. Loeb R. Fat pad sliding and fat grafting for leveling lid depressions. Clin Plast Surg 1981; 8(4):757–776.
12. Hamra S. The role of orbital fat preservation in facial aesthetic surgery: a new concept. Clin Plast Surg 1996; 23:17.
13. Tessier P. Le lifting facial sous périosté. Ann Chir Plast Esthet 1989; 34:193–197.
14. Coleman SR. Structural fat grafts: the ideal filler. Clin Plast Surg 2001; 28(1):111–119.
15. Coleman SR. The technique of periorbital lipo infiltration. Oper Techn Plast Reconstr Surg 1994; 1(3):120–126.
16. Fagien S. Advanced rejuvenative upper blepharoplasty: enhancing aesthetics of the upper periorbit. Plast Reconstr Surg 2002; 110:278–291.
17. Lambros V. Fat injection for the aging mid face. Oper Techn Plast Reconstr Surg 1998; 5:129.
18. Erol OO. Facial autologous soft tissue contouring by adjunction of tissue cocktail injections (micro-grafts and minigrafts mixture of dermis, fascia, and fat). Plast Reconstr Surg 2000; 106(6):1375–1385.
19. Terino EO. Three-dimensional facial contouring: utilizing upper-midface suspension technology and alloplastic augmentation. Facial Plastic Surg 2003; 19(2):171–184.
20. Ramirez OM. Full face rejuvenation in three dimensions: a "face-lifting" for the new millennium. Aesthetic Plast Surg 2001; 25(3):152–164.
21. Aiache AE, Ramirez OH. The suborbicularis oculi fat pads: an anatomical and clinical study. Plast Reconstr Surg 1995; 95(1):37–42.
22. Mendelson BC, Muzzaffar AR, Adam WR. Surgical anatomy of the mid cheek and malar mound. Plast Reconstr Surg 2002; 110(3):885–896.
23. Muzaffar AR, Mendelson BC, Adam WP. Surgical anatomy of the ligamentous attachments of the lower lid and lateral canthus. Plast Reconstr Surg 2002; 110(3):885–896.
24. Pessa JE, Garza JR. The malar septum: the anatomic basis of malar mounds and malar oedema. Aesthetic Surg J 1997; 17:1.
25. Youssif NJ, Gosain AM, Matloub HS. The naso labial fold: an anatomic and histologic reappraisal. Plast Reconstr Surg 1994; 93:60.
26. Trepsat F. Dermectomies palpébrales supérieures. Ann Chir Plast Esthet 1989; 34:251.
27. Januszkiewicz JS, Nahai F. Transconjunctival upper blepharoplasty. Plast Reconstr Surg 1999; 103(3):1015–1018.
28. Fagien S. Algorithm for canthoplasty: the lateral retinacular suspension: a simplified suture canthopexy. Plast Reconstr Surg 1999; 103(7):2042–2053.
29. Jelks JW, Glat PM, Jelks EB. The inferior retinacular lateral canthoplasty: a new technique. Plast Reconstr Surg 1997; 100(5):262–270.
30. Little JW. Applications of the classic dermal fat graft in primary and secondary facial rejuvenation. Plast Reconstr Surg 2002; 109(2):788–804.
31. Ramirez OM. Three-dimensional endoscopic mid face enhancement: a personal quest for the ideal cheek rejuvenation. Plast Reconstr Surg 2002; 109(1):329–340.

6 Skeletal Techniques for Achieving Three-Dimensional Facial Balance and Harmony

Kenneth E. Salyer, David G. Genecov, Yong-Chen Por, and Carlos Raul Barcelo
International Craniofacial Institute, Dallas, Texas, U.S.A.

INTRODUCTION

Facial beauty is perceived in the "eye of the beholder." The "beholder" is influenced by many objective as well as subjective factors. The objective factors include the proportion of the eyes, lips, nose, facial shape, projection, and volume. The subjective factors include culture, society, media, photography, art and artists, movie stars, models, surgery and surgeons, as well as makeup. The animated face with certain highlights and lowlights of the face and how they are presented with warm or cold light, as well as the surrounding ambiance all contribute to facial beauty.

The quantification and standardization of facial proportions have been studied extensively in skeletal cephalometrics and anthropological measurements of the soft tissues. The facial skeleton provides the structures and foundation for facial shape and projection and influences proportions underlying the jaws, teeth and their occlusion, as well as the nose, forehead, cheeks, and chin. These structures and their proportions are important in contributing to facial balance and harmony. The soft tissues—skin, muscle, fat, fascia, etc.—provide the cover. The animated facial features are provided by the composition, thickness, and quality of soft tissues. The nose is supported by bone and cartilage covered by the skin with various color and thickness that characterizes and highlights the face. Projection and volume of the facial skeleton, nasal structure, chin, jaws, forehead, and cheeks are key structures, which aesthetic skeletal surgery can alter and enhance, providing the surgeon with an expanded armamentarium.

Aesthetic balance and harmony of the face is created by the surgeon's perception of beauty and ability to create an attractive face given a certain set of circumstances. Faces can be beautiful even when a significant number of facial proportions are not normal. In an unpublished study, the authors looked at cephalometric and anthropometric studies of 20 fashion models. The authors found that most had many disproportions. Dallas's top model, out of 52 proportions, had 18 disproportions measured and yet was beautiful and distinctive. From this study, we determined that well-balanced faces can be beautiful even though they were proportioned differently.

It has been the authors' goal to use this concept of facial balance when performing reconstructive procedures as well as aesthetic surgery of the face. In reconstructive surgery especially, the authors' standard is not just to fix or correct the defect or deformity, but to create balance and harmony of the face resulting in "perceptual beauty."

Plastic surgery in the 21st century must include the ability to perform all techniques of bone as well as soft-tissue surgery. These techniques should be applied in both aesthetic and reconstructive facial surgery for achieving facial balance, harmony, and beauty.

ASSESSMENT

There is a continuous spectrum of facial imbalance and disharmony. On the extreme end are facial deformities that usually require major corrective osteotomies. In the middle are borderline problems that usually have microform or smaller versions of recognized syndromes. These patients may benefit from onlay grafts or camouflage procedures. On the other end of the spectrum are patients who have normal acceptable appearances but desire to enhance their aesthetic profile (1).

The references here will be made to the Caucasian face as individual ethnicities have unique facial proportions and aesthetic ideals. The assessment of the face is evaluated with reference to its width, height, and projection. The width and height of the face are assessed in the frontal view, while the projection of the face is assessed in the lateral profile. In the frontal view, the width of the face is divided into fifths by vertical perpendiculars from the inner and outer canthi of the eyes. The bitemporal, bimalar, and bigonial distances should be approximately equal. The widest point of the face is the bizygomatic distance. The bigonial distance determines the width of the lower face. The symmetry of the face is compared by making a midline connecting the forehead, tip of nose, center of upper lip, dental midlines, center of lower lip, and midpoint of chin (Fig. 1).

The height of the face in the neoclassical canons is divided into thirds, starting from the trichion to the glabella, the subnasale and the menton. Further assessment of the lower facial height is made by dividing it into thirds; from the subnasale to the stomion, the mentolabial sulcus, and the menton (Fig. 2).

It must be mentioned that although some authors have validated these proportions (2), others have found that the lower part of the face was longer in males (3). Bell and Jacobs (4) also felt that the nasion-to-subnasale height should normally be about 44% and the subnasale-to-menton height about 56% of the nasion-to-menton height. Of this total height, the upper lip length (subnasale to stomion) should be 18% and the distance between the stomion and the menton 38%. The vertical balance of the face is also enhanced when the distance from the outer canthus of the eye to the angle of the mouth is equal to the distance from the subnasale to the menton (5).

The lateral profile is assessed carefully beginning superiorly at the forehead to inferiorly at the chin (Fig. 2). The forehead begins to curve approximately 1 cm above the orbital rim and passes vertically and gently backwards towards the vertex. The mean forehead inclination in the male and female is -10° and -6.6°, respectively. The mean nasofrontal angle in the male and female is 130.5° and 134°, respectively (6). The columella-lip angle should ideally be obtuse with a mean of $98.9^\circ \pm 8^\circ$ in males and $99.1^\circ \pm 8.7^\circ$ in females (5,6), or $102^\circ \pm 8^\circ$ (2,5) and with the upper pole of the labial line tilted forward at the angle (meeting point of the two lines) (7). The upper lip cant should be $14^\circ \pm 8^\circ$ (8,9) and the upper lip should be slightly in front of the lower lip with both showing an equal full vermilion (Fig. 3) (5,10) The facial convexity angle measured between the glabella, subnasale, and pogonion should average 11° to 12° (2,5). The assessment of the lower face can also be based on a perpendicular line dropped from the glabella in the midline. This can serve as a guide to evaluate the relative protrusion of the maxilla and mandible to each other or to upper facial structures (11). The lower lip and anterior projection of the chin are ideally in almost the same vertical plane as the nasofrontal angle (1). In addition, the aesthetics of the lower face is determined by the shape and course of the mandible. The mandibular angle (gonion) is approximately 100° to 110°.

The assessment of the lateral profile must include the eyes as well. The protrusion of the eye in relation to the orbital margin is important. The anterior edge of the cornea should lie 8–10 mm posterior to the supraorbital rim (15–20 mm behind the eyebrow), 12–16 mm anterior to the lateral orbital rim, and 2–3 mm anterior to the inferior orbital rim (1).

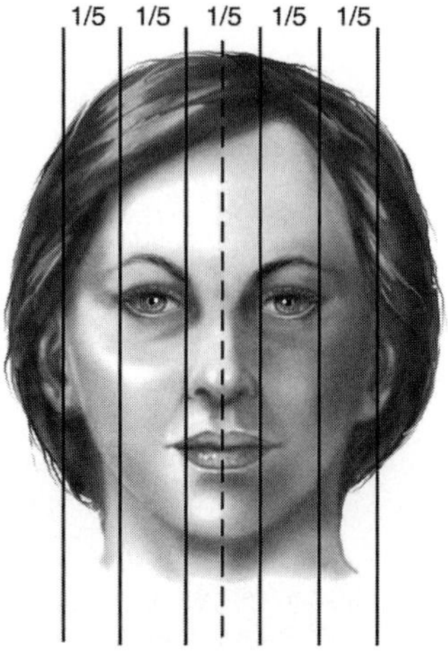

Figure 1 Frontal assessment of the face demonstrating the division of the facial width into fifths based on vertical perpendiculars dropped from the inner and outer canthi of the eyes, as well as the placement of a midline to assess facial symmetry.

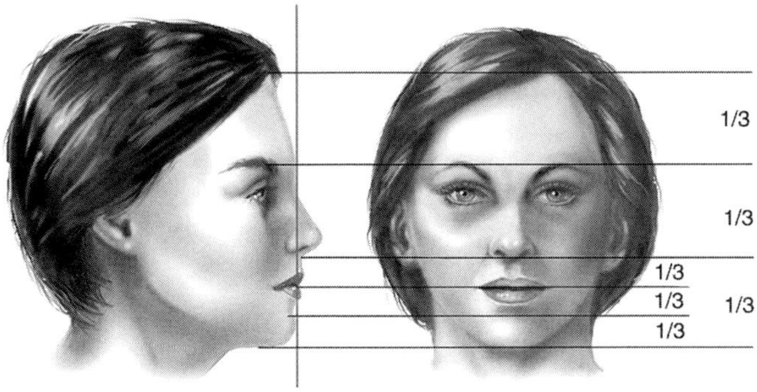

Figure 2 Facial proportions and assessment of the lateral facial profile with divisions of the facial height and the lower facial height into thirds. Note also the lateral profile of the face and the perpendicular line from the glabella used to assess the relative position of the maxilla, mandible, and upper facial structures.

In addition, the soft-tissue drape over the facial skeleton is converted into three highlight and four lowlight areas (12). The highlight areas are: (*i*) the supraorbital ridge–temporal ridge extension, (*ii*) the malar-midfacial complex, and (*iii*) the posterior mandible–chin region. Above and below as well as in between these areas are four lowlight regions: (*i*) the forehead superiorly, (*ii*) the orbit-temporal fossa inferior to the supraorbital ridge, (*iii*) the soft tissue of the cheek superficial to teeth and between the malar-midfacial complex and the posterior mandible–chin region, and (*iv*) the neck below the posterior mandible and chin (Fig. 4). The highlights and lowlights of the face are most prominent in the full-face view or in a 45° angle view.

Upon considering all the above factors in the face, it is important for the surgeon to take into account the overall balance of the face. As long as one portion of the facial pattern is not overemphasized at the expense of another, minor facial disproportion can still result in a beautiful face.

The surgeon's aesthetic facial preferences and experience is important in the decision-making process. The senior author's preference is for a protrusive, full volume, anteface enhancement (Fig. 5). During the clinical assessment, previsualization of the intended result is necessary before surgical decision making. Making aesthetic decisions should not be limited to looking at models, tracing X-ray films, or measuring lines and angles, but should call on the right brain as well.

The surgical process involves detailed preoperative planning with respect to osteotomies and advancement of bony segments plus bone augmentation and/or remodeling to achieve aesthetic enhancement of the face. Planning of skeletal movements must be carried out to within 1 mm accuracy. This is aided by life-size 1:1 ratio photographs, cephalometric posteroanterior and lateral X rays, iCAT of the maxillae and mandible, a panorex of the mandible, dental consult and dental study models, anthropological consult, computed

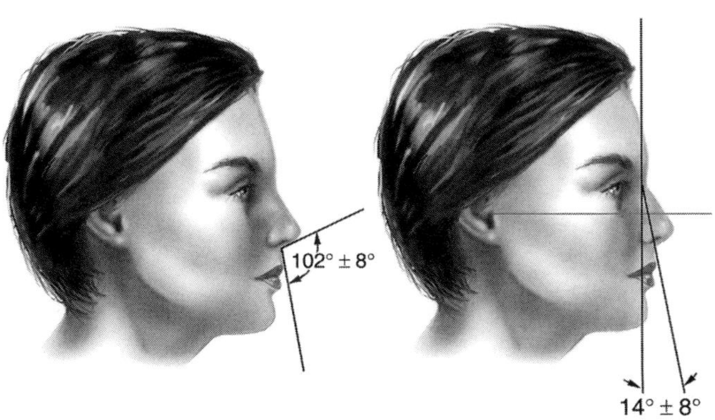

Figure 3 The columella-lip angle and the upper lip cant. The columella-lip angle describes the angle between the base of the nose and the upper lip. The upper lip cant describes the angle between the upper lip and the nasion perpendicular. *Source*: From Ref. 9.

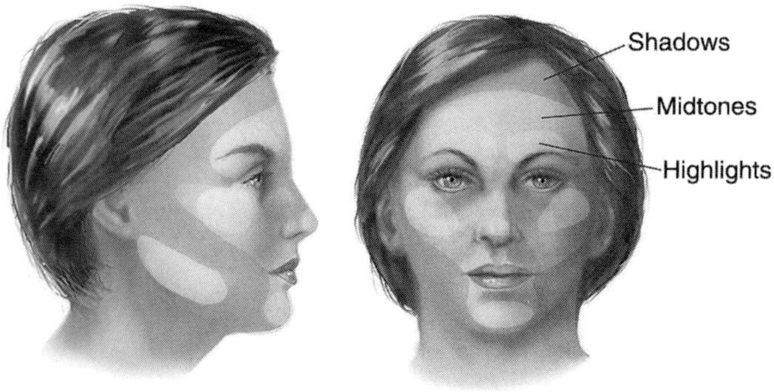

Figure 4 The three highlight and four lowlight areas of the face. The highlight areas are the supraorbital ridge–temporal ridge extension, the malar-midfacial complex, and the posterior mandible–chin region. The lowlight areas are the forehead, the orbit–temporal fossa inferior to the supraorbital ridge, the soft tissue of the cheek superficial to the teeth and between the malar–midfacial complex of the posterior mandible–chin region, and lastly, the neck below the posterior mandible and chin.

tomography (CT) with three-dimensional reconstruction, and stereolithographic models in cases where major skeletal detail is needed.

In the authors' opinion, the craniofacial skeleton can be divided into the following aesthetic skeletal units; in this modern era, the entire craniofacial skeleton is available for remodeling. The challenge is for the surgeon to use these techniques judiciously to achieve facial balance and harmony because being able to change soft-tissue volume only will not be enough to achieve optimal balance and beauty in many cases.

1. The cranial vault
2. The forehead
3. The supraorbital ridge, the brow-corneal distance, and the frontonasal angle
4. The orbits
5. The nose
6. The midface
7. The lower face
8. Lastly, the expected result comprising the height, width, projection, and volume of the face

Although many implants are available in the market for augmentation of various regions in the face, the authors feel that the use of autogenous or biologic material is the best as it is associated with the least complications and has the best long-term outcome. This is absolutely true if the face is still growing. In addition, the familiarity with the use of skeletal techniques that will be briefly discussed here will add to the repertoire of both the reconstructive craniofacial surgeon as well as the aesthetic plastic surgeon.

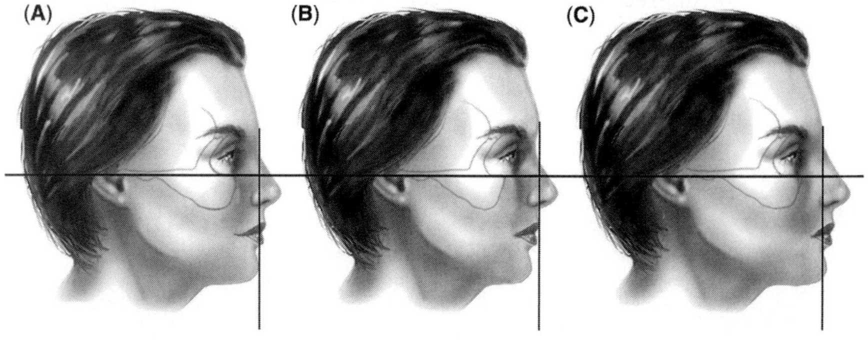

Figure 5 Normal (**A**), retrusive (concave) (**B**), and protrusive (convex) (**C**) facial profiles. Note the reference made to the glabella perpendicular, especially with regard to the facial outlines and the positions of the malar eminences.

OSTEOTOMY VS. DISTRACTION OSTEOGENESIS

In the past decade, the advent and popularization of distraction osteogenesis has changed the practice of craniofacial surgery. Distraction osteogenesis has become the treatment of choice in places with severe grades of craniofacial anomalies, limited bone stock, and soft-tissue deficiencies (13). Such cases include both unilateral hypoplastic mandible in hemifacial microsomia and bilateral hypoplastic mandibles in mandibular airway obstruction syndrome. In addition, distraction osteogenesis may play a major role in severe maxillary retrusion (more than 10–12 mm) where scarring and soft-tissue deficiency is present in the growing child. Orthognathic surgery in the form of intraoral segmental osteotomies of the maxillary, mandibular, and alveolar ridge, including widening of the arches may, in certain cases, be treated with distraction osteogenesis or classic osteotomy.

However, the use of the traditional osteotomy for procedures such as total cranial vault, frontocranial, and orbital remodeling using classic osteotomies offer the best modality for treatment of cranial vault asymmetries and deformities in all age groups. In addition, the classic osteotomies as described by Le Fort for fractures also have better results when compared to cases of distraction after growth is complete in certain cases (14). The advantage that the traditional osteotomy has over distraction osteogenesis is that it allows precise three-dimensional bony movements so the exact position and proportion can be achieved with precise fixation at the time of operation. This is necessary to prevent relapse and recurrence of the preoperative deformity. The segments at the time of osteotomy must be entirely free and mobile in all planes of movement to prevent relapse. When major movements are necessary and soft-tissue restriction exists, distraction osteogenesis is an alternative choice.

ONLAY GRAFTING VS. OSTEOTOMY

The use of onlay grafts is popular because of the reduced need for performing osteotomies. In certain areas in adults, the use of alloplastic material is preferred over bone by some surgeons because there is no necessity for a donor site and its ease of use. Autogenous material such as pericranial or frontalis muscle flaps can be used for 2- to 3-mm augmentation of the supraorbital ridge and temporal regions. If greater augmentation is required (4–8 mm), then bone grafts or forehead remodeling, or even alloplastic material can be used. However, contouring of the forehead-supraorbital ridge, altering of the infraorbital and lateral orbital projection are best achieved by the use of autogenous material. In areas where bone grafts have an unpredictable or high resorption rate (15), such as the zygoma, mandibular ramus, angle or body, or the dorsum of the nose, alloplastic materials can be considered. In the chin, the horizontal mandibular osteotomy is the authors' preferred method of choice. Alternatively, an alloplastic chin implant with the desired squareness may be chosen by other surgeons producing good results when the principles of alloplastic augmentation are well applied.

If minor procedures are unable to achieve the desired aesthetic goal, then an osteotomy is considered. For example, if more than 5–6 mm of augmentation of the supraorbital ridge in relation to the cornea is needed, frontal forehead advancement must be considered. If the desired increase in bitemporal distance is more than 5–6 mm, an intracranial expansion of the calvarium must also be considered. If the dental occlusion is class II or III, orthognathic surgery must be considered. If there is an asymmetric face or borderline abnormal face, a corrective osteotomy has to be considered. Before performing the necessary osteotomies, the patient must be counseled regarding the permanence of the bone changes.

GOALS AND TECHNIQUES

Cranial Vault

The use of intracranial techniques are usually reserved for pathologically deformed skulls in children or young adults. Extracranial augmentation or reduction procedures are used for aesthetic contour defects in fully grown patients.

In cranial synostosis, the abnormal shapes of the head are dependent on the sutures involved and can be classified into various categories: sagittal synostosis will result in scaphocephaly; metopic synostosis will result in trigonocephaly; coronal and lambdoid synostosis will result in plagiocephaly; and synostosis of all the sutures will result in a clover-leaf or Kleeblattschädel skull.

The cranial reconstruction is dependent on the site of deformity. We believe that cranial vault remodeling is the method of choice and can achieve good results consistently in nonsyndromic craniosynostosis.

In severe deformities affecting the entire cranial vault, where the total cranial vault is remodeled, the 3-bandeau technique is used to provide circumferential form to the reconstruction (16). The positions of the bandeau are placed as follows: horizontally at the forehead, vertically in the coronal plane at the vertex, and horizontally at the occiput. These three bandeaus will act as an external scaffold upon which to place the bone grafts and contour the cranial vault.

Distraction has been used by some with rapid expansion to keep the skull open during rapid growth to improve on the aesthetic appearance and balance of the head and face in syndromal craniosynostosis.

Forehead

The forehead has been aesthetically assigned to occupy the upper third of the face. In general, the frontal bones comprising the forehead can be osteotomized, reshaped, and repositioned on its own in anterior cranial vault remodeling or as part of a craniofacial procedure such as a monobloc advancement.

Ousterhout (17) had also addressed the gender specificity of the female and male forehead contours. There were three categories of masculine foreheads in women; in the first group were patients with normal or slightly anterior projection of the supraorbital rims, minimal to moderate contour deformities (bossing), thick skull bone over the frontal sinus, and/or absence of the frontal sinus. These deformities could be corrected by bone reduction alone. In the second group, the individuals had relatively normal or slightly anterior placement of the supraorbital rims but in whom the frontal bone was combined with relatively thin bone over the frontal sinuses, the sinuses being of normal size. Correction of the deformity in these patients required completing as much contouring of the bone as possible without entering the sinus and then augmenting the concavity above the frontal bossing with methyl methacrylate and contouring to the final desired shape. In the third group of patients, the patients had an excessive projection of the supraorbital rims that adequate bone reduction contouring was not possible without entering the frontal sinus. In these individuals, the frontal sinus had to be opened through a sinus osteotomy and the entire anterior sinus wall and associated supraorbital rim set back and wired into position.

To perform an enhancement of the forehead slope, bone grafts incorporated within a pericranial or frontalis flap can be used to augment the supraorbital ridges.

Supraorbital Ridge, Brow-Corneal Distance, and Frontonasal Angle

The bandeau or brow is the key architectural component of craniofacial reconstruction (18). It typically includes the supraorbital rim, glabellar region, and the nasofrontal angle, which together form the lower portion of the forehead.

The osteotomy is performed and the bandeau can be manipulated in various dimensions. Bending and contouring can be done with the Tessier bone-bender, which makes greenstick fractures in the bone, or with a lamellar split osteotomy. After remodeling, the bandeau is examined in many different orientations prior to advancement. It is not always replaced in its original orientation. It may need to be tilted slightly or rotated to one side or another. Occasionally, it is possible to obtain the proper nasofrontal angle by flipping the bandeau 180° on itself. Many times, multiple osteotomies in the bandeau allow reshaping to provide the proper aesthetic projection.

If the original bandeau cannot be used because of resorption, marked deformity, or sclerotic changes, it is replaced with a strip of biparietal cranial bone. The desired curvature can be preselected with the Marchac wire guide or by visual experience only, to eliminate the need for further recontouring of the bone.

In other cases where the frontal bone is of an appropriate shape, it can be lowered in one piece to form both the bandeau and the forehead. This method can also be used when the frontal bone is unsuitable for remodeling by replacing it in one piece with split cranial bone.

To achieve the desired aesthetic results the bandeau and frontal bone are usually treated separately to achieve the proper shape and orientation.

Orbits

Orbital hypertelorism is a condition in which the interorbital distance, as measured from dacryon (lacrimal crest) to dacryon, is greater than the expected age-appropriate normative values (adult normative values range from 25 to 30 mm). Tessier had classified the severity of adult hypertelorism based on the interorbital distance. In a grade I deformity, the medial osseous interorbital distance (MOIOD) was defined to be from 30 to 34 mm in length; grade II as a MOIOD of 35 to 39 mm; and grade III as a MOIOD greater than 40 mm (19). In addition, this is termed true hypertelorism when the increased MOIOD is associated with an increased lateral IOD (7.0 cm in the newborn and 11.3 cm in adults), or when the angle between the lateral orbital walls, as assessed by computed axial tomography, is greater than 90°.

The degree of hypertelorism and the severity of the comorbid deformities dictate the type of surgical intervention to be used. A single procedure can be used for simple deformities while staged procedures are necessary for severe deformities. In the latter setting, the first operation corrects the orbital hypertelorism, and subsequent operations are aimed at correcting the associated deformities. In general, excellent aesthetic results can be obtained using a three-wall or four-wall orbital osteotomy. These initial maneuvers involve medial and lateral canthal repositioning and correction of any existing enophthalmos or exophthalmos. At times, this initial correction will also encompass a frontocranial vault remodeling with an associated primary nasal reconstruction.

If the patient is young and the maxillary dentition is at risk, we will proceed with a three-wall, inverted U-shaped osteotomy or facial bipartition. If the patient is more mature, our method of choice is the classic four-wall correction as described by Tessier and later modified by Converse or again in certain cases a bipartition procedure. In mild cases of hypertelorism, those requiring less than 10 mm of medial orbital translocation, we perform bilateral medial orbital wall osteotomies with complete ethmoidectomy followed by bilateral medial canthopexy. In cases of facial dysraphia in which the maxilla is narrow, vaulted, and V-shaped, the facial bipartition procedure may be used successfully.

Nose

The nose is the most important structure of the central face on frontal and lateral profile views (16). Due to its proximity to the orbits, nasal deformity is associated with orbital hypertelorism. Excessive growth and development of the ethmoid air cells contribute to the nasal deformity by widening the upper one-third of the nose. This leads to lateral displacement of the nasal bones, the columella, and the lower lateral cartilages, thus creating a nose that is both short and wide. The nasolabial angle is obtuse and the nasal septum may be thickened with abnormal configuration of the alar cartilages. In these cases, nasal reconstruction is performed using osteotomies and repositioning of the nasal bones and frequently requires additional bone and/or cartilage grafting.

Skeletal surgery of the nasal bones is also an integral part of rhinoplasty. In reduction procedures, this involves rasping and infracturing of the nasal bones; or in augmentation procedures, this involves using autogenous bone or cartilage grafts. In extreme shortening of the nose, the use of frontonasal disjunction techniques provides the surgeon with an excellent method to elongate the nose substantially.

Midface

The midface is an important area of facial aesthetics and a challenging area to achieve balance and harmony because of the many structures found within it. Ranging from the glabella to the subnasale, it contains the orbits, the nose, the malar eminences, and the maxillae with the teeth. The positioning and volume of the basal bone of the maxillae is the key to facial beauty. If the base of the maxillae is recessive or protracted in proportion to the face, then it must be repositioned. The best procedure is the Le Fort I because it addresses the basal bone as the primary function of the osteotomy.

In the midface, the essential types of skeletal surgery involving facial aesthetics are the Le Fort I and III osteotomies. The process of planning such surgery involves not only facial aesthetics but also orthognathic harmony.

The Le Fort I osteotomy can be altered to provide advancement, rotation, impaction, elongation, or a combination of movements. The authors frequently use a separate 4-piece maxillae, which provides stability, better occlusion, and aesthetics. The angle of the osteotomy and the height of the osteotomy above the occlusive plane can be altered to change the impact on the facial contour. The alar bases widen with maxillary advancement and the alae flatten and narrow with impaction of the maxilla. The projection of the nasal tip can also be altered by including or excluding the anterior nasal spine in the movable segment. However, only the Le Fort III osteotomy can provide malar projection and alter the height of the radix. A Le Fort III osteotomy can be performed in conjunction with a Le Fort I osteotomy depending on the desired dental relationships.

The lamellar split osteotomy (20,21) is another option for augmentation of the craniofacial skeleton when the bone is of good quality. This procedure takes advantage of the cancellous plane between the two cortices of the bone to allow significant translocation of the outer table against the inner table, which remains as a reference point upon which to make precise skeletal advancement or widening of the face with easy fixation to achieve a superior aesthetic result without bone resorption of the segment. The lamellar split procedure was originally done as part of intracranial remodeling procedures; however, it can be performed as an extracranial procedure for malar contouring in the aesthetic patient. It requires experience and care to obtain symmetry, but may yield a superior cosmetic result.

Distraction osteogenesis has also been popular in the Le Fort I and III osteotomies and especially so in cases that require an extensive advancement of more than 10–12 mm. The combination of the traditional osteotomies with the use of distraction osteogenesis has been the most useful in cases with severe maxillary retrusion, scarring, and soft-tissue deficiency.

Lower Face

In the lower face, the surgeon must bring into consideration the upper and lower jaws and teeth, the chin, the bigonial width, and the mandibular angle and body.

The maxillae traverse both the midface and the lower face and, therefore, are especially important when considering the aesthetic aspects of both these facial portions. In addition, maxillary displacement has orthognathic implications because of its important occlusal relationship with the lower jaws and teeth. Therefore, when considering facial aesthetic surgery affecting the jaws, it is necessary to include orthodontic consults and treatment where applicable. Frequently, the positions of the maxillae are determined first in relation to the anterior cranial base, then the position of the mandible in both sagittal and frontal planes are assessed and the osteotomies made accordingly (Fig. 6) (22).

To redefine the chin, the method of choice is the horizontal mandibular osteotomy. In a male, a strong, square projecting chin, and in a female, a smaller projecting chin with a greater squareness of the gonial angle is preferred (23). This will create a harmonious projecting chin with proper labial chin crease and angle. This operation is ideal for those with inadequate chin projection and normal occlusion. In addition, it rejuvenates the appearance of the lower third of the aging face by providing a scaffolding to improve the drape of the jowl and the soft tissues of the neck. The main advantage of the horizontal mandibular osteotomy to the use of alloplastic implants is that, unlike an alloplastic implant, it uses autogenous material that will not erode the native bone. The osteotomy line should begin below the mental nerve and extend to the lateral body area of the jaw to obtain a smooth jawline after advancement.

To redefine the bigonial width, patients can have reduction osteotomy of the mandibular angles or augmentation by onlay bone grafting.

In cases with varying degrees of hemimandibular absence, the skeletal technique of choice for reconstruction is distraction osteogenesis. Current state-of-the art implants use multidirectional distracters that enable the surgeon to work in three vectors. The invention of better distractors will improve the surgical results concomitantly. The use of distraction osteogenesis in Pruzansky type III mandibles (agenesis of the ramus, coronoid, and temporomandibular joint) has not proven long term to necessarily give a stable result.

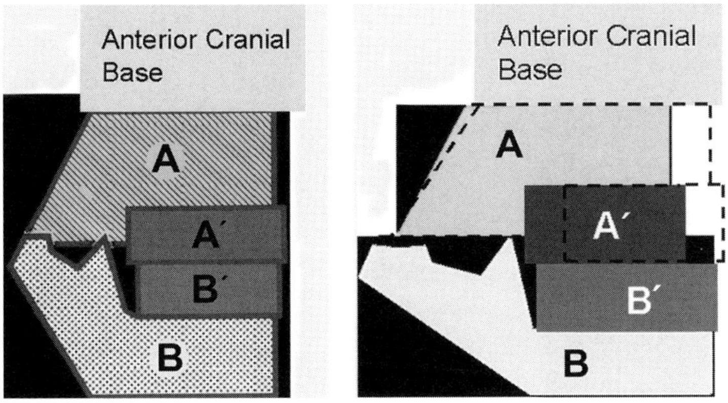

Figure 6 Demonstration of how the anterior cranial base is used as a reference point for determination of the maxilla, maxillary alveolus followed by the mandible and mandibular alveolus. The figure on the left demonstrates the normal positions of each element. The figure on the right demonstrates midfacial retrusion with an abnormal occlusion requiring repositioning of both the maxilla and maxillary alveolus individually to achieve aesthetic facial balance and normal occlusion. A: maxilla; A′: maxillary alveolus; B: mandible; B′: mandibular alveolus. *Source*: From Ref. 8.

Height, Width, Projection, and Volume

The results of surgery will depend on how the osteotomies may affect the facial appearance three-dimensionally: namely the height, width, projection, and volume of the face. Certain procedures will affect one more than the other, and the surgeon will have to use their experience to assess how many dimensions are affected in the face of the patient. This is the key to achieving balance, harmony, and an aesthetic improvement in the face.

EXAMPLES

Patient A

In the following example, the patient is assessed step by step to demonstrate the thought process of the authors during the consultation, the subsequent decision-making process, and the surgical procedure itself.

This is a 30-year-old female patient whom we treated for an asymmetric face, orbits, and oral commissures as well as vertical maxillary excess (Figs. 7 and 8). She had previous jaw surgery, which aggravated right temporomandibular joint popping sounds on jaw movement.

The patient was examined awake and a good idea of the aesthetically desired vertical height of the maxillae was determined preoperatively. The position of the maxillae should result in 2–3 mm of incisor exposure at rest, and the smiling lip line is generally located close to the gingival margin and shows a full upper arch of teeth (5).

The maxillae should be positioned to provide full support and enhancement of the soft-tissue facial mask of skin and muscles so that the upper lip is full and in front by a few millimeters of the lower lip. There should be no perioral soft-tissue deficiency. The columella-lip angle should be in the range of 99.1° (6). The width of the nose should be in proportion to the face, nasal dorsum, and lip projection.

To obtain facial symmetry, the maxillae must be level and of equal height on the horizontal plane of the face as reflected by the horizontal symmetry of both commissures of the mouth. In addition, the occlusal plane and the Frankfort horizontal plane bisect an angle of 6.2° and 7.1° in the male and female (24). This is determined and recorded preoperatively by visual examination and cephalometrics. Thus, the movement of the maxilla must be adjusted in four axes, namely in its vertical height, lateral movement, sagittal projection as well as rotation.

Preoperative planning included life-size drawings made by a professional artist to represent the idealized patient's face without deformity. This was then compared to similar life-sized photographs of the patient and the differences in soft-tissue landmarks noted. In this

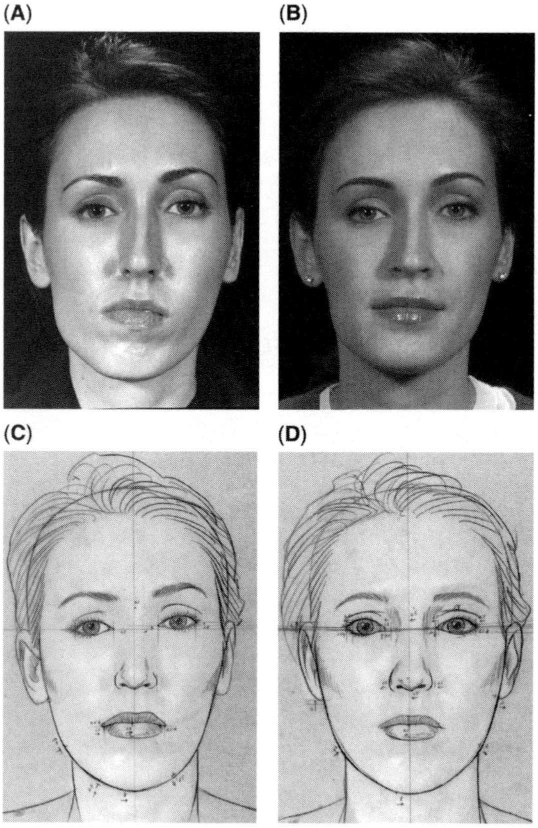

Figure 7 (**A** and **B**) Preoperative and six months' postoperative frontal views of Patient A. In the preoperative photo, note the asymmetric face, orbits, oral commissures, and vertical maxillary excess. This was corrected with a four-piece Le Fort I osteotomy, bilateral sagittal split osteotomy of the mandible, and horizontal mandibular osteotomy of the chin. Residual orbital dystopia was not corrected because she was satisfied with her improved appearance after the first surgery. (**C** and **D**) Life-size sketches of idealized features in the patient. Note that in the sketch without orbital repositioning (**C**) the midline was established 0.5 mm to the right of the nasion, through the subnasale, and 8 mm to the left of the gnathion. Thus, to obtain correction, the menton was moved 8 mm to the left, in addition to reduction of the right mandibular base and augmentation of the left mandibular base. In the sketch that shows complete correction of the facial scoliosis (**D**), the midline was established 2.5 mm to the right of the nasion, 1.5 mm to the right of the subnasale, and 8 mm to the left of the gnathion. In addition to the orthognathic surgery mentioned above, the left eye was lowered and the right eye was raised slightly, the intercanthal width was widened 2–3 mm, and the nose was moved to the right by 1–2 mm.

case, two separate frontal and a lateral drawing were made. One of the frontal drawings incorporated both orbital and orthognathic surgeries while the other included orthognathic surgery only. The reason for this was that orthognathic surgery was planned first followed by orbital surgery, and it was necessary to see the difference that would be achieved with one or both surgeries performed. The sketch that depicted correction of the jaw anomaly alone, established the midline to be 0.5 mm to the right of the nasion, through the subnasale, and 8 mm to the left of the gnathion. The appearance with orthognathic surgery alone would entail movement of the menton to the left by 8 mm, reduction of the right mandibular base, and augmentation of the left mandibular base (Fig. 7C). The sketch that showed correction of the facial scoliosis established the midline to be 2.5 mm to the right of the nasion, 1.5 mm to the right of the subnasale, and 8 mm to the left of the gnathion. Orbital repositioning was performed by lowering the left eye slightly and raising the right eye slightly. The intercanthal width was also widened 2–3 mm and the nose was moved to the right by 1–2 mm (Fig. 7D). Correction of the jaw anomaly was similar to that described above. The lateral sketch that showed the idealized profile of the patient indicated that the mandible itself was fine and that the lower lip protrusion required a set back of 2 mm (Fig. 8).

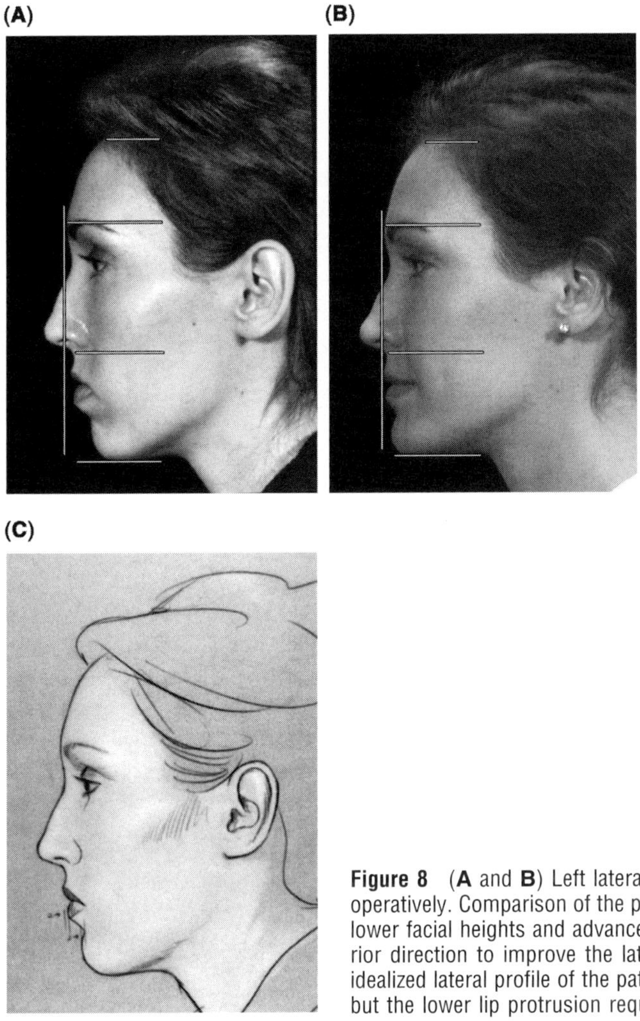

Figure 8 (A and B) Left lateral profile of Patient A preoperatively and postoperatively. Comparison of the photos demonstrates reduction of the mid- and lower facial heights and advancement of the maxilla and mandible in an anterior direction to improve the lateral facial profile. (C) Life-size sketch of the idealized lateral profile of the patient. Note that the mandible itself looked fine, but the lower lip protrusion required a set back of 2 mm.

At the same time, CT scans of the patient's skull were done and a stereolithographic model was made to obtain a better impression of the skeletal deformity and to enable accurate preoperative planning to correct the skeletal abnormalities (Fig. 9). In addition, the planning for corrective osteotomies was also based on the intended soft-tissue result as seen on the sketches.

The decision was made to do the correction in two stages. The first stage would involve a four-piece Le Fort I osteotomy, bilateral sagittal split osteotomy of the mandible, and horizontal mandibular osteotomy of the chin. The second stage was to do a correction of the orbital asymmetry. However, the patient declined orbital repositioning after satisfactory results were obtained from the first stage.

At the operating table, adjustments in height and symmetry and projection and teeth show, determine facial aesthetics, balance and beauty. A skeletal full-volume face is much more attractive than a retrodisplaced skeletal projection.

For aesthetic surgery, the face comes first followed by the occlusion. The operation was planned using a four-piece Le Fort I osteotomy. Once the osteotomy was completed, the four-piece osteotomy was defined using a space created between the premolars. The osteotomy went from the alveolus backwards on both sides of the septum to create a central portion that included the central and lateral incisors as a single block. Once the four segments had been created, an intermediate splint was secured in place to evaluate the intrusion, rotation, and reposition of the maxilla. The midline of the maxilla was translocated 2 mm to the left; the left hemimaxilla was moved superiorly by 6.5 mm, and the right hemimaxilla was moved

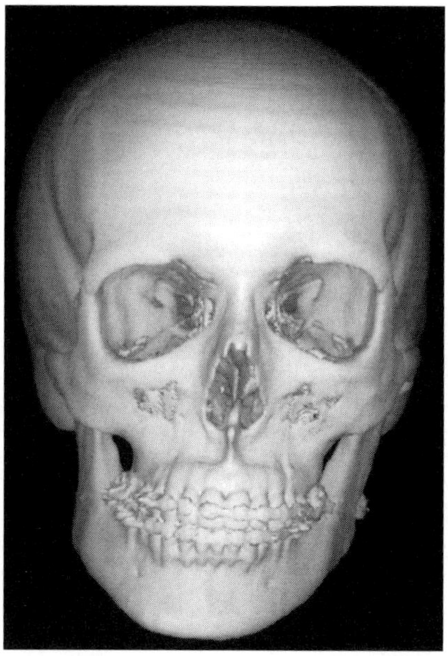

Figure 9 Three-dimensional computed tomography scan reconstruction of the patient demonstrating abnormal positioning of the orbits, maxilla, and mandible. Reproduction of this scan in a stereolithography model enabled accurate preoperative planning to achieve correction of skeletal abnormalities.

superiorly by 5 mm. Once the maxillae was fixed optimally three-dimensionally in space to give optimal show of teeth, projection and positioning of the upper lip, fullness of the perioral area, equal height of both commissures, then fixation was done with four 26 gauge stainless steel wires first for stability and then for fine adjustment. Semirigid fixation of the maxilla was then completed using low-profile 1.5-mm L-shaped titanium plates and screws.

A bilateral sagittal split osteotomy was then performed and the mandible was moved to the maxillae to achieve good occlusion. The volume and mandibular angle was aesthetically assessed and adjusted as planned to give optimal aesthetics. A horizontal mandibular osteotomy, with a 2-mm displacement of the chin to the left, completed the correction of lower facial asymmetry in this patient. Postoperative elastics were applied and allowed for a further 1- to 2-mm adjustment of the teeth for optimal stable results (Figs. 7B, 8B, and 10).

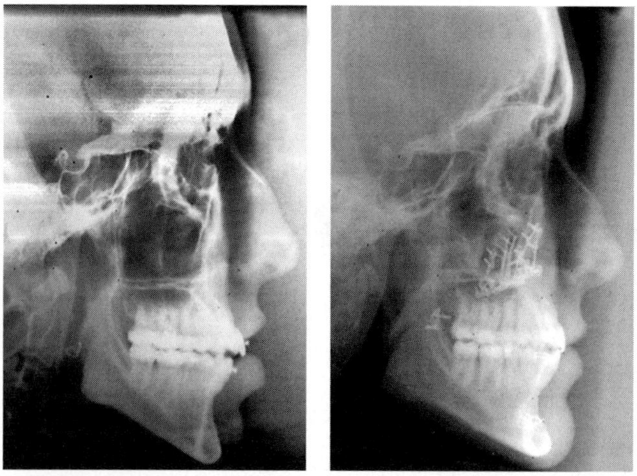

Figure 10 Lateral cephalograms of Patient A demonstrating the result of the skeletal surgery on both occlusion, facial profile, and facial aesthetics. A four-piece Le Fort I osteotomy was performed. The midline of the maxilla was translocated 2 mm to the left, the left hemimaxilla was moved superiorly by 6.5 mm, and the right hemimaxilla was moved superiorly by 5 mm. Bilateral sagittal split osteotomy of the mandible was then performed to achieve good occlusion. The chin was then repositioned with a horizontal mandibular osteotomy with reduction of the lower facial height and displacement of the chin 2 mm to the left.

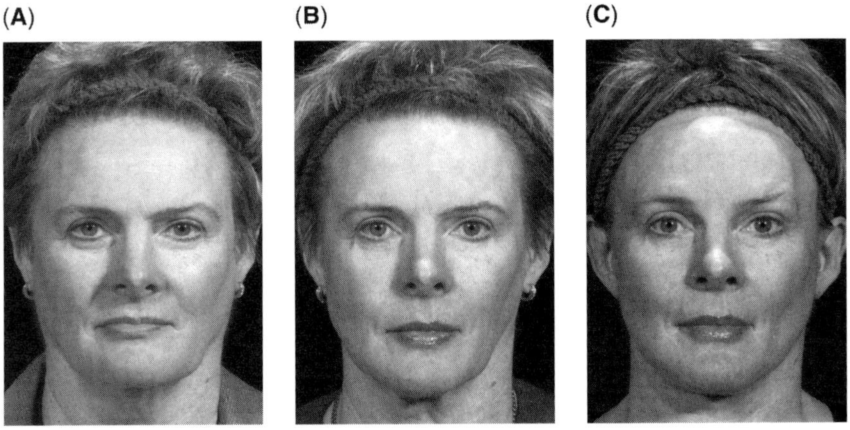

Figure 11 Patient B presented to the authors with previous orthognathic surgery performed elsewhere with an untold and unfavorable result (see text for more details) (**A**). She has since had two surgeries in the authors' care. The photos were taken four months after the first surgery (**B**) and seven months after the second surgery (**C**). The first surgery comprised a Le Fort I osteotomy, bilateral sagittal split osteotomy of the mandible, and horizontal mandibular osteotomy while the second surgery comprised a forehead-lift, brow-lift, midface-lift, cheek-lift, neck-lift, and onlay demineralized bone graft at the left mandibular angle. On the frontal profile, note the improvement of the facial proportions by increasing the lower facial height in the first postoperative photo (**B**). The second postoperative photo (**C**) shows improvement of the soft-tissue drape as well as the contour of the left mandibular angle.

Patient B

In this example, the patient was a 53-year-old female who had a Le Fort I osteotomy, mandibular advancement, rhinoplasty, and eyelid surgery done previously by a dental surgeon (DDS) for bad occlusion. However, she was unhappy with the result because although she had an improved occlusion, the resultant facial appearance was that she looked older after that surgery.

On the frontal assessment, it was noted that she had widened bigonial distances and on the lateral profile, the vertical line from the glabella showed a concave facial outline (Figs. 11A, 12A, and 13A). This was in accordance with the problem of a retrusive maxilla. In addition the upper lip was in an abnormal retruded position in comparison to the lower lip. It appeared that the initial surgery had failed to advance the maxillae sufficiently. Independent orthodontic assessment was that she needed preoperative orthodontic work in preparation for surgery.

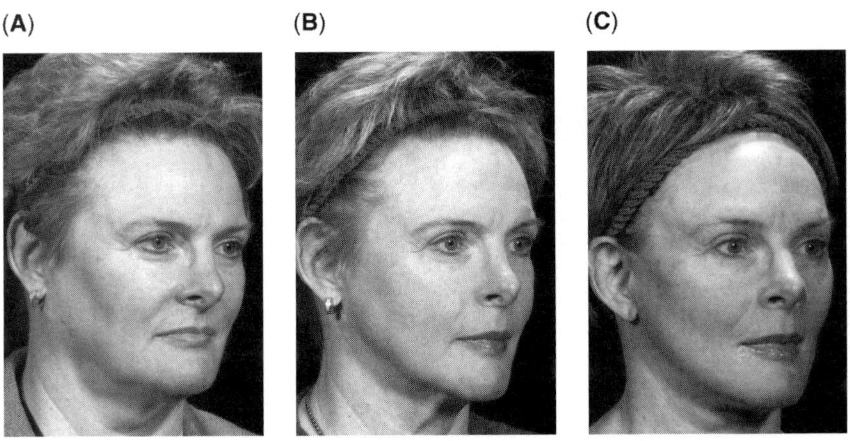

Figure 12 Right oblique view of Patient B, demonstrating the effects of skeletal repositioning of the maxilla before the first surgery (**A**), after the first surgery (**B**), and improved soft tissue drape over the craniofacial skeleton after the second surgery (**C**).

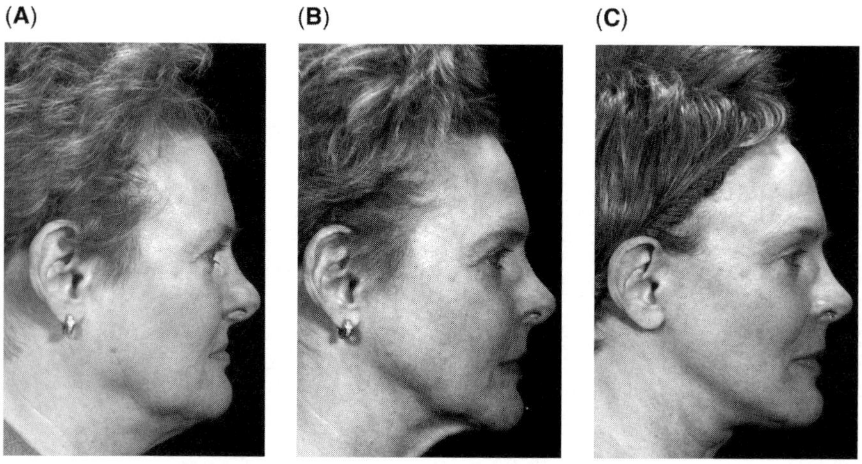

Figure 13 Right lateral profile view of Patient B demonstrating the improvement in facial proportions as the mid- and lower facial heights were adjusted (**A–C**). The anterior movement of the maxilla and clockwise rotation of the mandible downwards are also apparent. All this resulted in a change from a retrusive midface to become a more protrusive face on the lateral profile.

To correct the above abnormalities, she had a repeat Le Fort I advancement osteotomy with a maxillary movement of 8 mm anteriorly and 1 mm to the right. The Le Fort I osteotomy was inclined slightly cephalad posteriorly with the intention of increasing the mid- and lower facial heights as well as the mandibular plane when the maxilla was advanced. This was followed by bilateral sagittal split osteotomies of the mandible, bilateral turbinectomies, and a soft-tissue release of the chin. This enabled the correction of maxillary retrusion to one of protrusion and a volume-enhanced face. To further enhance the aesthetic appearance of the patient, she required soft-tissue surgery in the form of a forehead, brow, midface, cheek-lift, neck-lift, and onlay demineralized bone graft over the left mandibular angle, which was performed five months after the skeletal surgery.

Postoperative results revealed an improved lateral facial profile as well as lengthening of the upper lip, restoration of the normal columella-lip angle, and the position of the upper lip in relation to the lower lip (Figs. 11–14).

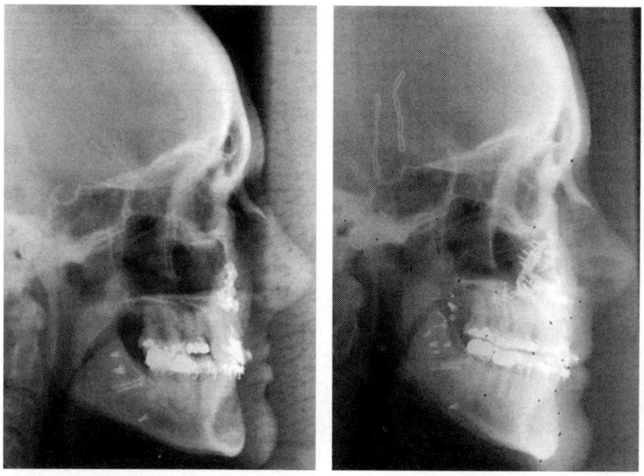

Figure 14 Lateral cephalogram of Patient B demonstrating results of Le Fort I advancement osteotomy of 8 mm and bilateral sagittal split osteotomy of the mandible. This resulted in improved facial proportions and balance.

REFERENCES

1. Whitaker LA. Facial proportions in aesthetic surgery. In: Farkas LG, Munro IR, eds. Anthropometric Facial Proportions in Medicine. 1st ed. Springfield: Charles C Thomas, 1987:103–117.
2. Legan HL, Burstone CJ. Soft tissue cephalometric analysis for orthognathic surgery. J Oral Surg 1980; 38(10):744–751.
3. Scheideman GB, Bell WH, Legan HL, Finn RA, Reisch JS. Cephalometric analysis of dentofacial normals. Am J Orthod 1980; 78(4):404–420.
4. Bell WH, Jacobs JD. Tridimensional planning for surgical/orthodontic treatment of mandibular excess. Am J Orthod 1981; 80(3):263–288.
5. Dagys AP. The use of proportions in planning surgical-orthodontic treatment in young adult patients. In: Farkas LG, Munro IR, eds. Anthropometric Facial Proportions in Medicine. 1st ed. Springfield, Illinois: Charles C Thomas, 1987:83–101.
6. Farkas LG. Anthropometry of the Head and Face in Medicine. New York: Elsevier, 1981.
7. Fanous N, Yoskovitch A. Premaxillary augmentation: adjunct to rhinoplasty. Plast Reconstr Surg 2000; 106(3):707–712.
8. McNamara JA Jr, Brudon WL. Cephalometric evaluation of the orthodontic patient. In: McNamara JA Jr, Brudon WL, eds. Orthodontic and Orthopaedic Treatment in the Mixed Dentition. 1st ed. Ann Arbor: Needham Press, 1993:13–54.
9. McNamara JA Jr, Brust EW, Riolo ML. Soft tissue evaluation of individuals with an ideal occlusion and a well-balanced face. In: McNamara JA Jr, ed. Aesthetics and the Treatment of Facial Form, Monograph 28, Craniofacial Growth Series, Center for Human Growth and Development, University of Michigan, Ann Arbor, Michigan, 1993.
10. Epker BN, Fish LC, Paulus PJ. The surgical-orthodontic correction of maxillary deficiency. Oral Surg Oral Med Oral Pathol 1978; 46(2):171–205.
11. Davidson WM. Anthropometrics, cephalometrics and orthodontics. In: Achauer BM, Eriksson E, Guyuron B, Coleman JJ III, Russell RC, Vander Kolk CA, eds. Plastic Surgery. Indications, Operations, and Outcomes. Vol. 2. 1st ed. St. Louis: Mosby, 2000:637–650.
12. Whitaker LA. Skeletal contouring. In: Vistnes LM, ed. Procedures in Plastic and Reconstructive Surgery: How They Do It. . 1st ed. Boston: Little, Brown and Company, 1991:13–29.
13. Salyer KE, Hubli E, Genecov DG, Agarwal R. Distraction osteogenesis vs primary osteotomy: Indications and contraindications. A clinical perspective from a busy craniofacial service. Proc 8th Int Congress of the International Soc of Craniofacial Surgery, 1999; 8:167–170.
14. Salyer KE, Genecov DG, Barcelo CR. 10 years experience: Distraction vs osteotomy in craniofacial and cleft surgery. Proc 4th Int Congress of Maxillofacial and Craniofacial Distraction, Monduzzi Editore, Bologna, Italy, 2003:341–346.
15. Enlow DH. Facial Growth. Philadelphia: W.B. Saunders, 1990.
16. Salyer KE. Salyer and Bardach's atlas of craniofacial surgery. In: Craniofacial Surgery. Vol. 1. Philadelphia: Lippincott-Raven, 1999.
17. Ousterhout DK. Feminization of the forehead: contour changing to improve female aesthetics. Plast Recon Surg 1987; 79(5):701–713.
18. Salyer KE, Hall JD. Bandeau—the focal point of frontocranial remodeling. J Craniofacial Surg 1990; 1(1):18–31.
19. Tessier P. Orbital hypertelorism. I. Successive surgical attempts. Material and methods. Causes and mechanisms. Scand J Plast Reconstr Surg 1972; 6(2):135–155.
20. Salyer KE, Hall CD, Joganic EF. Lamellar split osteotomy: a new craniofacial technique. Plast Reconstr Surg 1990; 86(5):845–853 (discussion 854–855).
21. Salyer KE. Malar augmentation using lamellar split osteotomy. J Craniofac Surg 1994; 5(2):116–123.
22. Enlow DH, McNamara JA Jr. The neurocranial basis for facial form and pattern. Angle Orthod 1973; 43(3):256–270.
23. Whitaker LA, Pertschuk M. Facial skeletal contouring for aesthetic purposes. Plast Reconstr Surg 1982; 69(2):245–253.
24. Burstone CJ, James RB, Legan H, Murphy GA, Norton LA. Cephalometrics for orthognathic surgery. J Oral Surg 1978; 36(4):269–277.

7 Simulating Facial Skeletal Osteotomies with Alloplastic Implants

Michael J. Yaremchuk
Massachusetts General Hospital and Harvard Medical School, Boston, Massachusetts, U.S.A.

INTRODUCTION

To correct severe deformities, which are disfiguring and may have functional consequences to vision, breathing, and mastication, craniofacial surgeons may find it necessary to perform skeletal osteotomies and rearrangement. These operations are significant undertakings. Many more patients have mild forms of these deformities, for example, "prominent eyes" due to midface hypoplasia or "receding chins" due to underdeveloped mandibles. Particularly in the lower face, some patients have had partial correction of mandibular deficiency through orthodontic treatment. In these patients with less severe abnormalities or those who already have had their occlusion normalized through orthodontic treatment, the appearance of skeletal osteotomies and rearrangement can be simulated through the use of facial implants. Implant surgery can provide the visual effect of certain LeFort I, LeFort III, and mandibular osteotomies.

RATIONALE FOR ALLOPLASTIC VS. AUTOGENOUS MATERIALS

Alloplastic materials have major advantages over autogenous tissue when used as facial skeletal onlays. Alloplastic implants avoid donor site morbidity, are of unlimited supply, save operating time, and are not susceptible to the contour changes seen with autogenous onlay bone grafts. Work done in our laboratory showed that the volume loss of onlay bone grafts was related to their rate of revascularization, thereby allowing access by osteoclasts for resorption. In that study, cranial bone resorbed more slowly than iliac crest bone because it had a greater proportion of cortical bone, which is more slowly revascularized than cancellous bone (1). Wolff's law states that bone placed in a different environment will respond to that environment by changing its internal architecture and external morphology. If extrapolated to the facial skeleton, Wolff's law will predict that any autogenous bone graft onlayed to the facial skeleton is predisposed to changing its shape and volume when it becomes revascularized.

SIMULATING THE LEFORT I OSTEOTOMY WITH ADVANCEMENT

The LeFort I osteotomy advancement is performed alone or in combination with other mandibular osteotomies to correct occlusal disharmonies and to correct lower midface concavity. Patients with satisfactory occlusion and midface concavity can have their aesthetic desires satisfied with skeletal augmentation. Implantation of alloplastic material in the paranasal area can simulate the visual effect of LeFort I advancement and other skeletal manipulations (2). Paranasal augmentation does not alter occlusal relationships and, therefore, avoids perioperative orthodontic treatment and limits surgical morbidity and hospital expense. Figure 1 shows how the visual effect of a LeFort I level osteotomy with advancement can be simulated by augmenting the skeleton at the pyriform aperture level with alloplastic implants. In patients with acceptable occlusion, implants can correct congenital, posttraumatic, and cleft-related midface retrusion. The most common indication for paranasal augmentation is a patient with relative midface deficiency. In patients with flat faces and large noses, implants placed adjacent to the pyriform aperture will camouflage the large nose. Patients with a "dish face" deformity after midface fractures may be candidates for these implants. Retrusion of the central midface may

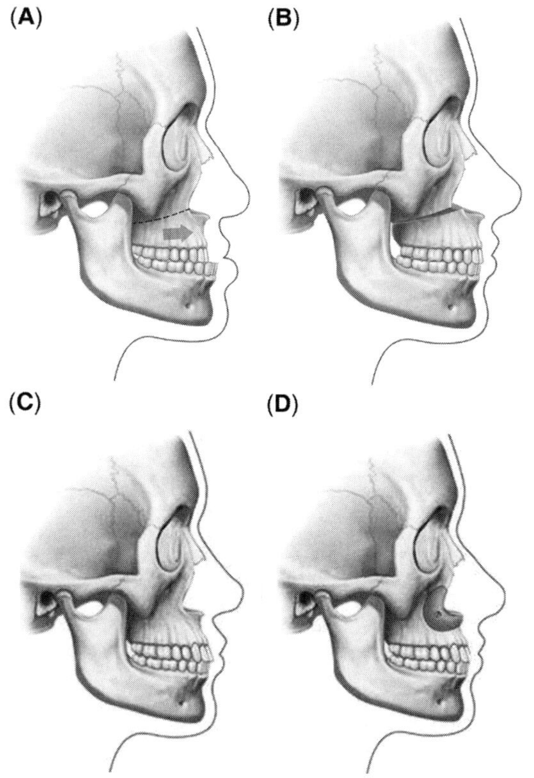

Figure 1 (**A, B**) Diagrammatic representation of LeFort I osteotomy with advancement. Note that a Class III dental relationship has been changed to a Class I relationship. Note that the lower midface soft tissues have been changed from concave to a convex appearance. (**C, D**) Diagrammatic representation of augmentation of the paranasal area with alloplastic implants. Note that the occlusal relationship remains unchanged, but that the midface soft-tissue envelope has been changed from concave to convex similar to the appearance obtained after LeFort I osteotomy with advancement.

occur when upper and lower jaw fractures are reduced with respect to occlusion only and not to the three-dimensional skeletal restoration. Patients who have had cleft repair often have a deficiency in lower midface projection due to the growth-restricting forces of surgical intervention and scarring. Augmentation of the alveolar and the lateral paranasal area will improve lip and nasal relationships in these patients.

THE IMPLANT

This author prefers to perform facial skeletal augmentation with porous polyethylene Medpor® (Porex Surgical, Fairburn, Georgia, U.S.A.) implants. This material's pore size (range 160–368 μm, average 240 μm) allows fibrous tissue ingrowth at the recipient site. This relative incorporation by the host minimizes the encapsulation provided by smooth implants. Encapsulation can lead to disfiguring soft-tissue changes, particularly when large implants are placed under relatively thin skin. Porous polyethylene material's properties also allow it to be carved with a scalpel or mechanical burr and to be fixed to the skeleton with a screw. Preshaped paranasal implants are available in two sizes and are custom contoured during surgery to the patient's aesthetic needs.

SURGICAL TECHNIQUE

Although facial skeletal augmentation can be done under local or general anesthesia, the author prefers a general anesthesia via nasotracheal intubation. Because most of the procedures are performed through intraoral incisions, nasotracheal intubation allows the best protection of the airway during surgery, ideal preparation of the oral cavity, and optimizes the surgical exposure. After sterile preoperative preparation and draping, a local anesthetic with 1:200,000 epinephrine is infiltrated at the surgical site. An upper gingivobuccal sulcus incision is made just lateral to the pyriform aperture to avoid placing incisions directly over the implant. An adequate cuff of mucosa is left to allow layered closure.

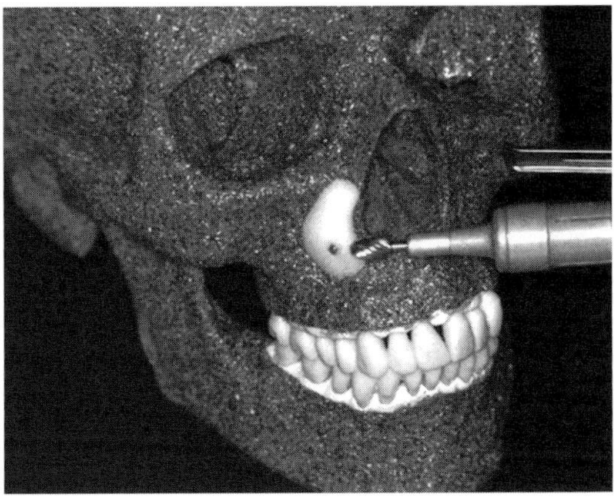

Figure 2 Porous polyethylene paranasal implants are designed to augment both the lateral and inferior aspects of the pyriform aperture. Implants can be carved to allow selective augmentation. Screw fixation prevents movement of the implant and allows in-place contouring. Intact screw-fixed implant about to be contoured with power equipment. Implant contoured and positioned to selectively augment maxilla lateral to pyriform aperture.

Wide subperiosteal dissection exposes the area to be augmented and facilitates placement of the porous implant to which soft tissues tend to adhere. The implant is positioned to sit flush on the bone. The patient's anatomy will determine whether the entire crescent or just the horizontal or vertical limb of the crescent will be used (Fig. 2).

Fixation with a single screw is useful for several reasons. It ensures precise placement of the implant, preventing any displacement with soft-tissue redraping. It allows in-place contouring of the implant with either a scalpel or cutting burr. This simplifies custom shaping and minimizes the soft-tissues manipulation inherent with implant placement and replacement. Finally, screw fixation applies the implant to the skeleton, obliterating any gaps between the implant and

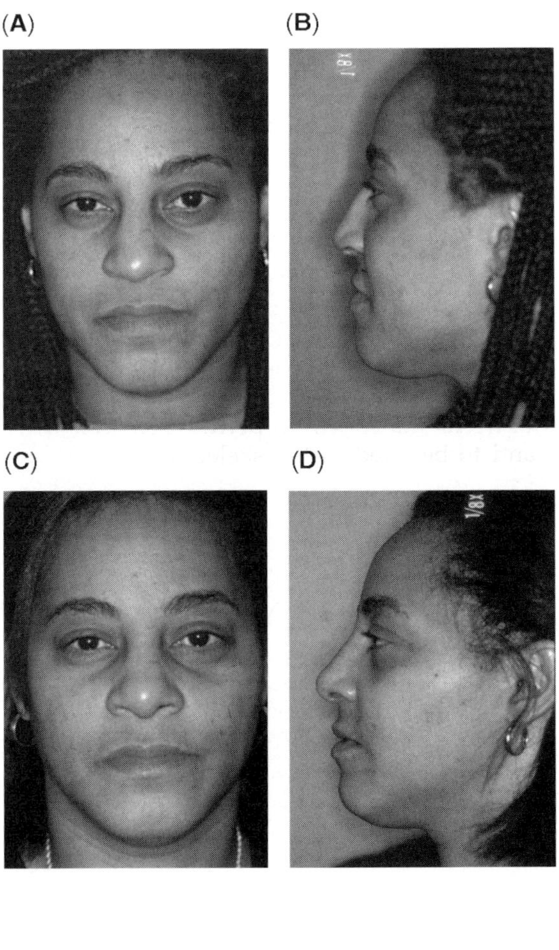

Figure 3 A 44-year-old woman presented for rhinoplasty. An open rhinoplasty with tip graft, submucous resection, and paranasal augmentation was performed. The implant was placed in the manner shown in Figure 1, above. (**A**) Preoperative frontal view. (**B**) Preoperative lateral view. (**C**) One-year postoperative frontal view. (**D**) One-year postoperative lateral view. *Source*: From Ref. 2.

the skeleton. Gaps between the implant and skeleton effectively increase the amount of augmentation provided by the implant making the outcome less predictable and precise.

The wound is closed in two layers. Perioperative antibiotics are used. The implant is not impregnated with any antibiotics at the time of surgery. Figure 3 shows a patient who underwent paranasal augmentation at the time of the aesthetic rhinoplasty.

SIMULATING THE LEFORT III OSTEOTOMY WITH ADVANCEMENT

The LeFort III osteotomy is usually employed to treat the craniofacial dysostoses of Crouzon and Apert syndromes. These patients have severe midface deficiency resulting in Class III malocclusion, exorbitism and, in extreme cases airway compromise. Infraorbital rim augmentation alone, or in combination with paranasal and medial malar augmentation, can provide the visual effect of LeFort III advancement as shown (Fig. 4).This can be effective treatment for patients with mild midface hypoplasia.

Lack of central midface projection, particularly the infraorbital rim, results in several stigmata. The eyes are prominent with scleral show. The lack of skeletal support results in premature cheek descent often allowing lower lid fat compartments to be visible—giving "early bags." In addition, the midface concavity makes the nose appear large. It has long been known that patients with midface hypoplasia are predisposed (or "morphologically prone") to lower lid descent after lower lid blepharoplasty (3).

Jelks and Jelks categorized globe–orbital rim relationships and the tendency for the development of lower lid malposition after blepharoplasty (4). On sagittal view, they placed a line or vector between the most anterior projection of the globe and the malar eminences and lid margin. A positive vector relationship exists when the most anterior projection of the globe is posterior to the lid margin and the malar eminence. A negative vector relationship exists when the most anterior projection of the globe lies anterior to the lower lid and the malar eminence. They warned that, patients whose orbital morphology has a negative vector relationship are prone to lid malposition after lower blepharoplasty.

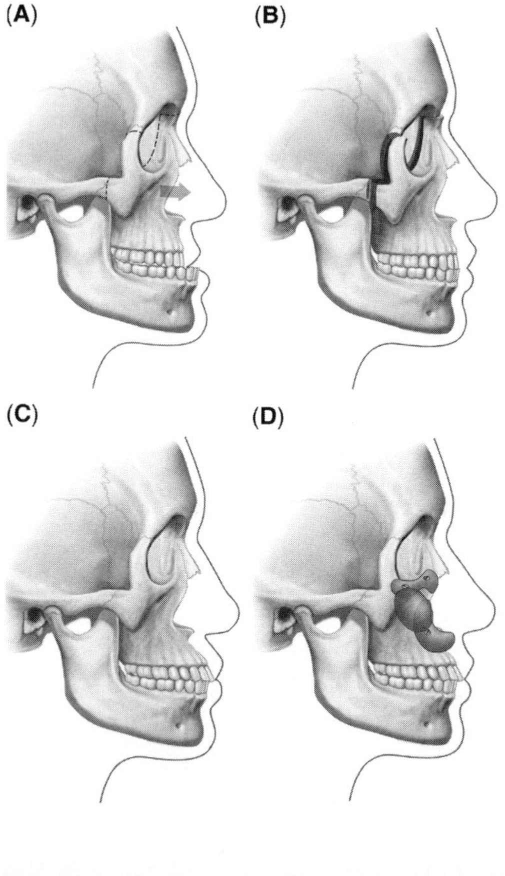

Figure 4 (**A, B**) Diagrammatic representation of LeFort III osteotomy with advancement. Note that a Class III skeletal relationship has been changed to a Class I relationship. Note that the midface soft tissues have been changed from concave to convex appearance. (**C, D**) Diagrammatic representation of augmentation of the infraorbital rim, the paranasal area, and medial malar area with alloplastic implants. Note that the occlusal relationship remains unchanged, but that the midface soft-tissue envelope has been changed from concave to convex, similar to the appearance obtained after LeFort III osteotomy with advancement.

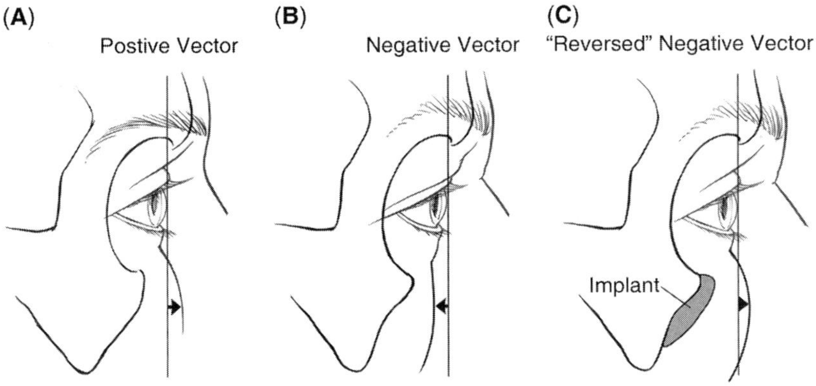

Figure 5 Diagrammatic representation of globe–rim relations on sagittal view. (**A**) A positive vector relationship exists when the most anterior projection of the globe is posterior to the lid margin and cheek prominence. (**B**) A negative vector relationship exists when the most anterior projection of the globe lies anterior to the lid and cheek prominence. (**C**) Infraorbital rim implant can effectively "reverse the negative vector" relationship.

Augmentation of the infraorbital rim with an alloplastic implant can effectively reverse the negative vector (Fig. 5). Subperiosteal freeing and elevation of the midface soft tissues and an augmented skeletal infrastructure reduce the prominent eye appearance, lessen scleral show and premature bags, as well as correct premature cheek descent. This skeletal augmentation not only normalizes skeletal morphology, but also has a rejuvenating effect (5–7).

SURGICAL TECHNIQUE

Implants are available, which are specifically designed for infraorbital rim augmentation. They can provide up to 5 mm of anterior projection. They are custom carved to fit the specific needs of the patient. A small flange on the implant allows it to rest on the most anterior aspect of the orbital floor. This flange allows easier positioning of the implant and a possible area for screw fixation to the skeleton.

The infraorbital rim and adjacent anatomy must be exposed sufficiently to assure ideal implant placement, smooth implant facial skeleton transition, and screw fixation. Direct, subciliary skin or skin–muscle flap incisions can provide this exposure. A transconjunctival incision alone is inadequate for implant placement and screw stabilization. A transconjunctival retroseptal incision, if used, requires lengthening with a lateral canthotomy or an intraoral incision. Figures 6 and 7 show clinical examples of patients who underwent midface augmentation with several implants as well as subperiosteal midface-lift.

SIMULATING MANDIBULAR OSTEOTOMIES WITH IMPLANTS

Skeletal mandibular deficiency resulting in a Class II occlusal relationship is a common clinical problem. The majority of these patients can have their dental relationships normalized through orthodontic tooth movement. Patients with severe malocclusion usually require sagittal split osteotomies, often with horizontal osteotomies and advancement of the chin. Those patients who have had their malocclusion treated with orthodontics alone are left with mandibular skeletal deficiencies, which may be deforming. The skeletal anatomy associated with mandibular deficiency, which can be camouflaged with implants designed to augment the ramus and body of the mandible, includes the obtuse mandibular angle with steep mandibular plane, as well as decreased vertical and transverse ramus dimensions (9). The addition of an extended chin implant will camouflage the poorly projecting chin (10). Figure 8 shows how mandibular and chin implants can mimic the appearance of mandibular osteotomies with repositioning.

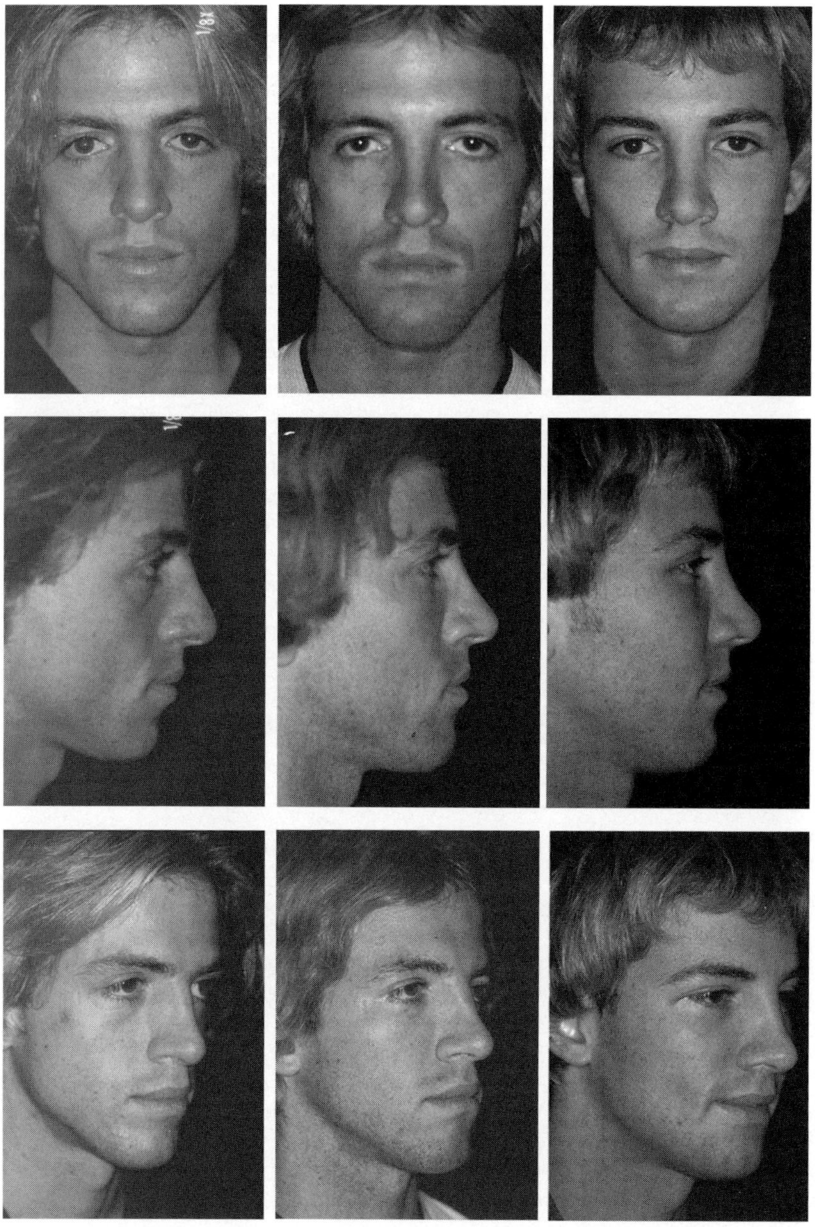

Figure 6 A 24-year-old male patient who requested several changes in his facial contour. Two operations were performed, 18 months apart. In the first operation, malar and infraorbital rim implants were placed and a rhinoplasty was performed, through bicoronal, intraoral, and intranasal incision. In the second operation, paranasal and mandibular body implants were placed, the rhinoplasty was revised, and a midface-lift and lateral canthopexies were performed. Frontal, lateral, and oblique views (*left*) before the operation, (*center*) after the first operation, and (*right*) after the second operation. *Source*: From Ref. 8.

MANDIBULAR BODY AND RAMUS IMPLANT

An implant is designed to augment the congenitally deficient mandible (Fig. 9) (9). This implant increases ramus, as well as anterior and posterior body width. Its tapering projection beyond the inferior edge of the mandible (C and E) allows it to change the inclination of the plane of the mandibular border. Because it also projects beyond the posterior border, in addition to extending beyond its inferior edge of the ramus, it can lessen the obliquity of

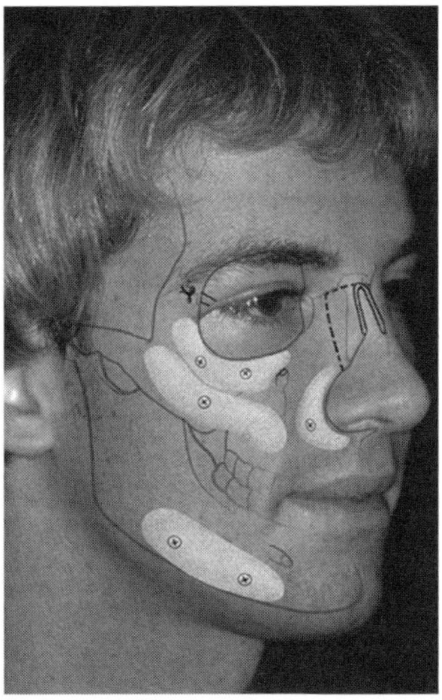

Figure 6 (*Continued*) Diagrammatic representation of the combined procedures.

the mandibular angle. All dimensions of the implant may be trimmed to meet the aesthetic needs of the patient.

SURGICAL TECHNIQUE

A generous intraoral mucosal incision is made to expose the ramus and the body of the mandible. It is made at least one centimeter above the sulcus on its labial side. The anterior ramus and the body of the mandible are freed from their soft tissues. The mental nerve is visualized as it exits its foramen to avoid its injury. It is important to free both the inferior and posterior borders of the mandible of soft-tissue attachments to allow implant placement.

As determined by preoperative assessment, the implant is trimmed with a scalpel before its placement on the mandible. To ensure the desired placement of the implant and its application to the surface of the mandible, the implant is fixed to the mandible with titanium screws. In most individuals the screw fixation can be performed through intraoral access. If intraoral access does not allow screws to be placed perpendicular to the implant and the anterior mandibular surface, stab-wound incisions (2–3 mm) are made in the neck skin beneath the inferior border of the mandible. The screwdriver is then gently manipulated through the intervening soft tissues and into the operative field. This allows strategic unicortical screw fixation of the implant to the mandible. Usually two to three screws are used to obliterate any gaps

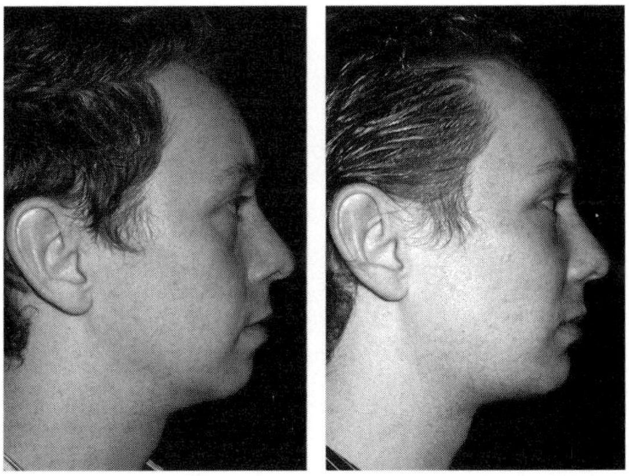

Figure 7 A 24-year-old man who underwent paranasal infraorbital and medial malar augmentation as well as subperiosteal midface-lift. He also underwent mandibular angle, body, and chin augmentation.

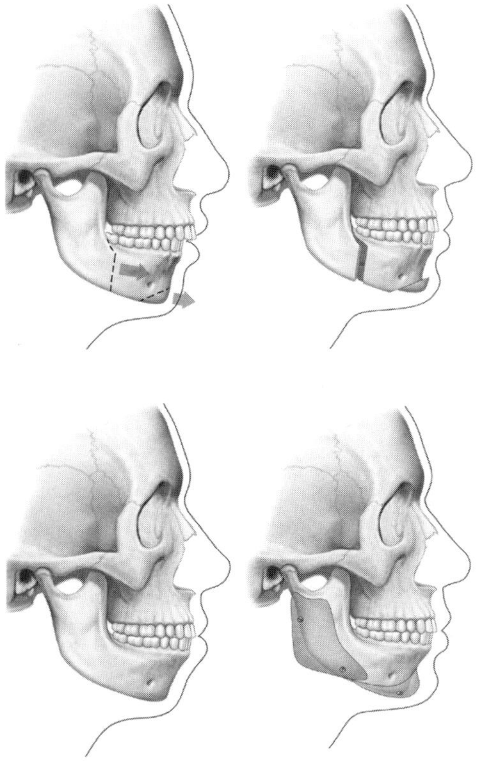

Figure 8 (*Upper*) Diagrammatic representation of sagittal split osteotomy to correct Class II malocclusion with horizontal osteotomy advancement of the chin to increase chin projection. Note that the occlusion has been corrected from Class II to Class I. (*Lower*) Diagrammatic representation of the visual effect of sagittal split osteotomy and horizontal osteotomy of the chin with advancement has been simulated with mandible and chin implants. Note that the Class I occlusion is unchanged. Notice also that the border regularities inherent with skeletal osteotomies are avoided when implants are used.

between the mandible and the implant. Screws are placed to avoid the anticipated path of the inferior-alveolar nerve before it exits from the mental foramen. The wound is closed in layers to provide a watertight seal.

If the mental area is being augmented, a submental incision is made for access and exposure of the anterior mandible. This approach avoids damage to the mentalis muscle and subsequent lower lip descent. It also allows a panoramic view of the area to be augmented. The preferred chin implant is a two-piece design with right and left halves. The two-piece design allows the lateral extension of the implant to follow the inclination of the mandibular border (This is usually not possible with an "extended" one-piece chin implant) (10). Figure 10 shows a patient who had previously undergone orthodontic correction of her Class II malocclusion. Mandibular body and chin augmentation was performed as well as reduction rhinoplasty.

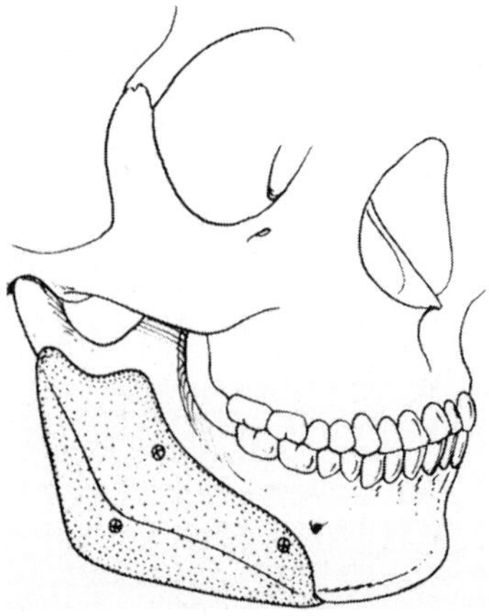

Figure 9 Configuration and dimension of mandibular ramus and mandibular body implant used to augment the deficient mandible. Because it extends beyond the posterior border of the ramus and inferior edge of the ramus and body, it closes the mandibular angle and lessens the plane of the mandibular border. Screw fixation guarantees position and ensures application of implant to skeleton. *Source*: From Ref. 9.

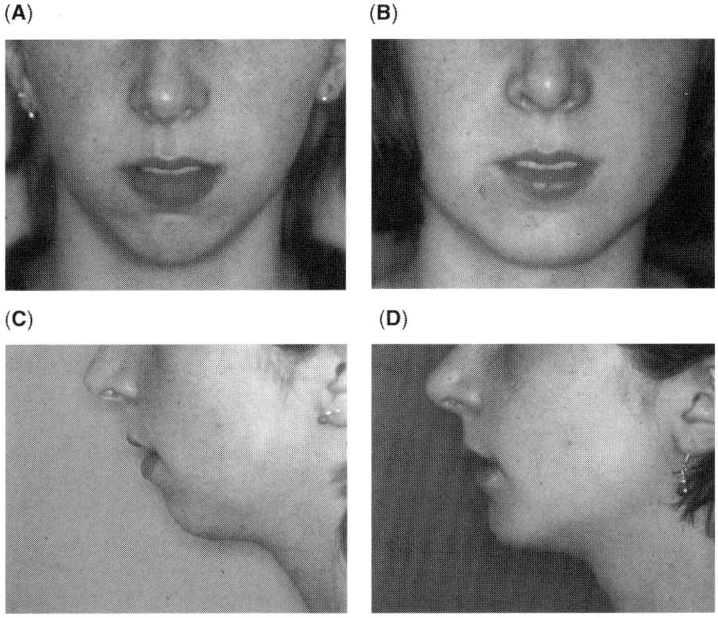

Figure 10 A 21-year-old woman who had undergone orthodontic correction of her Class III malocclusion desired improved nasal and mandibular contour. Reduction rhinoplasty and mandibular augmentation with mandibular ramus and body implants were performed, together with an extended anatomic chin augmentation. (**A**) Preoperative and (**B**) six-month postoperative frontal views. (**C**) Preoperative and (**D**) six-month postoperative lateral views. *Source*: From Ref. 9.

SUMMARY

Patients with skeletal deficiencies and normal or orthodontically corrected occlusion can have their aesthetic needs satisfied with alloplastic augmentation of the facial skeleton. Implants and combinations of implants can simulate the visual effects of LeFort III and Lefort I advancements as well as certain mandibular osteotomies. This surgery is safe and effective.

REFERENCES

1. Chen NT, Glowacki J, Bucky LP, Hong HC, Kim W-K, Yaremchuk MJ. The role of revascularization and resorption on endurance of craniofacial onlay bone grafts in the rabbit. Plast Reconstr Surg 1994; 93:714–722.
2. Yaremchuk MJ, Israeli D. Paranasal implants for correction of midface concavity. Plast Reconstr Surg 1998; 102:1676–1684.
3. Rees TD, LaTrenta GS. The role of the Schrimer's test and orbital morphology in predicting dry-eye syndrome after blepharoplasty. Plast Reconstr Surg 1988; 82:619–626.
4. Jelks GW, Jelks EB. The influence of orbital and eyelid anatomy on the palpebral aperture. Clin Plast Surg 1991; 18:193–201.
5. Yaremchuk MJ. Infraorbital rim augmentation. Plast Reconstr Surg 2001; 107:1585–1592.
6. Yaremchuk MJ. Restoring palpebral tissue shape after previous lower blepharoplasty. Plast Reconstr Surg 2003; 111:441–450.
7. Yaremchuk MJ. Improving periorbital appearance in the "morphologically prone". Plast Reconstr Surg 2004; 114:980–987.
8. Yaremchuk MJ. Facial skeletal reconstruction using porous polyethylene implants. Plast Reconstr Surg 2003; 111:1818–1827.
9. Yaremchuk MJ. Mandibular augmentation. Plast Reconstr Surg 2000; 106:697–706.
10. Yaremchuk MJ. Improving aesthetic outcomes after alloplastic chin augmentation. Plast Reconstr Surg 2003; 1121:1422–1432.

8 The RARE Technique: The Renaissance of the Aging Face and Neck

Thierry Besins
Plastic Surgeon, Paris, France

INTRODUCTION

The aging process of the face depends on three main factors: muscular contractures, loss of volume of each tissue layer, and gravity. The concept of this "Renaissance" technique is to act on these different factors, and to produce the least surgical damage possible. The "fixed areas of the face" have been well studied (1). The stronger attachments, as evidenced during extended dissection of the face, are the zygomaticomasseteric and the mandibular ligaments, the so-called Furnas' ligaments (1), (Fig. 1). Therefore, the logical question becomes: Are we allowed to destroy those natural fixations during surgery, and, if we do so, is the sliding process instead possibly increased later on? This could account for the short-lasting results occasionally observed with some classical face-lift procedures.

If we agree that gravity is one of the main factors responsible for tissue drooping of the face during the aging process and that some retaining zones are potentially dedicated to inhibiting this inevitable process, a new surgical concept becomes available: The face must now be looked at as consisting of three separate vertical zones, or sectors (Fig. 2). In our concept, only one sector of the face is "moving," and the other two are "fixed." Thus, maybe we should dedicate our attention and surgical efforts to focus more specifically on the anatomical movements of the age-related segment and to attempt an actual reversal effect.

The challenge of this technique is to move all the face tissues (of only this sector) en bloc, back upwards, in a "homothetic" way (Fig. 3), by repositioning of the volumes where they were before, first, and adding volumes where they are missing (the "shadow tracking"). An interesting comparison could be that of the sagging of the aging breast, which we correct by a surgical reversal concept (Fig. 4) to achieve a real impression of rejuvenation.

Following the same concept, the aging process of the neck is completely different, and must be treated in the same etiologic manner: The posterior oblique sliding (due largely to the shrinking and bending of the cervical column) must be repaired by a posterior oblique repositioning vector, in a total divergence with the vertical facial one. As a result, the area anterior to the ear should not necessarily require surgery, other than as a minimal dissection for harmonious repartition of the excess tissues, as in a simple "dog ear" treatment. We should always keep in mind that any skin undermining creates undesirable skin excess.

CONCEPTUAL AND ANATOMICAL CONSIDERATIONS

A new aesthetic unit: The "Time Sector 2." In considering the aging process, the face can be divided into three vertical sectors, and the previous concept of three horizontal parts of the face (upper, mid, and lower) should be abandoned (Fig. 2).

1. Sector 1 is the center of the face (pro-face of the embryology): nose, middle part of the lip, chin, and middle part of the forehead, which are fixed and maintained by bony eminences and short, strong muscles.
2. Sector 2, or "Time Sliding Sector" (meso-face) is the muscular and adipose part of the face, from the temporal area (including the tail of the eyebrow), down to the jowl. It represents the "sliding face," which is involved in the drooping of facial aging, because it is free from almost any retaining structures. The mobile facial tissues droop vertically, and only within the "moving" zone of Sector 2.
3. Sector 3 (meta-face) is the fibrous embryologic sector, with deep entanglement of all the layers of the face: Furnas' ligaments and the fibrous part of the superficial muscular

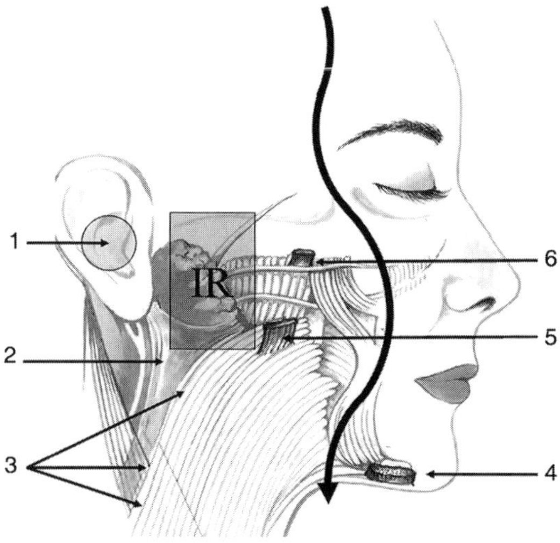

Figure 1 Main fixed zones of the face and the neck. (**1**) Fixed conqua of the ear. (**2**) Auriculoplatysmal ligament. (**3**) Fixed adherences between the posterior border of the platysma and the Sterno-Cleido-Mastoidien muscle (per T. Besins, personal communication). (**4**) Mandibular ligament. (**5**) Cutaneoplatysmal anterior ligament. (**6**) Zygomatic ligaments. *Abbreviation*: IR, identity rectangle. *Source*: From Ref. 1.

aponeurotic system (SMAS) firmly adherent from the preauricular area, down to its crossing with the Sterno-Cleido-Mastoidien (SCM) muscle. This sector is more physiologically "fixed," and should be substantially preserved.

As with some other authors (2), but with a different approach, we advocate that only deep subperiosteal detachment of the soft tissues of the face and upward repositioning allows an efficient, natural (antigravity), harmonious (homothetic), and probably longer-lasting result. We want to avoid any disconnection and/or distortion between the different layers, and we accomplish this by repositioning them through two separate actions: The first one is a reestablishment of the relationship of those layers by a transfixion "intralayer scarring" procedure after manual repositioning; and then, the second action is a deep en bloc remounting of the restructured cheek mass. As a consequence, three different actions must be performed: repositioning, imbrication, and elevation.

The main surgical implications of our anatomical studies of the premalar area are as follows: (*i*) The safer approaches to prevent nerve injury are either the external orbital or the vestibular route; (*ii*) The main lymphatic drainage of the lower lid goes up vertically into the orbit, deep into the muscle and over the periosteum (3), where two to four main pedicles

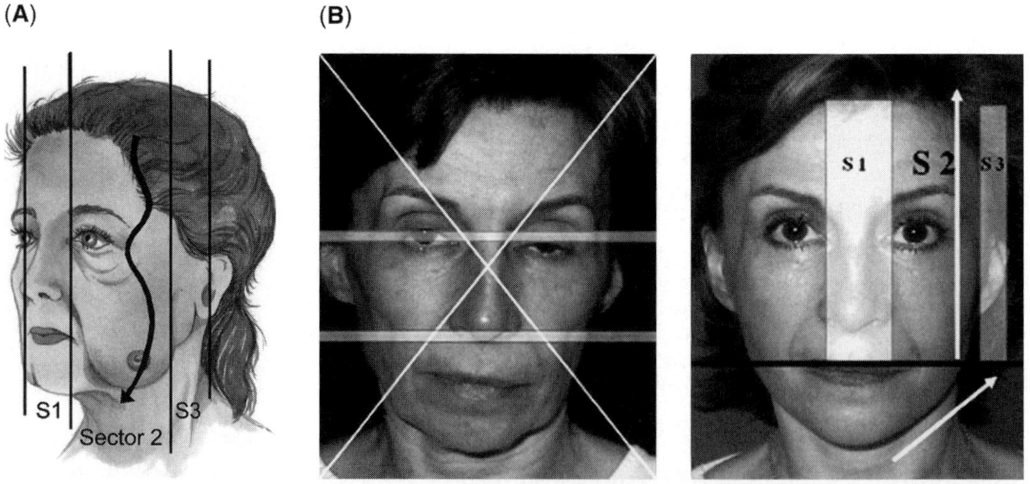

Figure 2 (**A**) Drooping of the volumes of the Sector 2 (meso-face), compared to the superimposition of drooping of the aging breast. In this simulation, the inner part of the inframammary fold of a ptotic breast represents the nasolabial fold (wherein treatment is similarly accomplished by raising the mass in an upward direction). (**B**) The three "traditional" horizontal delineations of the face should be turned to the three vertical sectors. Time-related drooping involves only Sector 2, which is the only one needing to be repositioned.

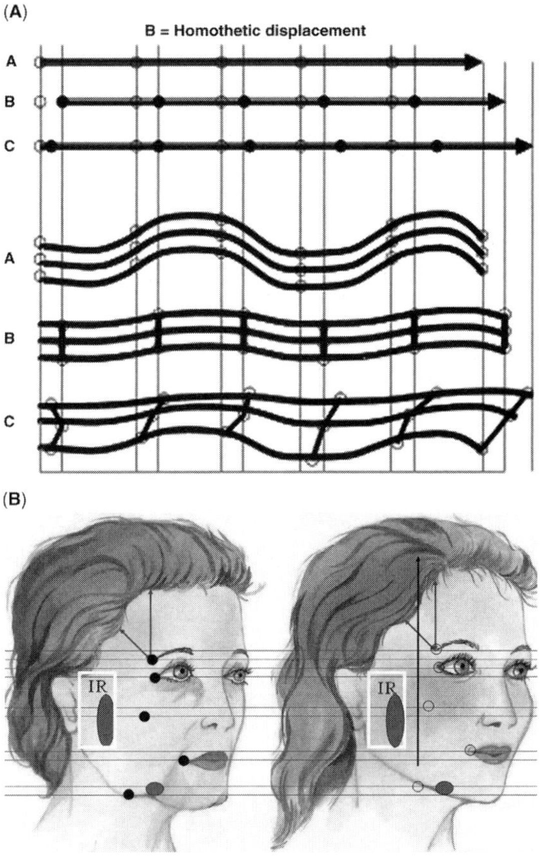

Figure 3 (**A**) Homothetia displacement theories: (*i*) Initial baseline and "three layers model," (*ii*) harmonious and homothetic displacement (the relationships between the different points are preserved), and (*iii*) disharmonious displacement as encountered in superficial techniques (stretching) or multilayer and multidirectional deep techniques. (**B**) Simulation of a homothetic displacement of five identity points, shown at left. The forced figure, on the right, could be the same, but rejuvenated about 20 to 30 years. Homothetia yields conservation of the identity. A few millimeters of elevation, in a "homothetic" movement, can offer an almost "generational" effect in terms of facial rejuvenation. *Abbreviation*: IR, identity rectangle.

are usually visible during anatomical dissections; and (*iii*) The motor nerves of the lower orbicularis oculi musculus run obliquely and vertically upward, deep into that muscle (4).

Based upon the three considerations mentioned above, we absolutely avoid a subciliary approach (down to the periosteum), which otherwise would have transected the muscle, the lymphatics, and the motor nerves of the lower eyelid. As a result, we now solve many common complications such as persistent lymphoedema, lagophthalmos (due to hypotonia), and deep-tissue retractions (involved in ectropion formation) (5). Concurring with the work of Mendelson (3), we advocate that firm structures are constantly present. Within our technique, these structures insure effective grasping, elevation, and suspension of the cheek volumes. The seven key structures are as follows:

1. The orbicularis oculi: The very wide orbicularis oculi, firmly attached to the skin, becomes a very effective skin tensor and interlayer sliding repositioning tool, but only if it has been widely liberated by a premalar subperiostal dissection. This is the only way of being able to efficiently displace the malar portion of the orbicularis oculi, which spreads downward very low to the upper part of the nostril, reinforced by the levator malaris (6) (Fig. 5);
2. The prezygomatic membrane separating the suborbicularis oculi fat (SOOF) from the prezygomatic fat;
3. The orbital retaining ligament, which limits the palpebromalar hollow and the visible tear trough;
4. The periosteum;
5. The levator labi of upper lip and the zygomatic minor;
6. The SOOF;
7. The premalar fat, the sliding of which accentuates the nasolabial folds.

METHODOLOGY

Facial surgery (Fig. 6A) with the reverse and repositioning effect (RARE) technique involves a nonendoscopic deep and subperiosteal face dissection with the following multistage fixations

(A)

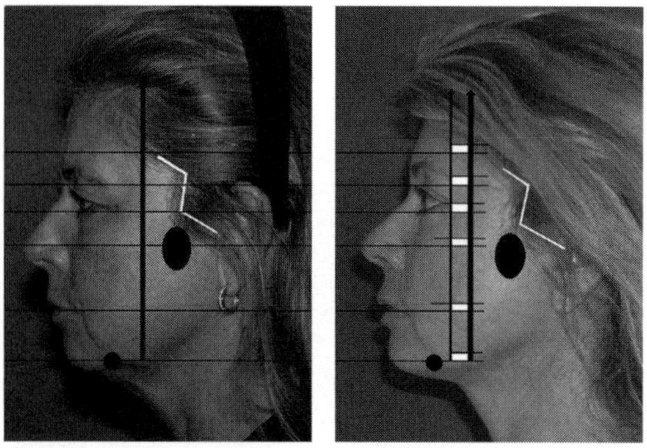

(B)

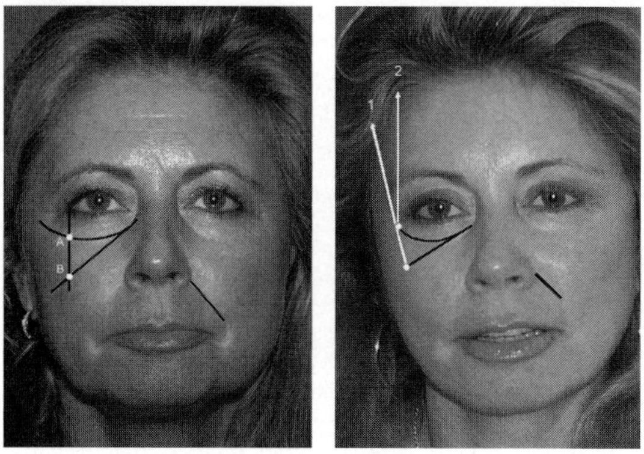

Figure 4 (**A**) Clinical application of reverse and repositioning effect technique on a 55-year-old patient at 18 months' post-op: profile reproduction of the deep "en bloc" upwards homothetic repositioning. The black spots represent the original "fixed" zones. (**B**) Same patient, with front view showing the rejuvenation effect of the homothetic elevation, without any modification of the hairline, and without any "face-lift look."

to the temporal area: cheek, orbicularis, and then temporal tissues. No "typical" lower eyelid dissection is performed, but only a lower eyelid skin resection, at the end of the surgery.

Then the distinctly separate neck surgery (Fig. 6B) is performed, with a limited preauricular undermining (to preserve the fixed areas), but an extended low-neck dissection, preserving as much as possible of the attachment to the SCM muscle. Plication of the platysma is performed on its muscular part, to prevent detachment and dissection of the fibrous posterior part (which is a deep fixed area), on the crossing zone of the mandibular angle and the SCM. The main stitch anchors the ideal point of the platysma (with the non-undermined skin) upward and backward to the very strong auriculo-platysma ligament, then three to four stitches are placed between the posterior border of the platysma and the SCM, in a posterior *vector, on site, without traction*, for two main reasons: traction enhances muscular contraction, and the lying position during surgery naturally replaces the platysma in its original position.

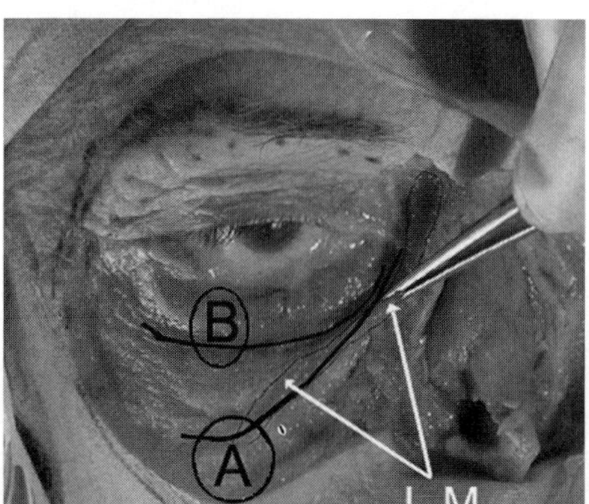

Figure 5 Dissection of the inferior orbicularis oculi area, which shows: (A) the huge inferior spreading of the orbicularis oculi malaris (OOM), nearly reaching the level of the alar groove and (B) the levator malaris (LM), which can be considered as a thick reinforcement of the inferior border of the OOM, crossing anteriorly the medial canthus. The two key "grasping" points A and B have been drawn onto the photo.

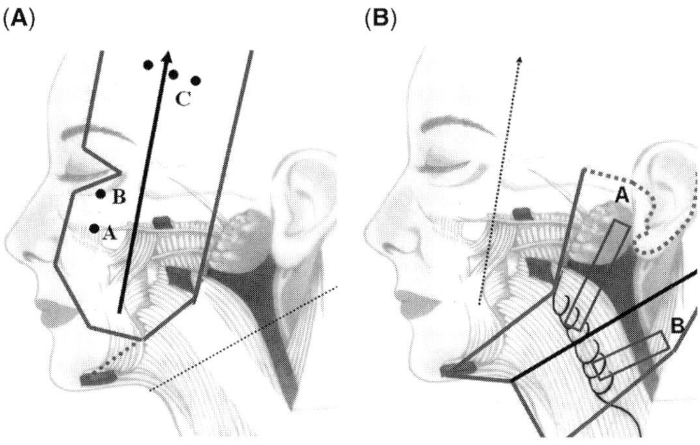

Figure 6 (**A**) Face portion of the surgery. (**B**) Neck portion of the surgery. Notice the posterior vectors and preservation of the attached fibrous border of the platysma.

Much of the SMAS was inherently elevated and anchored as part of the RARE (facial) technique and liposuction of the neck is performed when necessary, and in a routine manner.

Lipofilling is added in about 50% of the cases, at the end of surgery, when indicated for the temporal, internal, and medial premalar, or any other areas. It is easy to perform and very effective, especially because this superiostal and nondissociative technique avoids any undermining between the facial tissue layers.

SURGICAL PROCEDURE

The key to the RARE method of facial rejuvenation is the release and repositioning of the cheek mass (en bloc), which had held down the lower eyelid, the lateral canthus, and the tail of the eyebrow, all in an homothetic way. These elements mentioned above are thus repositioned, without any other specific surgery. Skin and hair resection are avoided, and the relationships between the different facial identity structures are preserved. Thus this homothetic lift (meso-lift of Sector 2) of the face preserves the original youthful proportion and identity, providing a natural look, which is highly appreciated by patients (after their slightly "different" postop period). Also, it should be noted that the entire procedure is routinely done without the endoscope.

Preoperative Markings Done in a Standing Position

The key point A is generally located a bit below the crossing point of the vertical outer canthus line, the extension tear trough line on the jowl, and a horizontal line crossing the inferior border of the nostril (Fig. 7A). One must always keep in mind that this point A is considerably higher in the supine position, and thus not too far from the desired location. This entire procedure has been completed via a limited lateral transorbicularis approach. This essentially "closed surgical process" also generally precludes any persistent bleeding.

The proper marking spot of point A is easy to locate and verify, using an extreme forced smile. This specific maneuver gives an idea of the rejuvenation look after the predicted ascension of the jowl, and provides a good preoperative evaluation of the amount of skin to be removed on the lower eyelid, at the end of the overall face surgery.

The key point B is located at the crossing point of a vertical line coming from the external canthus, and the line of the palpebromalar hollow. This point will determine the limit of the mandatory skin eyelid dissection, now reaching the thick and strong orbicularis oculi malaris (OOM) muscle.

Other useful markings are also done (Fig. 7A): temporal crest, V-nerve pedicles, incision lines, and VII-nerve position, at the junction of the middle and posterior third of the zygomatic arch.

The step-by-step procedure is as follows:

STEP 1: Deep dissection of the cheek: This is carried out through an external 10-mm transorbicularis incision, at the same place as a routine lower eyelid incision; but only in the lateral third (and very obliquely downward), as the final scar will be lifted into a horizontal position. A deep transecting incision is made, down to the external periorbital periosteum. Two different size Obwegeser elevators are then used: a narrow, 4-mm-wide elevator to start

(A)

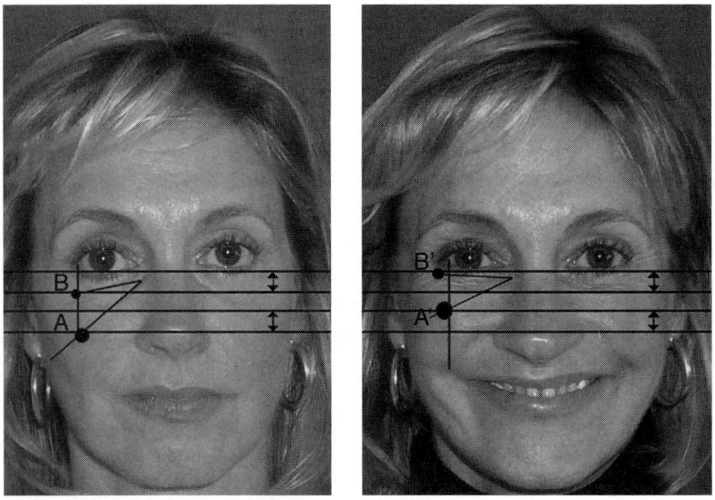

(B)

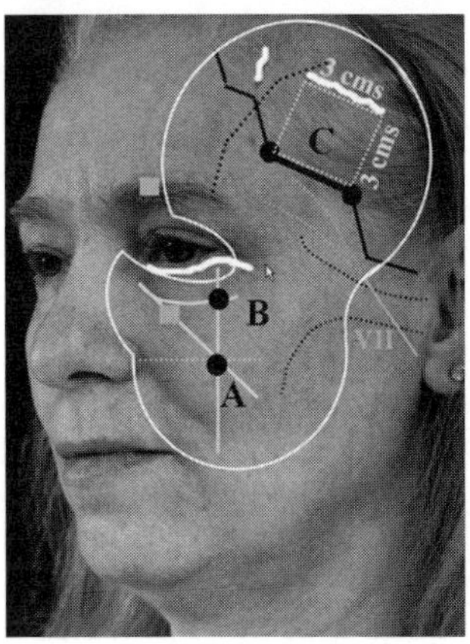

Figure 7 (**A**) Appreciation of the potential postoperative result, by movement of the points during forced smile; notice the homothetic relationship of points A and B. (**B**) Preoperative markings (Fig. 5). Point A denotes the intersection of the extended tear trough line with the vertical projection of the lateral canthus. Point B denotes the intersection of the infrapalpebral sulcus with the vertical projection line of the lateral canthus. Then the bold black line shows the three steps of a normal hairline. Bold white lines designate the incision markings. Dotted black lines show the temporal crest and zygoma. The white extended line shows the limits of the deep undermining.

the subperiosteal malar dissection downwards and medially on the infraorbital rim (arcus marginalis), reaching the nasal bone above the internal canthus. This maneuver is essential in order to obtain a significant yet "light" elevation of the internal part of the cheek and the nasopalpebral hollow. Then a larger, 8-mm-wide elevator achieves the dissection down to the vestibule, pyriform orifice, lateronasal area, and back to the anterior part of the zygoma.

Important points must be mentioned at this stage: Elevators must be very sharp to be sure to stay under the periosteum. Smooth or noncutting elevators are very dangerous, as they can induce a false sensation of being in a correct plane. A careful dissection at the beginning can prevent injuries to the temporomalar pedicle(s), when existing. Frequently, three, four, or five very thin, mixed pedicles exit from the malar bone and cannot be seen (and preserved). The thin elevator is useful to prevent injury of the infraorbital nerve during the orbital rim _dissection. A finger, placed between the globe and the inferior orbital rim, allows a perfect control of the elevator progression up to the nasal bone. The distance between the nerve and the orbital rim is always approximately 8 mm.

The lateral canthus must not be detached, if we do not wish to change the patient's look. Thus the original youthful location will be naturally obtained, by the upward lifting, which discharges the canthus area from the weight of the cheek. The orbicularis septum is routinely preserved; yet (though not recommended) we retain the option to open it, for spreading or removing the fat bags.

The periosteum must be entirely detached, and this is most easily done medially, because here it is very thin; and then it has to be perfectly elevated and completely transected in the whole vestibular area. The elevator must be seen, in a transparent way, in the mouth, all along the mucosa of the vestibule of the entire superior maxilla bone. Slight elevation movements, such as performed for supraorbital nerve dissection with endoscopic control, must be used to dissect the infraorbital nerve carefully. Periosteal detachment means detachment of the origin of the medial musculature of the mouth.

The preservation of the fixed prezygomatic area means that only zygomatic minor and levator muscle of the upper lip are detached from their bony insertion and will be tightened up with suspension. If limited medial zygomatic dissection is safe for the frontal branch of the facial nerve, the midorbital branch is very close. It runs deep under the zygomatic muscles, and over the levator muscle of the upper lip, ending in the medial part of the orbicularis muscle. The main area exposed to nerve injury involves the lateral part of the malar bone dissection.

STEP 2: Cheek suspension: A multistep transcutaneous procedure (Fig. 8A–G). The different steps are drawn on the series in Figure 8. Two important points must be underlined for succeeding in this maneuver: (*i*) To lift manually the malar fat pad up above the orbicularis muscle, before transecting the cheek, because this allows the repositioning of the sliding fat into an appropriate position before imbrication and elevation. (*ii*) To make a very wide grasping of the cheek structures, by progressing parallel to, yet under the dermis, for a distance of at least 1.5 cm. (Fig. 9).

STEP 3: Orbicularis (malaris) suspension (Fig. 9 and Fig. 10A, B): In this step, an extended subcutaneous dissection of the entire lateral third of the lower eyelid is performed, down to the palpebromalar hollow, avoiding completing the subciliary incision at this time. The complementary medial subcutaneous palpebral dissection (depending on the amount of skin to be removed) should only be performed at the end of the procedure, to avoid unnecessary undermining, and to limit complications and bruising.

In front of the inferior extension of the skin dissection, corresponding to the level of the junction of the eyelid with the cheek, the OOM and periosteum are firmly grasped with a 5-mm bite, to allow vertical and solid transposition of the premalar soft tissues, via the orbicularis oculi. Thus, we create a very strong adherence between the connections of the uppermost part of the muscle flap and the external orbital bone (with the periosteum removed). This is one of the keys of the long-lasting adherence and/or improvement of the rejuvenation, as well as of the skin appearance around the orbit. Concurring with Hamra (7), we advocate the continuity/imbrications of the orbicularis oculi with the cheek fat, which together (in continuity) constitute a key anatomic and surgical layer. The concept of the improvement of the skin tension comes as a result of the skin-muscle and/or periosteal adhesion, as has been advocated by others (8) as well.

We use either 2/0 Gore-Tex® (W.L. Gore, Flagstaff, Arizona, U.S.A.) or Vicryl (Ethicon, Somerville, New Jersey, U.S.A.) needled sutures (Fig. 11). The two ends of the symmetrical sutures are grasped with separate forceps, and pulling is exerted to check symmetry and effectiveness in absorbing the excess amount of tissue caused by the ascension of the cheek mass. This maneuver is essential before passing the sutures through the temporal incisions, and then fixing them on the skull and/or the temporal aponeurosis (depending on the most effective vertical pathway). Thus, Step 3 must absorb the excess wave created by Step 2. Steps 2 and 3 together now represent the biorbcularis oculi malaris (BOOM) suspension technique, which is one of the main steps of the RARE procedure.

STEP 4: Temporal or temporofrontal elevation and fixation (the mandatory final step for treatment of excess tissue following BOOM action): Temporofrontal dissection is performed in the same way for every case. The degree of final adjustments, such as extent of elevation of the eyebrow or upper eyelid skin resection, is dependent on the patient's (and the surgeon's) wishes and examination. A 35-mm incision is made 3 or 4 cm behind the hairline (Fig. 7A) and parallel to it. Ideally, this incision line must be drawn perpendicular to line AB (Fig. 12A, B), which means nearly horizontal. Its medial end must be 1 cm lateral to the temporal crest, to be certain to find a strong temporal aponeurosis support. Obviously, a very lateral position of the temporal crest may modify the vector direction and the vertical translation of the tissues. If a temporal aponeurosis is not available for a good vertical elevation, we then proceed to skull bone fixations.

If bone fixation becomes necessary to maintain orbicularis oculi (and cheek) elevation, holes in the frontal bone become required. A rotating 2-mm burr is used to create two oblique 45° communicating tunnels through the external cortical bone. This tunnel can easily support, if necessary, the two orbicular and/or malar fixation sutures (and also the eyebrow elevation fixation, if it has

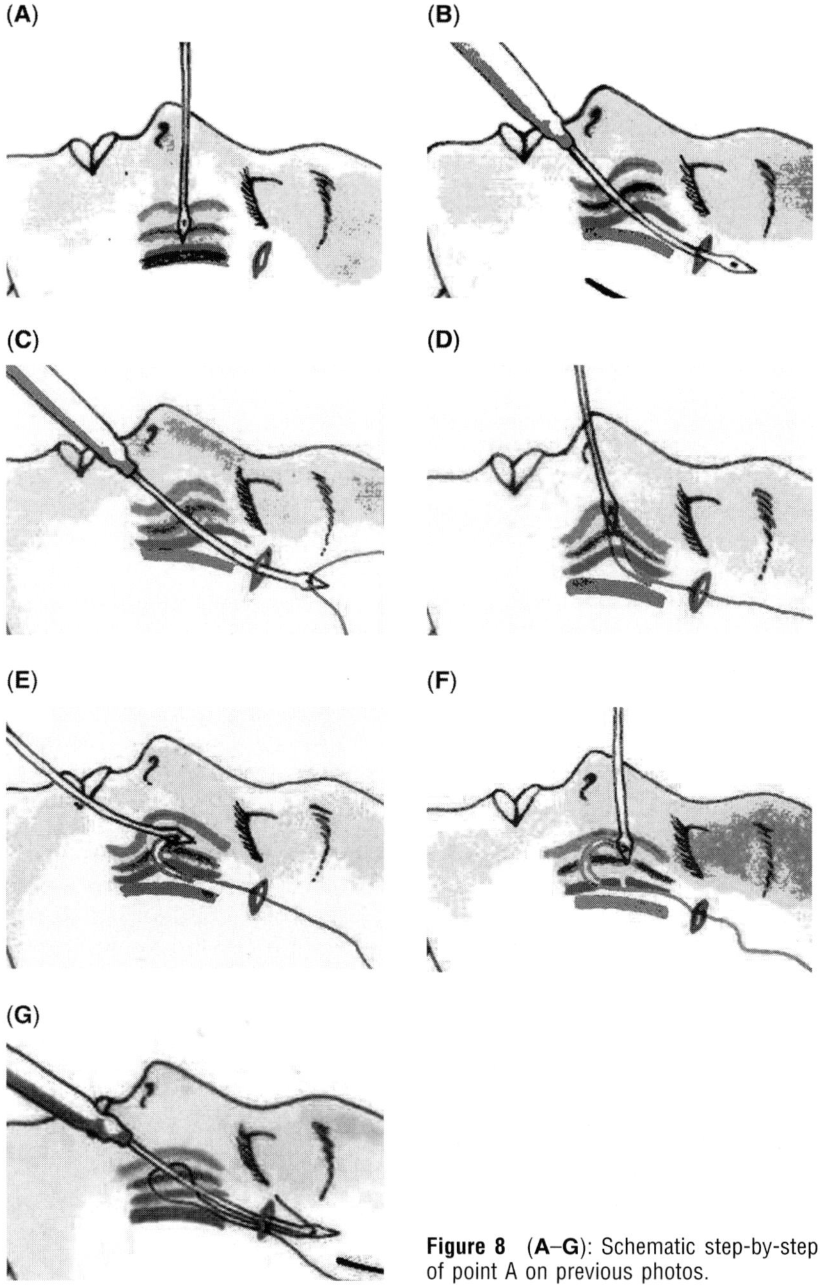

Figure 8 (**A–G**): Schematic step-by-step explanation of the fixation of point A on previous photos.

been planned). At the present time, we must note that the recently available ENDOTINE fixation devices (by COAPT™ system) have greatly facilitated the entire RARE procedure. The Endotine Midface Device for point A elevation "en block" of the cheek and the triple Endotine Device for the temporal and frontal wave elevation (C step) make the procedure safer and easier.

The temporofrontal dissection is performed without endoscopic control because we have gained experience from numerous open subperiosteal or "mask-lift" procedures. The dissection must be very extensive medially and posteriorly. Medially we must obtain a complete release of the temporal crest and the orbital rim. The periosteum must be incised and completely separated to easily reach the deep aspect of the orbicularis oculi. Preserving the preop-located supraorbital nerve is easy by a smooth elevation, as during an endoscopic approach. Posteriorly, somewhat extensive undermining is necessary to absorb the excess

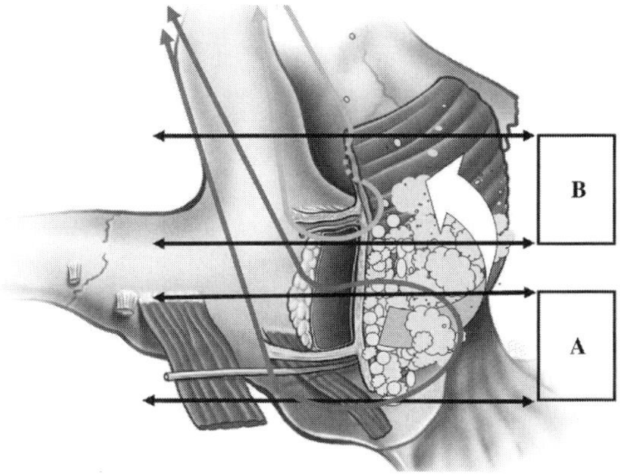

Figure 9 Representation of the grasped elements in each point A and B. The arrow simulates the manual repositioning of the volumes before transfixion.

of soft tissues coming from the elevation of the face, because skin and hair excisions are completely avoided in this technique.

The subsequent bump-like excess in the temporal region (Fig. 13B) will disappear within a few weeks. If it is not necessary to modify the direction of the palpebral fissure, the strong posterior insertion of outer canthus must not be detached. Alternatively and if required, a complete canthopexy may be performed, as described in the original Tessier's mask-lift technique (9).

In our RARE procedure, the purpose is to attain the complete repositioning of the soft tissues, back to the original youthful position, without any canthal procedure. Periosteal elevation of the half posterior lateral aspect of the zygoma is not done, to thus preserve this very fixed area of the face. And fortunately, this partial dissection prevents facial nerve injury to the frontal nerve branch.

The overall temporal incision concept allows the temporal fixation of the tissues coming from elevation of the cheek, in the homothetic manner previously described. Three 2/0 Vicryl sutures will fix the elevated galea to the temporal aponeurosis. To enhance a longer-lasting adherence process, we always remove some patches of the aponeurosis. As a result, the deep ascension of the tissues is effective without the appearance of any modification of the relationships and proportional distances within the face. This phenomenon explains why the hairline seems to have not been elevated at all.

(A)

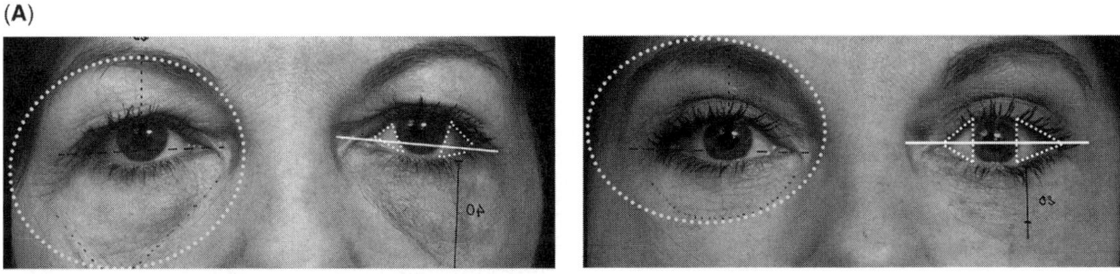

(B)

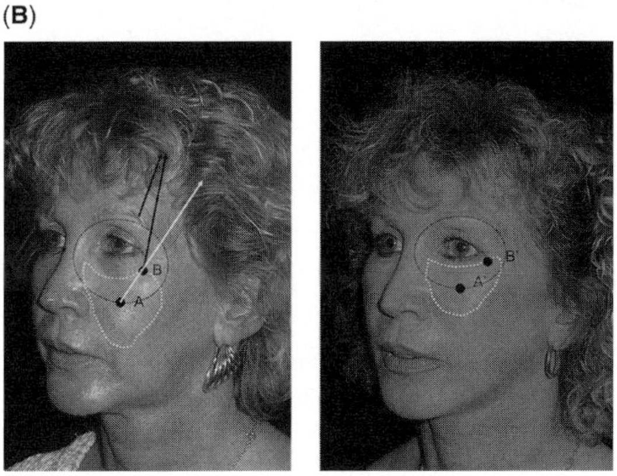

Figure 10 (**A**) Rejuvenation of the entire facial expression by repositioning of the orbicularis muscle (*dotted circle*) in a biorbicularis oculi malaris suspension technique, plus a discrete upper eyelid surgery. Notice the rejuvenation effect of the bicanthus line repositioning, and the "renaissance" of the two white dotted triangles of the eye. (**B**) Representation of the results of the repositioning of the orbicularis (*black circle*) and the malar fat pad (*white dotted areas*) in a 52-year-old patient.

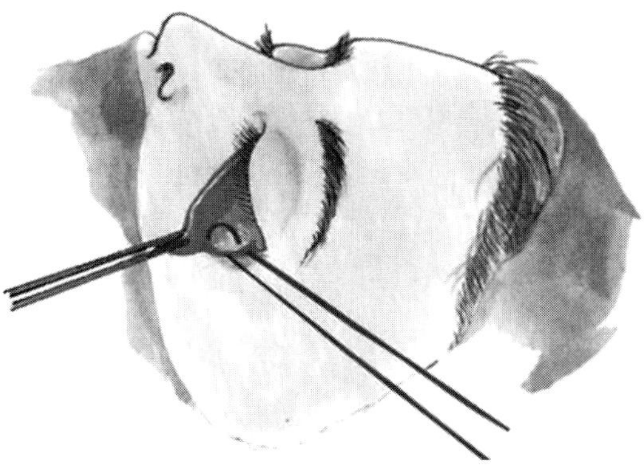

Figure 11 Details of grasping the premalar portion of the orbicularis oculi malaris and the periosteum (relative to points B and B' on previous photos).

In our RARE procedure, we have no need to remove any excess skin in the temporofrontal area. We close the temporal incision with three or four staples, which are removed on postoperative day 4, at the same time as we remove the lower eyelid sutures. Note that any excess tissue "wave" created during Step 3 has now been absorbed within Step 4.

STEP 5: The two final adjustments: eyebrow positioning and lower eyelid skin excision.

Eyebrow positioning: The entire lateral two-thirds of the eyebrows have been released during dissection in Step 3. It is easy to effect the changes we want to achieve by employing the standard upper fixations. In many cases, no changes were preplanned; the eyebrow release alone (plus the weight release of the cheek mass) produces a light yet natural and "homothetic" elevation.

Lower eyelid skin excision becomes mandatory within the RARE technique: we usually remove an impressive skin excess, which generally corresponds to the previous stretching of the cheek, related to the tissues sliding as part of the facial aging process. In unique opposition to the more conservative degree of resection [typically advocated to prevent complications (5)], we are convinced that we must completely remove this skin excess caused by our elevation of the cheek. We have three specific reasons: (*i*) the strong secondary adherence between orbicularis oculi and the underlying lateral orbital bone; (*ii*) safety given by tarsus hyperelevation; and (*iii*) integrity of the innervation of the orbicularis oculi, which retains its tone.

The patient's entire look is rejuvenated without aggressive eyelid surgery. We usually do not remove fat bags and never transect the orbicularis oculi in its pretarsal or subciliary area. The only surgical dissection necessary involves subcutaneous undermining, strictly limited to excess skin that must be removed at the end of Step 5. In doing this, we have preserved all the lymphatics, nerves, and blood pedicles of the fragile lower eyelid.

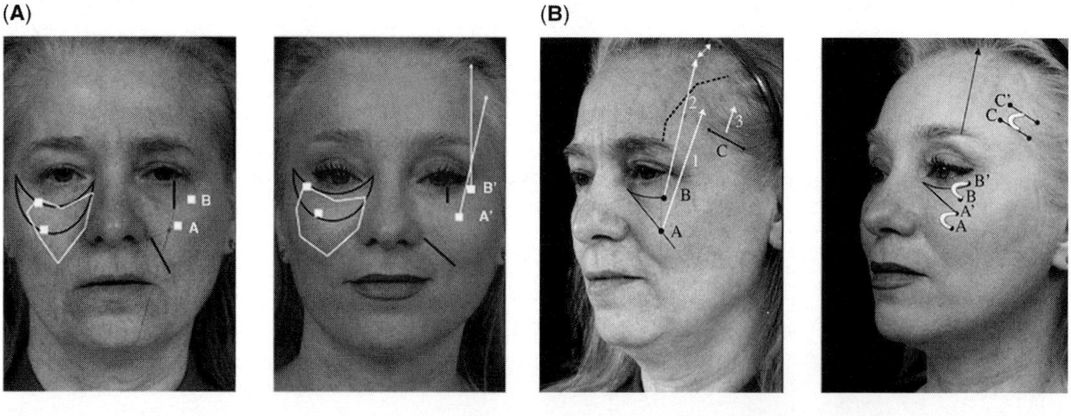

Figure 12 (**A**) 65-year-old patient, 18 months after reverse and repositioning effect (RARE) technique. Repositioning of the cheek, improvement of the contours, and luminosity of the face with lipofilling not required. Note the improvement within the polygonal figure drawn around six naevi (*white shape*), plus improved angle of the nasolabial groove. (**B**) Same patient, explaining points of movement and fixation of the "homothetic wave" in the RARE technique.

(A) **(B)**

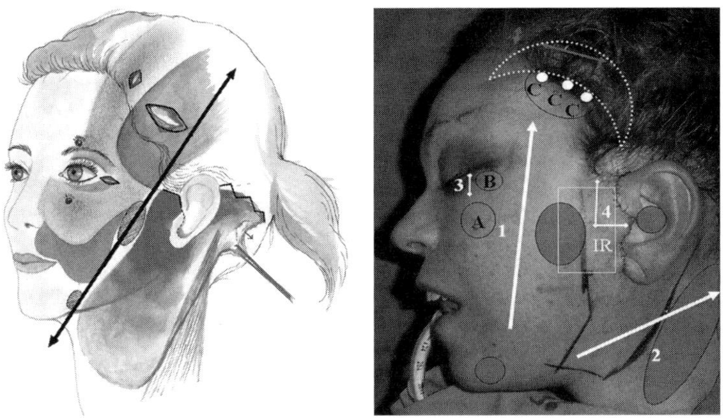

Figure 13 (**A**) Drawing showing incisions points for the complete rejuvenation of the face, and then separately the neck, preserving the fixed areas. (**B**) The white line 3 designates the amount of the mandatory skin incision and removal resulting from surgery 1 (*arrow 1*, facial elevation procedure). The suture line (referenced as line 4) designates the line of optional excision, if surgery 2 (neck procedure) delivers an amount of excess skin requiring removal. The "W" symbol represents the final wave of excess tissue (in the temporal area), which is not removed. The white rectangle is the identity rectangle. The large grey oval in the neck area represents the site of very strong natural attachments between skin and sterno-cleido-mastoidien muscle, which should be preserved as much as possible.

STEP 6: Neck surgery (Fig. 13A, Fig. 6B): The neck slides obliquely between the lateral fixed points of the face and the medial border of the SCM. Thus the horizontal (submental) segment of the neck is mainly related to the sagging of the face, and the vertical segment to the oblique sliding of the neck itself. As we have just seen in Figure 12, neck and facial surgeries are treatable as two completely separate procedures. Whereas the rejuvenation of the facial area (including a part of the sagging of the jowl area) was performed using the RARE technique (which elevated all the soft tissues, including the SMAS), neck surgery now requires an oblique/posterior tissue repositioning.

Platysma surgery is indicated if it provides satisfaction to the surgeon; but we are convinced that, here again, deep fixed areas should be preserved. Therefore, certain important concepts should be applied. The platysma slides without any dissection, by grasping and pulling it at the level of the angle designed by the SCM muscle and the mandible. Once this fixation is done, two simple running sutures, vertically and horizontally, are performed to maintain this muscular repositioning. The preauricular skin undermining should not exceed a few centimeters, sufficient only to absorb the amount of excess skin, resulting from the neck surgery and thus also preserve the identity rectangle (IR) (Fig. 13B) of the zygomaticomasseteric fixed area (1). By continuing our research concerning this area, we have recently even been able to entirely avoid any incision in front of the ear, where tissue excess conditions were favorable.

The posterior border of the platysma is fixed and does not move at the level of the gonion; thus undermining of the platysma must be as conservative as possible. A simple double continuous suture, running vertically in front of the posterior border, appears to be a more effective and conservative technique (Fig. 6B). Of course, any submentally accessed treatment of the platysma bands can still be performed if required or desired, as well as the submaxillary gland excised. The SMAS in Sector 3 is fixed and fibrous, whereas it is muscular and mobile in Sector 2. For these reasons, undermining of the fibrous SMAS is unnecessary, and only its muscular distension has to be treated.

RESULTS

Over 200 such procedures have been performed. A total of 124 patients who have undergone the RARE technique (116 females and 8 males) were included in the study because they underwent exactly the same procedure and have been seriously followed up, each for a period exceeding six months. Half of the patients required an associated neck-lift, which did not change the facial result because of the separateness of the procedure, disassociated from the facial rejuvenation. The average age of our patients was 55, with the ages ranging from 38 to 88 years (Figs. 4, 10, 14–20).

The most satisfying aspect of this technique is a dramatic facial rejuvenation and preservation of the patient's original youthful identity. This is very noticeable from both the surgeon's and the patient's perceptions. Of our 124 patients, we noted 112 good, very good, or excellent results; and 12 poor results (eight from the patient's point of view, and four from both patient's and surgeon's point of view). This is possibly accounted for by the patient's inadequate preparation for interim results, as well as our initial hesitations during the earlier cases.

We are now convinced that an excellent understanding of the concept of the procedure, plus a thorough explanation of the postop appearance, are two important prerequisites. Generally, three weeks are necessary to recover a normal facial appearance, and six to eight

(A)

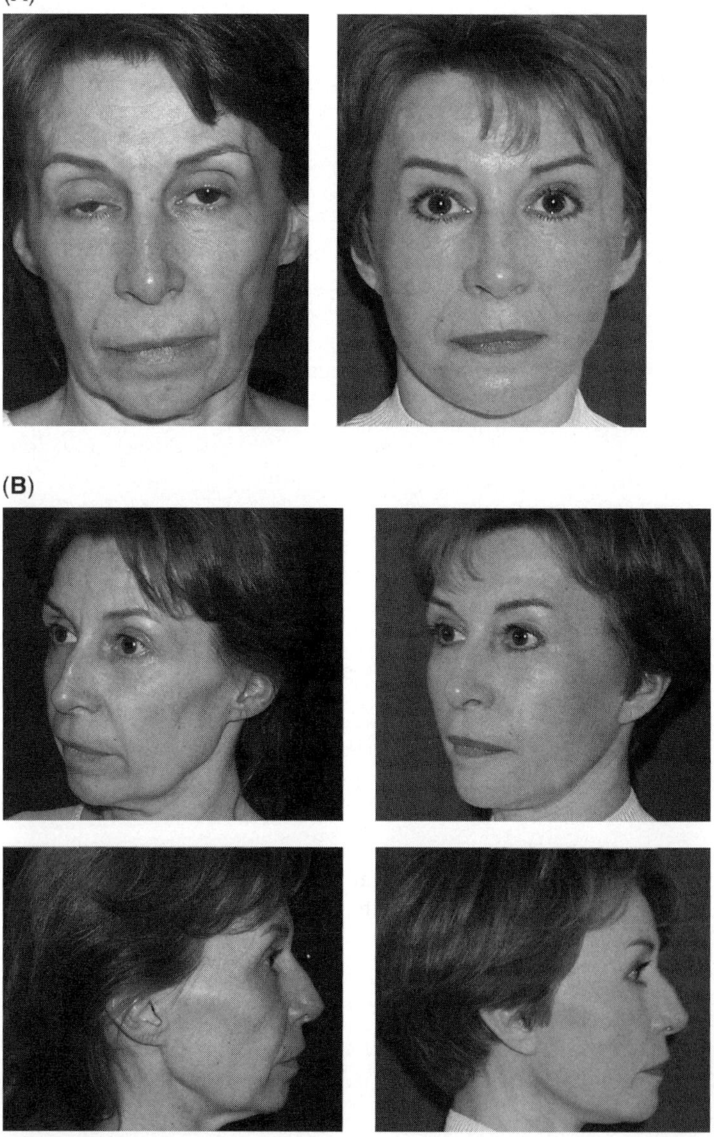

Figure 14 (**A**) Front view, (**B**) three-quarter view and profile: 56-year-old patient. Result at 11 months after reverse and repositioning effect technique plus lipofilling.

(A)

(B)

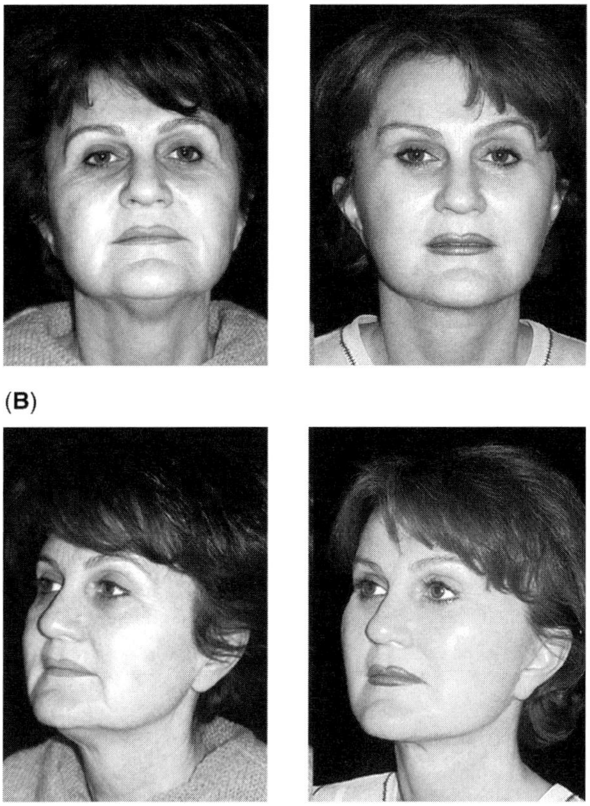

Figure 15 (**A**) Front view, (**B**) three-quarter view: 58-year-old patient with heavy skin. One-year result without any filling. Notice harmonious features on the three-quarter view.

weeks for the patient to be happy and to feel comfortable with the result. Please note that when (in younger patients) we perform a "face only" procedure (without the neck), the entire recovery takes place faster, occasionally in as little as three weeks (see case shown in Fig. 21).

COMPLICATIONS

This technique is applicable at any age, but results are best in middle-aged patients of normal weight. The main temporary complication is the extent of edema (and resultant distortion of features) during the early postoperative period (average two to three weeks). In every other respect, the technique seems to be very safe, and the morbidity very low. Our experience of other complications is as follows:

Hematoma: None. Drains have never been used in this face-lift surgery. Most of this surgery is closed, with little bleeding, and a good occlusive dressing seems to be very effective if duration of surgery is not too long.

Infection: One case. We have no explanation, except that it was a local orbital infection, which diminished by itself with local and systemic treatments; this is a very minor complication compared to major infections sometimes encountered with transvestibular approaches.

V-nerve Injury: None. Good knowledge of anatomy, as well as experience gained from endoscopic subperiosteal dissection, prevents injuries to the V-nerve in a closed surgery.

Ectropion: None. This normally would have been the major complication of this technique, but we have not observed any ectropion in our series. The possible explanations for the lack of ectropion issues might be: Wait and it will occur? Muscular and nerve supply integrity of the lower eyelid at the end of the procedure? Only the skin, which will be removed, is undermined (which means no scar retraction)? Dramatic new adherences between periosteo-orbicularis flap and external orbital bone? The very firm fixations of the cheek and the orbicularis oculi, due to the three stages and "en bloc" transecting stitches? Overcorrection

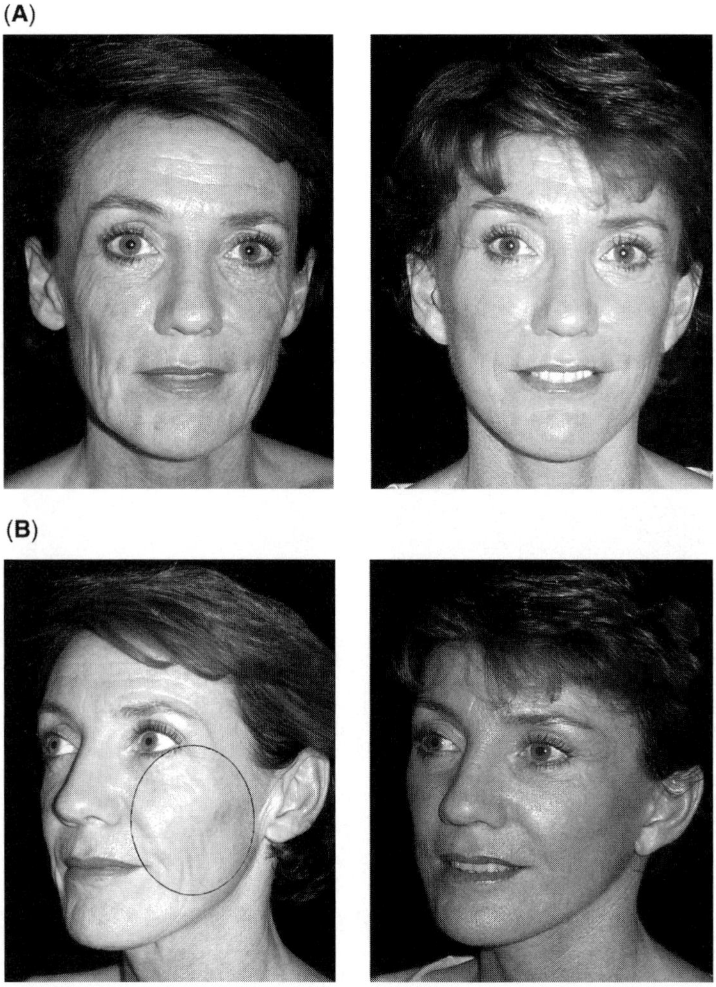

Figure 16 (**A**) Front view, (**B**) three-quarter view. 54-year-old patient with very thin skin, 14 months after reverse and repositioning effect technique without lipofilling. Notice improvement of skin with orbicularis oculi malaris muscle retensioning.

of elevation of the lower eyelid, which provides a few millimeters of security? Efficiency and durability of the suspension of the cheek?

Asymmetry: Transcutaneous cheek fixation, with very precise preoperative markings, largely prevents the risk of asymmetry. A possible cause of asymmetry can be a difference in the degree of traction, which gradually becomes easy to determine and correct during the procedure. Under direct view control, placement of the orbicularis malaris suspension suture is easy to perform. In all of our cases, slight temporary asymmetry was a constant finding, but only due to asymmetrical edema of the temporo-orbital region. We must keep in mind that any real asymmetry could be corrected under local anesthesia in the early postoperative period, if necessary.

Dimples: Three different sorts of dimples may occur. During the procedure, a cutaneous dimple is due to an overly superficial suspension, taking the dermis. It must be avoided by a correct utilization of the enlargement mark of the passer, which enables saving 5 mm of superficial tissue over the stitch. Any dimple due to excessive traction is easily avoided with experience. We prefer to get maximum traction on the orbicularis oculi before fixing the jowl suspension at its optimal tension, and before a dimple becomes evident. During the follow-up period, the four suspension points may create some temporary "edema dimples" during the first two to three weeks, and patients must be informed about this possibility. In any event, the problem can be resolved by removing any of the suspension suture(s), under local anesthesia,

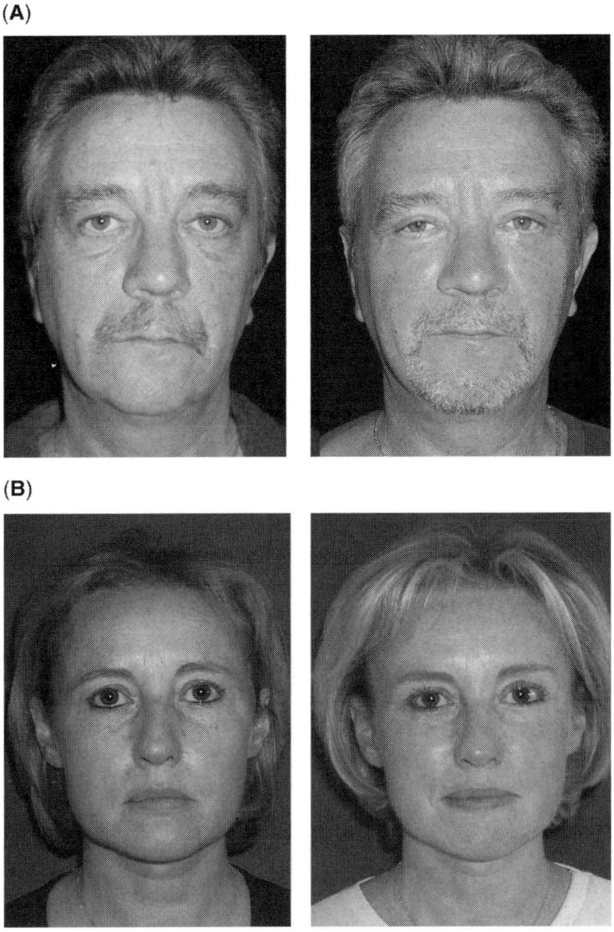

Figure 17 (**A**) 50-year-old male patient. Reverse and repositioning effect (RARE) technique with light superior eyelid surgery. Note the improvement of the midface and the expression. (**B**) Inherent correction of a poor result from a prior eyelid surgery, using only RARE technique (vs. additional eyelid surgery). Results at one year.

after two months. However, correct dimples, which are already evident at the end of surgery, and correct them *immediately*, to prevent their aggravated appearance in the standing position.

VII nerve injuries: Fortunately, we have never encountered any serious or permanent injury to the frontal branch of VII. Three explanations can be suggested: no retractors, very sharp elevators perfectly scraping the temporal aponeurosis, and no subperiosteal dissection of the posterior half of the zygoma. Nevertheless, we observed three minor temporary issues, possibly concerning the medial branch of VII (two temporary upper lip asymmetries and one possible medial lagophthalmos); yet in such cases, recovery is complete after a few days, as has been confirmed by others (10). The two problems could have the same explanation: the distension (during dissection) of the zygomatic branch of VII, under the zygomatic minor muscle. As we never observed that kind of incident with the vestibular approach, it seems that the convexity of the malar bone makes the dissection from the top more difficult, because of the need for greater elevation of the tissues when accessed from above.

Touch-up: On one patient, we had rare "expanded polytetrafluoroethylène" (PTFE) intolerance, and two other patients experienced persistent dimples. We waited two months to proceed with atypical suture removal (under local anesthesia) through the original temporal incision. The Gore-Tex remained well visible and swept very easily. Thus, the suspension stitches were able to be removed without any damage to the aesthetic result. This confirms for us that no difference exists for the result between absorbable or nonabsorbable suspension sutures. But in our experience, Gore-Tex seems to be the more favorable material, for the following reasons: (*i*) Adjustability of the stitches, because the knots sweep very easily during surgery and for touch-up after a few weeks as well. (*ii*) The white color permits very easy recognition when necessary. (*iii*) The elasticity and smooth texture reduces cutting problems of the tissue suspensions and facilitates patient facial movement after surgery. (*iv*) The

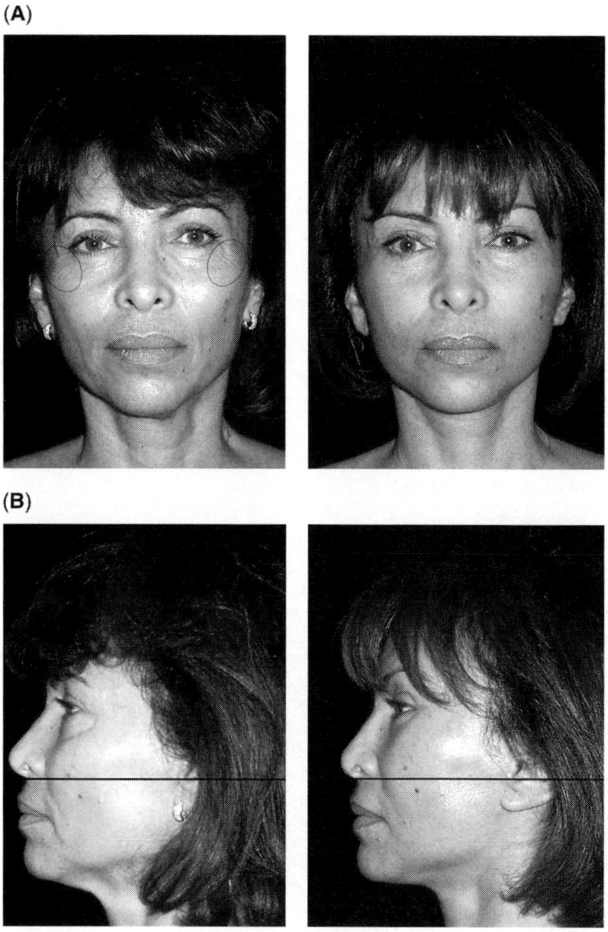

Figure 18 (**A**) Front view of a 52-year-old patient, two years' postop. (**B**) Profile view of the same patient, showing the vertical and homothetic repositioning of the two naevi of the cheek and of the external part of the palpebral malar groove.

inflammatory process around the suture creates stronger deep beneficial "scarring" as part of the transsection of the layers during the en bloc fixation.

SUMMARY OF COMPLICATIONS

Temporal depression, when and if a too-deep dissection damages the aponeurosis. This happened during our first cases and was successfully treated by deep muscular lipofilling.

Semipermanent dimples (in some early cases), which are now easily avoided with experience and/or treated by suspension removal.

Possibility of hypertrophic and persistent (three months) redness, at the aspect of the lateral scar of the lower eyelid. The explanation could be the difference in thickness of the two edges of skin (after removing the excess portion). We have not yet found any solution for this problem, but we inform our patients of the possibility of temporary redness.

DISCUSSION

The RARE technique concept seems to provide solutions to many questions we have encountered during 20 years of face-lifting practice.

Is anatomical layer undermining useful or not? In our former typical face-lift, the effects of the huge process of multiple separations almost always gave the illusion of good results for a few months. The unnatural temporary adherences of the healing process soon dissipated and the desired fixation effects were lost. Thus we now choose to leave the layers of the soft tissue intact and connected, only separating the cheek mass from the bone below. As a result, the definitive adherences (from inflammatory nonsurgical plane dissection) are created by

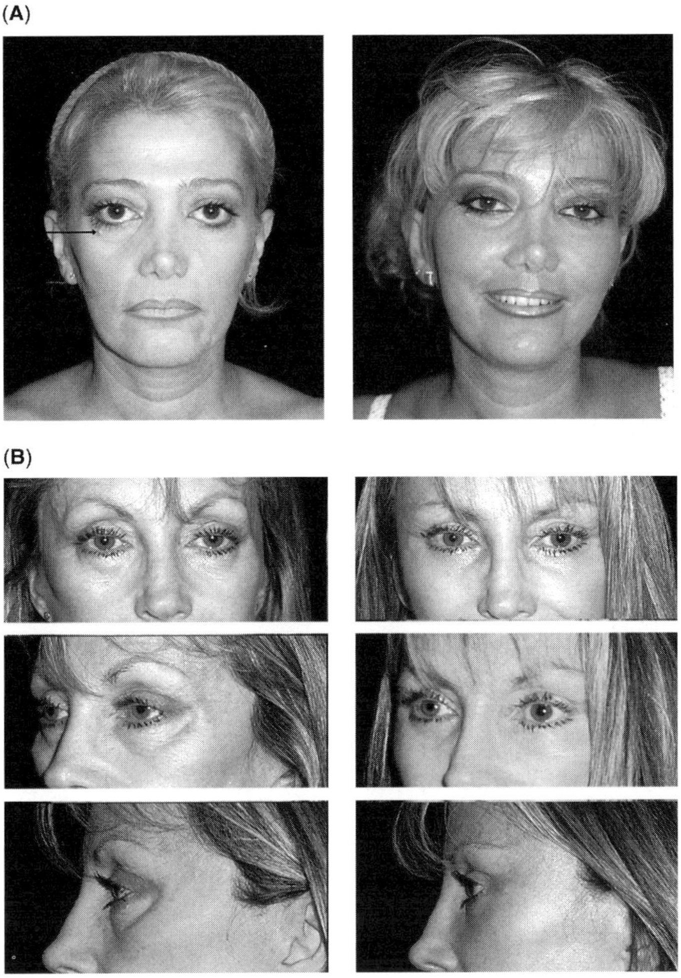

Figure 19 (**A**) Reverse and repositioning effect (RARE) technique plus lipofilling on a 44-year-old patient with prior poor lower eyelid surgery. (**B**) Rejuvenation of the midface by RARE technique and lipofilling. Notice the improvement of the tear trough.

a subperiosteal surgical dissection, which produces desirable permanent adherences. In addition, voluntary "trauma" of the temporal aponeurosis (plus the transection during "en bloc" fixation) now enhances permanence of the adherences.

Is it necessary to destroy the very useful fixed areas (natural antiaging anatomical structures) by the surgical procedure? We now think it is not; moreover, we are convinced that this is the key point of natural and harmonious results, as was explained above.

Is major subcutaneous dissection beneficial for the skin, as previously advocated? We don't think so. Consequently, the skin undermining should be performed only for the resection of mandatory skin excess.

Is it possible to avoid frontal hair resection and hairline modification? Yes, and this change precludes so much of the scarring, which otherwise was one of the main side effects of face-liftings.

Is it possible to rejuvenate the lower eyelid and still preserve its anatomical integrity? Yes, which is important due to the natural fragility of that area.

Is it possible to have more natural, predictable, and long-lasting results? Certainly, because in aging, all the tissues (in Sector 2) move downward in the same way and keep their relationship. In the RARE method, the natural and integral layer attachments are preserved, and thus the entire sagging volume can be lifted "en bloc," without any unnatural disturbances between the different layers.

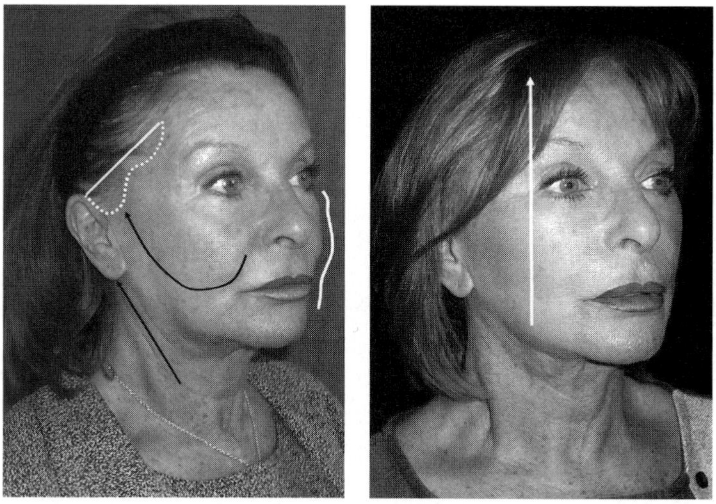

Figure 20 Typical disharmonious look on a 62-year-old patient after two previous face-lifts (*left*). Improvement and natural aspect after a reverse and repositioning effect procedure (facial zone only) (*right*). Note the enhanced features on the three-quarter view.

SUMMARY OF CONCEPTS

This technique does not specifically present anything entirely new in terms of surgical processes, as almost every individual portion has been performed before. Instead, our main innovation comes from the application of our alternative concepts, as follows:

- Separate corrections of vertical sliding of the face and oblique horizontal sliding of the neck.
- Fixed points, which are the areas that have to be preserved to maintain static and dynamic identity (IR: ear, hair, middle of the zygoma, and gonion).
- The "homothetic wave tissue repositioning," which means a harmonious result and a more true facial rejuvenation.
- A substantial conservation of the lower eyelid structures where fat bags are now reintegrated, and not removed, by OOM retensioning.
- Minimization of typical face-lift aftereffects, with no hair removal required, and the advantages of very short scars.
- Avoidance of undermining in surgical planes, and detachment of fixed areas, which can otherwise affect the stability of the result. The integrity of the different layers allows lipofilling anywhere during the same procedure.
- The beneficial use and effect of transecting internal suspension "scars," which can now produce useful permanent adherences through the different layers.
- The strong and resistant OOM is the only possible "expression" and cheek-repositioning vector, compared to the very weak and fragile pretarsal or preseptal portions of this muscle, which cannot be used for this main action, but only for additional refinements.
- By avoiding important superficial undermining on the face and the neck and preserving the integrity of the inferior eyelid, this technique is usable on almost any patient, at virtually any age. Furthermore, the comparative lack of substantial skin undermining allows the technique to be used for more aged and/or fragile patients, and for heavier smokers as well.

CONCLUSION

Gradually, over the past four years, we have recommended using our RARE technique on more and more cases. In reality, we feel comfortable proposing this option to a majority of our patients. Yet, we recognize that it will take time to acquire a greater percentage of patients willing to accept a new form of procedure.

We find that there is only one facial aging process related to the effects of time and gravity, wherein all the different structures are similarly subject to a sliding motion. Thus, each

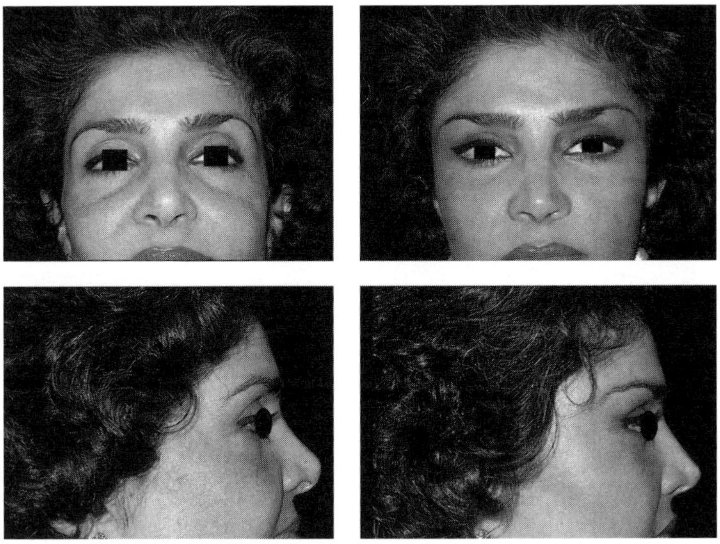

Figure 21 Postoperative aspect at *10 days* on a 49-year-old female. Reverse and repositioning effect technique with COAPT Endotine midface and triple Endotine Devices, with slight tip of the nose surgery, but without any lipofilling. Note the speed of recovery, versus that for standard eyelid surgeries.

component of the aging face is dependent on the one above it, and all of them (en bloc) should be repositioned by being treated homothetically. Thus this concept defines what we have called "the homothetic wave of the time"; otherwise, disharmony can occur whenever Sector 2 is not treated as an indivisible entity. This technique has dramatically improved our results over the past four years, including a more unified positive appreciation of the result from patients, their "entourage," and the surgeon. We must keep in mind that a repositioning of a few millimeters of the drooping volumes of Sector 2 can offer a true rejuvenation effect of one decade!

The OOM has now become our key tool for facial rejuvenation. If its integrity is preserved, its vertical retensioning produces a combination repositioning of the skin, muscle, and fat volumes; these longer-lasting results are rather clearly due to the new and strong bony adherences, which we have induced in the periorbital areas.

By preserving the identity structures and the relationship between the main points of the face, this technique produces a true rejuvenation by its homothetic movement, and thus a reversal and repositioning effect on the sliding aging tissues is achieved for a long time to come....

RARE technique's purpose is to achieve a repositioning of each part of the face and the neck where it was before, by a better understanding of the aging process, and adapting to it an etiologic "reverse and repositioning" procedure, keeping always in mind the two main elements of the aging process: the loss and sliding of the various volumes. The repositioning and adding of volumes releases the muscular contractures "ipso facto" and a new "well being" of the face is noticeable, month after month.

From our critical point of view, the results of many former techniques were sometimes less than hoped for, in terms of full rejuvenation and longer-lasting results. Maybe this is one of the reasons that so many papers about alternative face-lift procedures are published every year. In critically observing our RARE outcomes, it clearly appears that the patient's face has recovered a more luminous and harmonious appearance, conveying an impression of facial rejuvenation, without loss of the important youthful facial identities. Distances and relationships involved in the facial personality are preserved, and this is now evident with the face in either static or dynamic mode. Preservation of fixed areas, conservative surgery, and homothetic tissue repositioning of the face and then the neck, probably all account for this favorable result, and the perception of a true "renaissance."

REFERENCES

1. Furnas D. The retaining ligament of the cheek. Plast Rec Surg 1989; 83(1):11–16.
2. Ramirez O. Full face rejuvenation in three dimensions: a ''face-lifting'' for the new millennium. Aesth Plast Surg 2001; 25:152–164.
3. Mendelson B. Fat preservation technique of lower-lid blepharoplasty. Aesth Surg J 2001; 21:450–459.
4. Ramirez O, Santamarina R. Spatial orientation of motor innervation of the lower orbicularis occuli muscle. Aesth Surg J 2000; 20(2):107–113.
5. Carraway J, Mellow C. The prevention and treatment of lower lid ectropion following blepharoplasty. Plast Reconst Surg 1990; 85(6):971–981.
6. LeLouarn C. Botulinum toxin A and facial lines: the variable concentration. Aesth Plast Surg 2001; 25:73–84.
7. Hamra ST. Composite Rhytidectomy. St Louis, Missouri: QMP Inc., 1993.
8. Casagrande C, Saltz R, et al. Direct needle fixation in endoscopic facial rejuvenation. Aesth Surg J 2000; 20(5):361–365.
9. Tessier P. Lifting facial sous periosté. Ann Chir Plast Esthet 1990; 34:193–197.
10. Dardour JC, Ktorza T. Endoscopic deep periorbital lifting: study and results based on 50 consecutive cases. Aesth Plast Surg 2000; 24:292–298.

9 Evolution of the Midface-Lift: Thought and Process

Malcolm D. Paul
Department of Surgery, Aesthetic and Plastic Surgery Institute, University of California, Irvine, California, U.S.A.

INTRODUCTION

Face-lift techniques proceeded for many decades utilizing techniques that repositioned ptotic soft tissues of the lower one-third of the aging face with single-direction advancement, and with little or no improvement in the midface. Basically, the skin was elevated and repositioned with lateral tension. Only later did one appreciate the value of bivector correction at multiple planes [skin and submuscular aponeurotic system (SMAS)]. Procedures that utilized a superior vector for SMAS repositioning and a posterior vector for skin redraping provided a quantum improvement in the long-term appearance of patients undergoing a face-lift. Maneuvers that included a high SMAS dissection and composite face-lifting were developed to reliably reposition ptotic midface tissues. Only recently has the combination of multivector correction and soft-tissue augmentation provided results that truly approach three-dimensional facial rejuvenation. With evolution comes challenges that, when approached in a logical way, provide safe, reliable rejuvenation of the aging face.

PERSONAL HISTORY

Stimulated by the work of many in this important area of esthetic plastic surgery (1–11), I began my journey in midface rejuvenation with the "periosteal hinge flap" (12). The development of this technique was stimulated by the pioneering work of Hester et al. who, in 1996, published their approach to rejuvenating the middle third of the aging face by directly attacking the problem through the lower eyelid. Certainly, I had to visit the anatomy of this area. The components of the midface that one must think about when planning procedures in this area are as follows:

1. Lower-eyelid skin
2. Malar fat pad
3. The three components of the orbicularis oculi muscle
4. Suborbicularis oculi fat (SOOF)
5. Retroseptal fat pads
6. SMAS
7. Periosteum
8. Levator labii superioris muscle
9. Infraorbital nerve
10. Tendon of the masseter muscle
11. Lateral canthal tendon
12. Infraorbital rim
13. Zygomatic arch
14. Malar eminence
15. Anterior surface of the maxilla
16. Buccal fat pad

PHASE ONE: THE PERIOSTEAL HINGE FLAP TECHNIQUE

The goal was to incorporate Hester's philosophy of vertical midface correction utilizing the subperiosteal dissection plane via a lower-eyelid incision. The end point would be a

90° rotation of the central oval of the face producing a horizontally wider and vertically shorter-appearing orbit. Adding the periosteal hinge flap at the level of the arcus marginalis seemed a natural fixation point for the elevated composite flap. The procedure was performed as follows (Fig. 1):

1. A standard lower-eyelid blepharoplasty incision was made lateral to the lateral canthus.
2. Several millimeters of pretarsal muscle were left attached to the tarsal plate to preserve lid innervation.
3. Subseptal orbital fat was largely repositioned and only reduced when in excess.
4. The inferior orbital rim was identified and the periosteum was incised a few millimeters below the arcus marginalis.
5. Posterior dissection, as one would perform in exploring an orbital floor fracture, provided a firm periosteal hinge to which the soon-to-be-elevated midface could be anchored.
6. Dissection proceeded carefully along the malar eminence and the anterior surface of the maxilla to raise a composite flap including all structures from the periosteum to the skin.
7. The infraorbital nerve, typically 7 mm below the inferior orbital rim, was identified by first visualizing the levator labii superioris muscle, a marker adjacent to the nerve.
8. Wide dissection medial and lateral to the nerve mobilized the flap, which typically required additional release for vertical movement. This included dissection over the anterior 30% to 40% of the zygomatic arch.

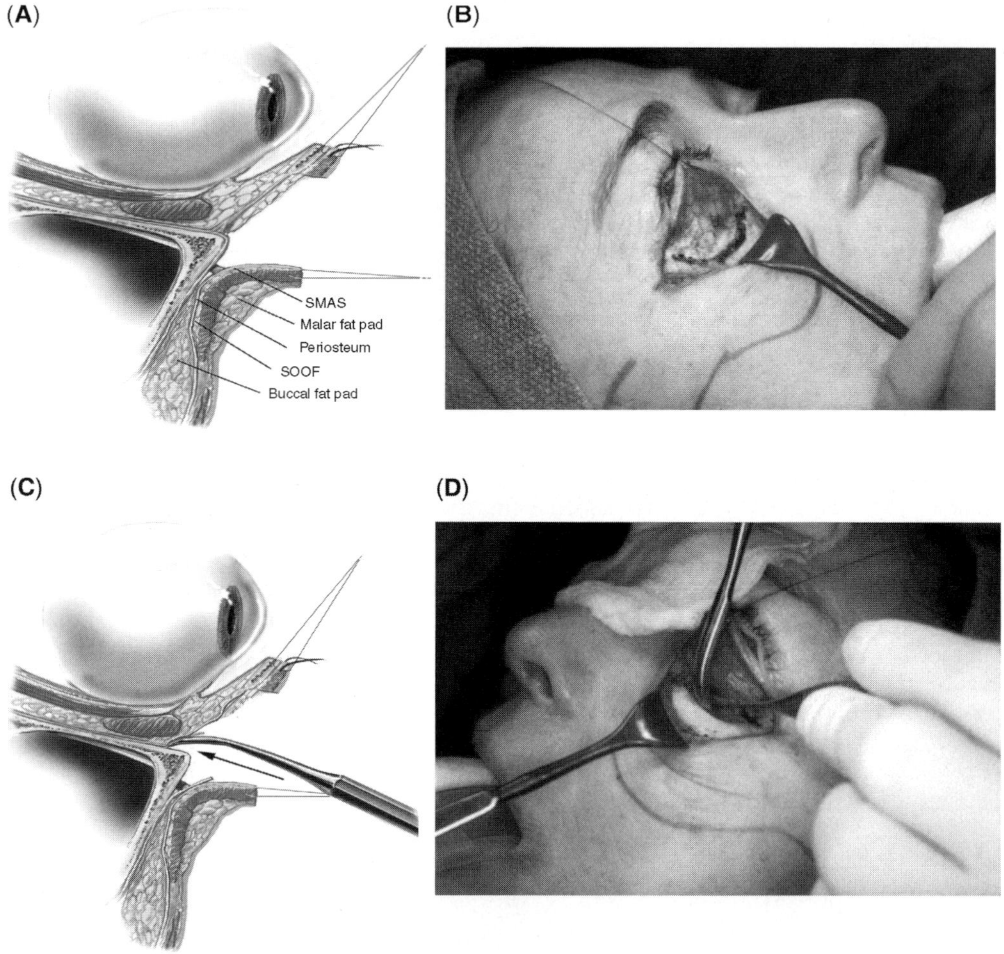

Figure 1 Periosteal hinge flap: dissection of periosteal hinge flap and suspension of composite flap to periosteal hinge flap. *Abbreviations*: SOOF, suborbicularis oculi fat; SMAS, submuscular aponeurotic system.

(E)

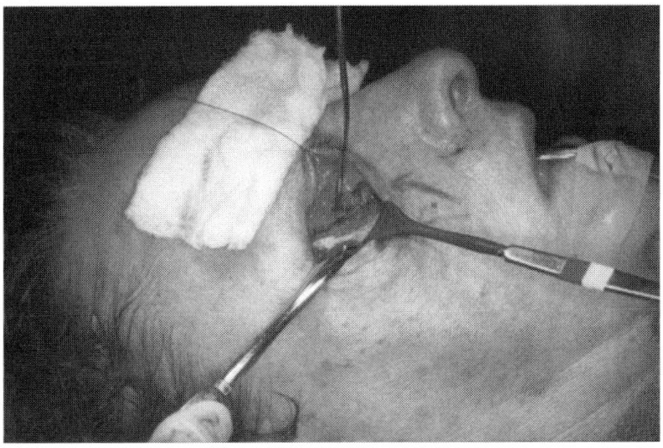

(F)

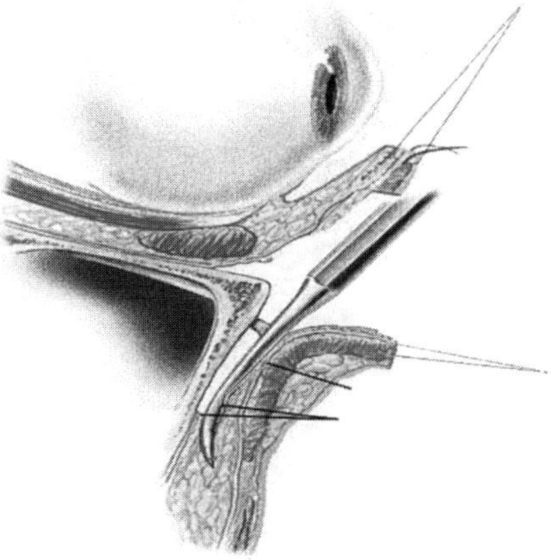

(G)

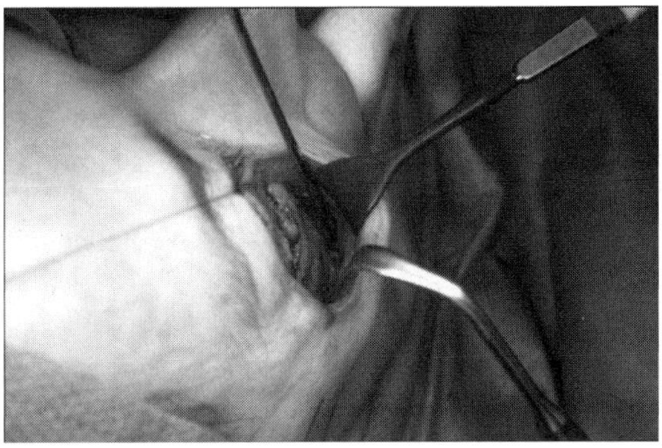

(H)

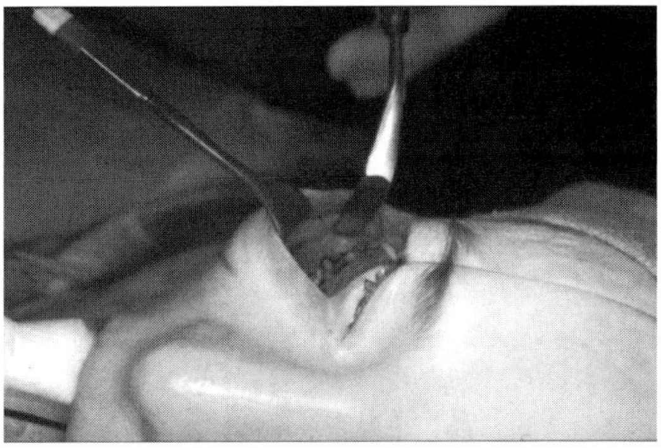

(I)

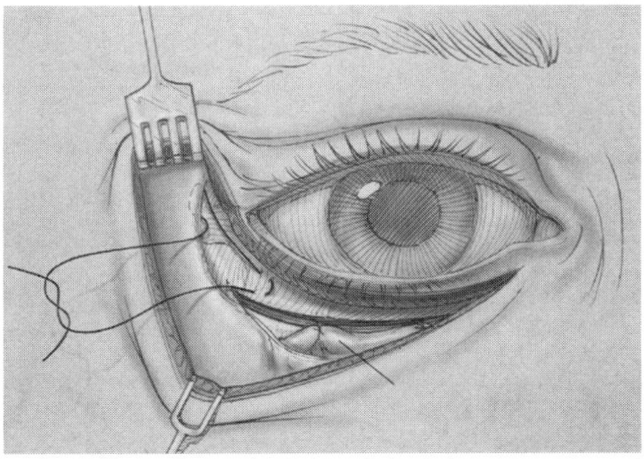

Figure 1 (*Continued*)

9. The composite flap was advanced in a pure vertical direction, repositioning ptotic midface soft tissue with several 3–0 PDS sutures (Ethicon, Somerville, New Jersey, U.S.A.) to the periosteal hinge flap.
10. A slight lateral vector could be obtained with additional sutures.
11. Malar augmentation was not utilized with this technique.
12. Lower-lid support included an inferior retinacular lateral canthopexy or a more aggressive lateral canthoplasty as indicated by the morphology.
13. The orbital septum was divided horizontally if there was evidence of inferior traction resulting from tension of the repositioned soft tissues on the lower eyelid.
14. Conservative trimming of redundant lower-eyelid skin and muscle.

PROBLEMS WITH THE PERIOSTEAL HINGE FLAP

Any discussion of techniques must include a listing of and a distinction between sequelae and complications. Sequelae are frequent events that occur in the early postoperative period and usually do not alter the final result. Sequelae of transblepharoplasty midface surgery are as follows:

1. Swelling
2. Chemosis
3. Ecchymoses
4. Lagophthalmos
5. Decreased tear production (dry-eyes)
6. Temporary asymmetry
7. Suture reaction
8. Minimal-edema–related lid malposition
9. Sensory and motor deficits (periorbital hypesthesia, muscle weakness)

Complications

Early in the use of this technique, lower-lid malposition, the major complication of transblepharoplasty subperiosteal midface-lifting, occurred with unacceptable frequency. An analysis of the technique provided several possible etiologies.

1. Manipulation of the midlamella was identified as a major cause of lower-lid malposition with accompanying dry-eye symptoms.
2. Prolonged edema of the lower lid and subconjunctival edema provided a volume load to the lower eyelid that could not overcome the gravitational force.
3. Failure to completely release the periosteum in the midface dissection produced a tethering of the flap with inferior tension-based displacement.
4. Long-lasting absorbable sutures may have produced more reaction and, therefore, a tendency for more inferior flap traction.
5. Lower-eyelid stabilizing techniques could not overcome aggressive removal of lower-eyelid skin and muscle. Although planned as a conservative removal, the powerful vertical advancement of the composite flap often seduced the surgeon to remove more skin and muscle than would have been customary with a "standard" lower-lid blepharoplasty. Limiting the skin and muscle removal to that which could be assessed before flap dissection and advancement could have prevented this problem.
6. The length of the lower-eyelid incision was, by necessity, longer than the incision utilized in a traditional lower-eyelid blepharoplasty. Although well accepted in older patients, younger women with minimal crow's-feet were less accepting of incisions that crossed the lateral orbital rim.
7. Asymmetries that did not improve substantially within four to six weeks were not well tolerated by the patient or the surgeon.

Sequelae and complications can be substantially reduced in frequency and severity with the following maneuvers:

1. Meticulous dissection to avoid postoperative hematomas that can produce cicatrical lid retraction, exposure keratopathy, and permanently impaired vision.
2. Use of a microcautery needle using the lowest effective current to decrease chemosis.
3. Addressing lid laxity with appropriate horizontal lid shortening techniques or incorporating a canthopexy or a canthoplasty for prevention of postoperative lower-eyelid malposition.
4. Utilizing a frost suture for lateral lid apposition thereby decreasing exposure, chemosis, etc.
5. Liberal use of eye lubrication (drops during the day and ointment during the night).

Although the above maneuvers are valuable, the morbidity associated with aggressive midlamellar surgery convinced me to abandon the transblepharoplasty subperiosteal approach to midface rejuvenation.

PHASE TWO: RECOGNIZING THE IMPORTANCE OF GENDER AND MORPHOLOGY ON DECISION MAKING IN MIDFACE SURGERY

Searching for a more trouble-free approach to midface rejuvenation, I directed my attention to surgical methods that respected gender and morphologic-based decision making (13). It became obvious to me that oblique vectors utilized in midface rejuvenation may not be appropriate in some cases. Specifically, most men did not desire the look that was produced with an oblique vector. Some women, specifically those with round, full faces, did not achieve an acceptable appearance with application of an oblique vector that further widened their midface. Therefore, the approach used in men and women differs in the selection of the appropriate vector for midface rejuvenation.

A comprehensive preoperative consultation is performed that includes a discussion of the goals of the procedure(s). Frequently, a midface-lift is one component of panfacial rejuvenation that may include:

1. Endoscopic brow-lift
2. Upper- and lower-lid blepharoplasties
3. Lower–face- and neck-lift (bidirectional with a vertical SMAS vector and a posterior skin vector)
4. Submental suction lipectomy
5. Open neck platysmaplasty and fat contouring including direct defatting above and below the platysma muscle, possibly adding a platysma muscle myotomy
6. Silastic chin augmentation
7. Perioral dermabrasion
8. Placement of soft-tissue fillers (autogenous or allogenic)

I have found computer imaging extremely valuable in understanding the patient's goals, morphing their images to simulate the effect(s) of the planned procedure(s), comparing photos taken at least 10 years before the consultation, and agreeing on the surgical plan. Concomitant alloplastic malar and/or submalar augmentation is planned when preoperative photos taken at a younger age indicate midfacial skeletal deficiency or the patient desires more midface volume that can be achieved with soft-tissue repositioning alone. There is enormous benefit in sitting side by side with the patient as opposed to the typical face-to-face approach. Patients are comfortable with the consultation and believe that the surgeon has a vision for their rejuvenation that matches the patient's goals. Frequently I am surprised when patients indicate that their goals are much different than our discussion would have indicated. Obviously, the time to learn about this is preoperatively.

MIDFACE REJUVENATION IN WOMEN

Whether performed as an isolated procedure, or with other facial esthetic procedures, the midface-lift is performed under general anesthesia. Local anesthesia in the form of 1% lidocaine with epinephrine is infiltrated into a planned 4-cm temporal incision that is mostly oblique behind the temporal hairline. The anterior end of the planned incision is in line with the nasal ala and lateral to the temporal line of fusion. A 2-cm buccal sulcus incision, also infiltrated with 1% lidocaine with epinephrine, is planned at the canine running obliquely from the canine to the malar eminence (transverse incisions in the buccal sulcus would likely be closed under tension as the flap is advanced over the malar area and therefore have been replaced with the oblique incision). I have found it quite helpful to use a liposuction infusion pump set at a high speed to thoroughly infiltrate the areas to be dissected. The formula that I use is as follows:

500 cc lactated Ringer's solution,
1 cc epinephrine,
50 cc of 1% lidocaine plain, and
10 mg triamcinolone

This produces a solution containing 0.1% lidocaine with epinephrine 1:500,000. Liberal infiltration with an infusion pump substantially decreases bleeding allowing for rapid dissection.

The temporal incision is made behind the hairline parallel to the follicles. Dissection is performed between the superficial and deep layers of the temporal fascia to the orbital rim. The orbital rim dissection includes release of the orbital ligament and the periosteum along the rim for a varying distance, depending on the findings in the upper eyelid and brow. Frequently the midface-lift is combined with an endoscopic brow-lift, in which case the brow-lift is completed at this time. Proceeding around the orbital rim, dissection is between the superficial and the deep layers of the deep temporal fascia until the malar eminence is seen with the endoscope or "felt" with the periosteal elevator. The buccal sulcus incision is made and the periosteum is elevated off the maxilla in the direction of the malar eminence as one would do in performing a malar or a submalar augmentation. A breakthrough tunnel to the temporal pocket is made with the periosteal elevator. Medial dissection is performed under direct vision to visualize and avoid injury to the infraorbital nerve. When this technique was first employed, more aggressive dissection along the pyriform aperture was routine. This was discontinued as it did not improve flap mobility nor oblique and vertical vector correction, but did prolong the recovery and often produced temporary weakness in lip elevation. The arcus marginalis can be incised intraorally and the periorbital fat allowed to flow over the infraorbital rim in cases of protruding, pseudoherniated fat pads. The index finger, rotated 180°, will quickly find areas of adherent fascia that prevent flap mobility. Adhesions frequently are at the masseter tendon, orbital ligament, and malar septum along the inferior orbital rim. The release of these points of adherence is essential to allow the flap to be advanced freely. Determining the proper placement of the cable suture(s) is critical to achieving the goals of the midface-lift. Moving the malar fat pad while looking at the effect will provide a guide as to where to place the suture(s). Low placement in line with a perpendicular dropped from the lateral canthus intersecting a horizontal line from the nasal ala will improve upper-lip position. A second suture placed more superiorly will have a direct effect on the malar fat pad, moving it higher on the zygoma. When the desired suture position(s) are determined, passing a 25-gauge, 1.5-in. needle, from the skin through the full thickness of the flap will show the surgeon where to place the suture(s) intraorally. The point is marked with a marking pen and a 2–0 PDS suture on a UCL needle (Ethicon, Somerville, New Jersey, U.S.A.) is placed in the flap and passed through the tunnel to exit at the temporal incision. The strength of this needle prevents it from detaching from the suture while passing through the temporal pocket. A small window of deep temporal fascia is excised away from the planned anchor point to allow adherence of the superficial temporal fascia to the temporalis muscle in hopes of stabilizing lateral brow position. The cable suture(s) is anchored as a figure of 8 to the deep temporal fascia with placement determined by visualizing the amount and direction of flap elevation. Typically, incisor show will indicate an adequately released and repositioned flap. To prevent the suture(s) from detaching from the deep temporal fascia, a figure of 8 suture of 3–0 PDS is used to lock the cable suture(s) in place. Spanning sutures of 3–0 PDS are placed between the superficial and the deep layers of the temporal fascia to smooth the temporal area and, along with adequate temporal pocket dissection, prevent bunching (Figs. 2–7). The pocket is well irrigated with dilute povidone-iodine solution before closure with skin clips. Symmetry is checked with the opposite side before closing the temporal incisions. Careful evaluation of preoperative photos will demonstrate preexisting asymmetries that may require cable suture adjustment for optimal improvement.

The use of barbed sutures has replaced single suture fixation and has dramatically facilitated the accurate placement of suspending sutures while adding the benefit of stacking the soft tissue for volumetric augmentation of the midface. The intraoral incision is also irrigated with dilute povidone-iodine solution. If alloplastic malar and/or submalar augmentation is planned, the implant is inserted at this time. Typically, the flap advancement diminishes the size of the remaining inferior pocket, which would allow inferior migration of the implant. If, however, the implant seems unstable, options to prevent malposition include: temporary nonabsorbable sutures passed through the temporal pocket and tied over bolster dressings behind the incision or the use of fibrin glue (Tisseel, Baxter Healthcare) to secure the pocket. A new generation of Silastic implants that have a ribbed surface (Implantech, California, U.S.A.) discourage implant malposition as the surface promotes implant stability. The intraoral incision is closed with 4–0 Chromic catgut leaving room for a ¼ inch penrose drain sutured in place at the inferior end of the incision. The drain is removed in 72 hours.

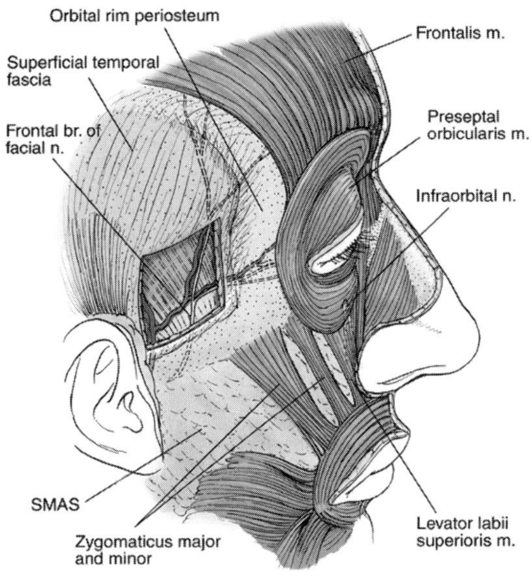

Figure 2 Subperiosteal midface-lift: sagittal anatomy of the midface. *Abbreviation*: SMAS, submuscular aponeurotic system.

Attention is next directed to the lower eyelid. Options include the following:

1. No treatment in younger patients who do not demonstrate skin redundancy when the flap is advanced, or older patients who have had a prior lower-eyelid blepharoplasty and have minimal "excess" skin
2. A skin pinch lower-lid blepharoplasty avoiding any dissection through the muscle and the midlamellar structures
3. Lateral fat pad reduction in those patients who show protruding fat when in upward, medial gaze
4. In those patients that require a bit more dissection to contour the lower eyelid, perform a tarsal tuck to support the lid against the orbital rim and a medially based orbicularis oculi flap to further support the lid (Fig. 8)

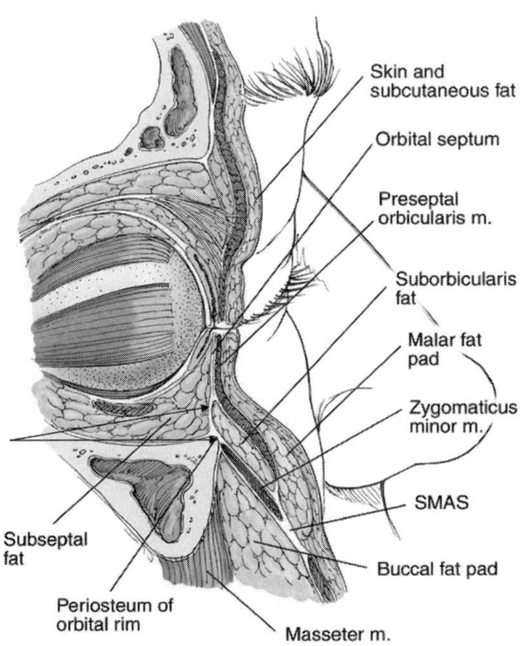

Figure 3 Subperiosteal midface-lift: sagittal anatomy of plane of dissection. *Abbreviation*: SMAS, submuscular aponeurotic system.

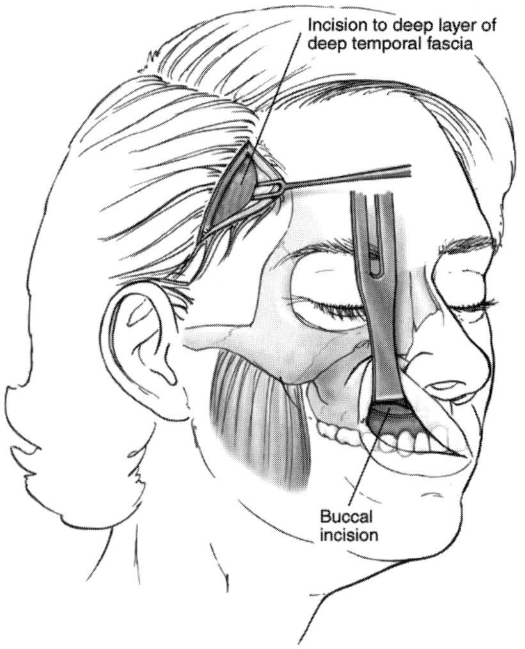

Figure 4 Subperiosteal midface-lift: temporal and buccal access incisions.

5. Horizontal lid shortening may be indicated with a wedge resection just medial to the fissure if there is bowing of the lid and the lateral canthus is at or above the level of the medial canthus
6. A formal canthoplasty may be necessary in poorly supported lower eyelids in which the lateral canthus is below the level of the medial canthus
7. Steri-strips™ (3M, Rochester, Minnesota, U.S.A.) that are elasticized, are placed from the lower lid obliquely to the temporal skin for five days of support.

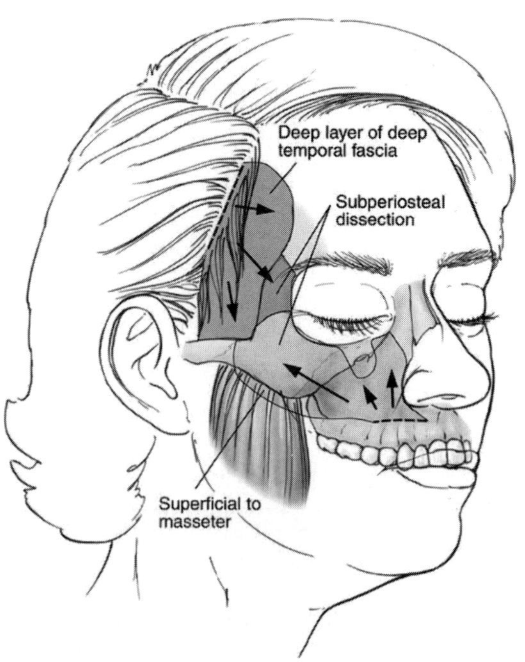

Figure 5 Subperiosteal midface-lift: temporal plane of dissection and buccal plane of dissection.

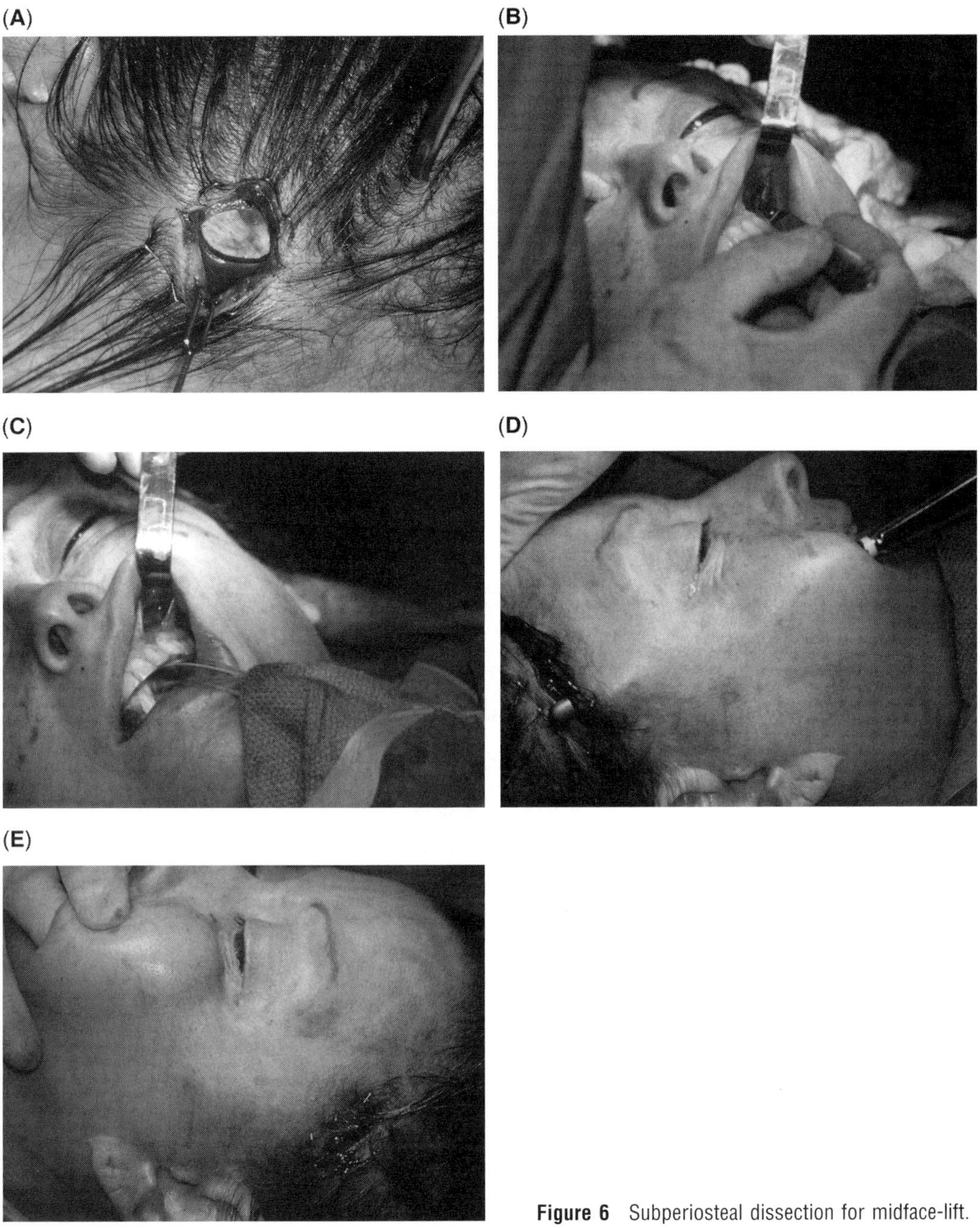

Figure 6 Subperiosteal dissection for midface-lift.

My regimen includes the following: preoperative and 24 hours of postoperative intravenous steroids (Decadron 10 mg preoperatively and 4 mg every eight hours for two or three more doses), six days of antibiotic coverage with a cephalosporin, liquid diet for one day followed by a soft diet, decreasing doses of prednisolone (20 mg, day 2; 15 mg, day 3; 10 mg, day 4; and 5 mg, day 5), intermittent ice goggles as tolerated, eye lubrication, head elevation, careful monitoring of and adjustment of blood pressure, pain management for comfort and to keep the blood pressure within normal limits, intraoral drain removal on day 3 and skin clip removal on day 7. Fast-absorbing 5–0 or 6–0 catgut eyelid sutures avoid the discomfort of suture removal.

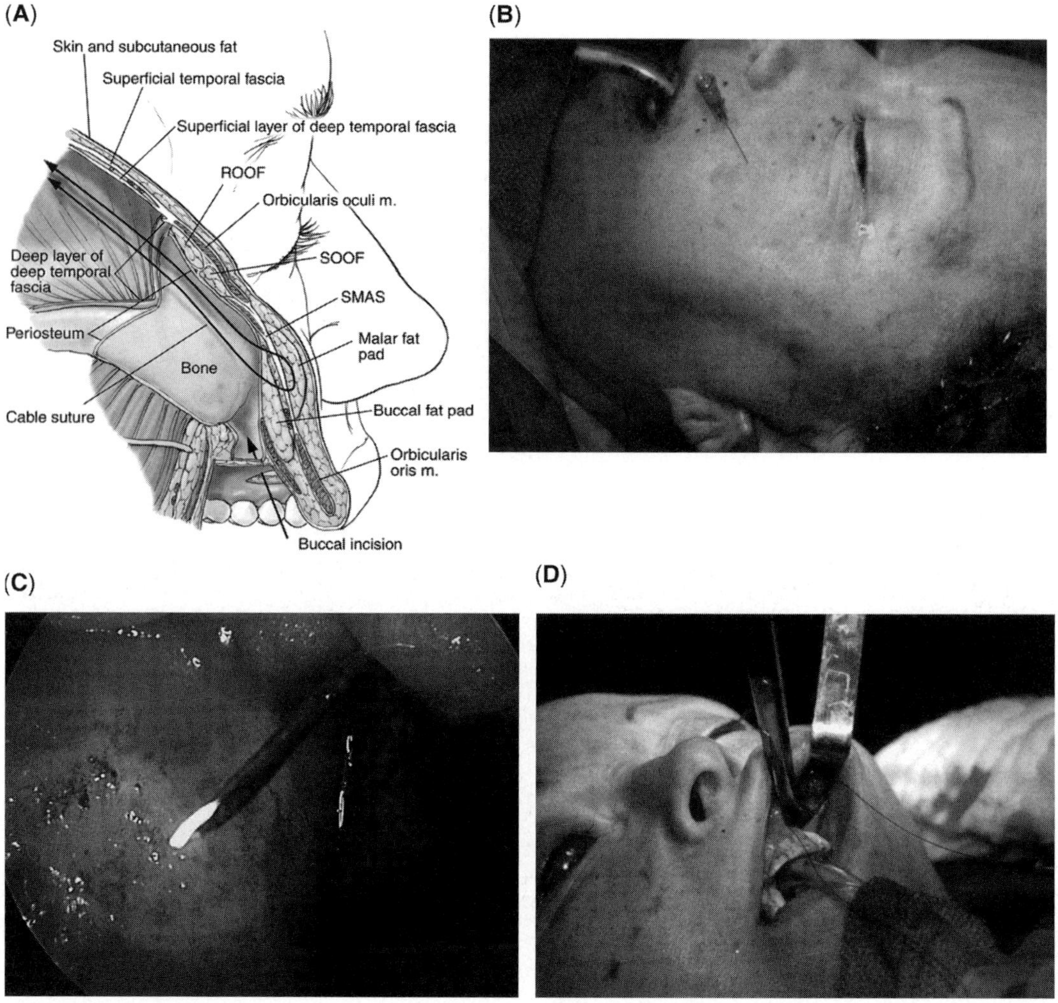

Figure 7 Suture placement for midface suspension. *Abbreviation*: SOOF, suborbicularis oculi fat; ROOF, retroorbicularis oculi fat; SMAS, submuscular aponeurotic system.

MIDFACE REJUVENATION IN MEN

Aesthetic goals in men typically are different than those desired by women with regard to the midface. An oblique vector in men may produce undesirable malar fullness and an increased interzygomatic distance. Therefore, I use a pure vertical vector in men and accomplish this in one of two ways. Depending upon the work to be done on the lower eyelid and the bony morphology of the area, I work either through the lower eyelid or the mouth. If there is no need to address the lower eyelid in more than the skin-pinch technique, I will perform the intraoral dissection as mentioned above and merely advance the tissues vertically without developing a tunnel to the temporal area. Working only through the mouth, the vertical flap advancement is supported with the use of a fine mist spray of fibrin glue. Steri-strips help to maintain a tension-free vertical correction for five days. The fibrin glue maintains soft-tissue fixation for about two weeks, which seems to be of sufficient duration to allow attachment of the flap that has also been supported with Steri-strips.

When I have planned to address the lower eyelid in a more aggressive way, I may approach the midface in the following way:

The procedure is performed precisely as mentioned for the periosteal hinge flap technique with important modifications. I do not develop a periosteal flap. Rather, after

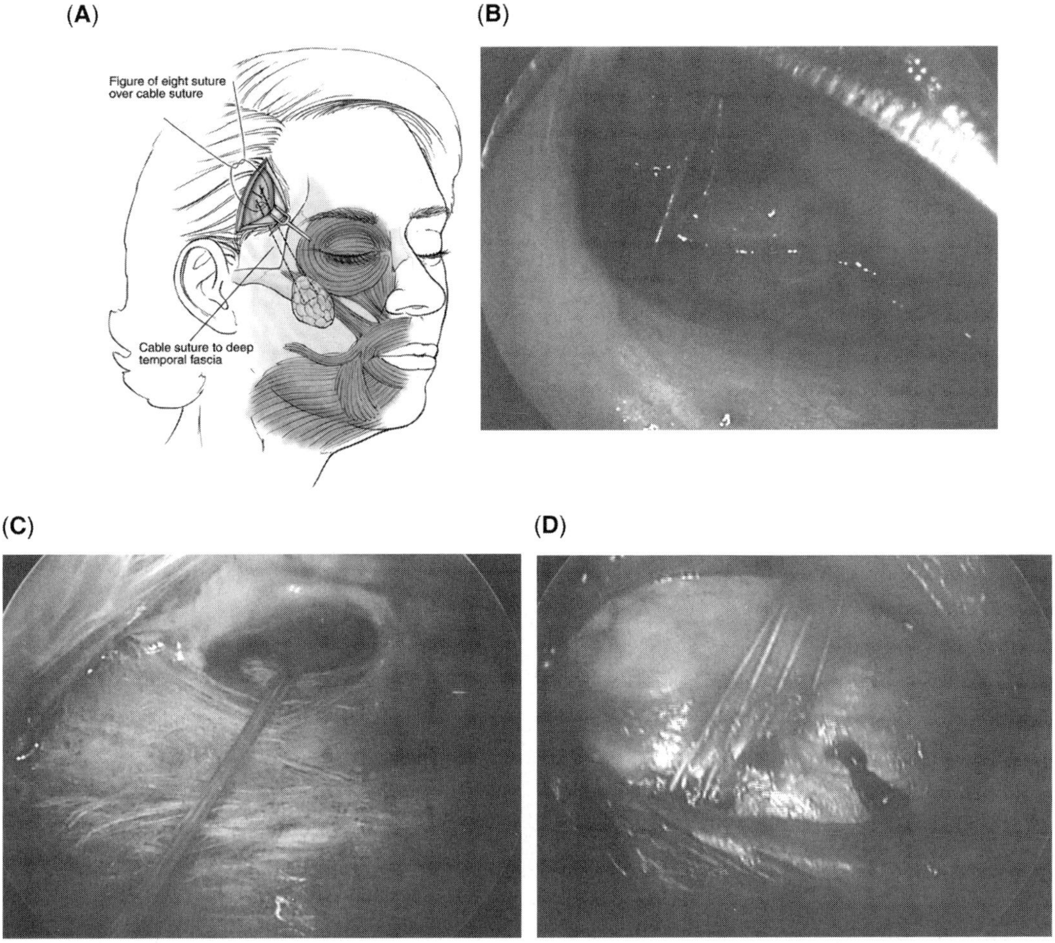

Figure 8 Suspension of midface.

elevating the skin/muscle flap to the level of the inferior orbital rim, I treat the subseptal fat with either light cautery, modest reduction, and/or advancement of the orbital septum to the inferior orbital rim to reposition the fat behind the orbital rim with 5–0 Vicryl sutures (Ethicon, Somerville, New Jersey, U.S.A.). I then proceed to dissect beneath the orbicularis oculi muscle, through the malar ligament, above the zygomaticus major muscle. The flap, consisting of skin, malar fat pad, muscle, SOOF, and SMAS, is elevated to the midnasolabial fold or lower if necessary to achieve the desired correction. The flap, advanced to the inferior orbital rim, is anchored to the arcus marginalis with sutures of 5–0 Vicryl. I spray the dissected area with 0.25% Marcaine with epinephrine and triamcinolone 10 mg/cc. Two cubic centimeters of the mixture is sufficient for both lower eyelids. Horizontal lid laxity may be treated with a wedge resection or a canthoplasty as indicated by the clinical findings (e.g., position of the lateral canthal tendon relative to the medial canthal tendon, preoperative findings on lid snap-back, and lid distraction tests). When a lateral canthoplasty is not indicated, a tarsal tuck (lateral canthopexy) and a medially based orbicularis oculi flap are always added to enhance lid support. Malar hypoplasia, both congenital and developmental, may be corrected with the concomitant intraoral placement of a malar, submalar, or combined shell. I tend to avoid placing the implant through the lower eyelid when performing a midface-lift to decrease the chance of postoperative cicatrical lower-eyelid retraction that may accompany wound healing.

Avoiding the subperiosteal plane diminishes edema, providing for a faster recovery, and reduces the chance of producing lower-eyelid retraction.

LESS AGGRESSIVE PROCEDURES THAT PRODUCE MIDFACE REJUVENATION

Some patients are not in need of or will not consent to aggressive midface rejuvenative procedures. They may simply want a refreshed appearance with minimal "downtime." Frequently, these patients present with pseudoherniated lower eyelid fat pads, a prominent arcus marginalis, and tear trough (nasojugal fold) deformities. Approaching the problem from the lower eyelid, I proceed as I would for a supraperiosteal midface-lift. In those patients in whom I wish to merely improve the convexity of the pseudoherniated fat pads, I lightly cauterize the bulging fat pads or minimally reduce them. I then advance the orbital septum to the inferior orbital rim with 5–0 Vicryl sutures (Figs. 9–14). To obtain a blending of the lid/cheek junction, I completely release the orbital portion of the orbicularis oculi muscle from the inferior-medial orbital rim with a microdissection needle and a freer or a similar elevator. I continue the dissection for a short distance below the muscle medially and the muscle and SOOF laterally. The orbital septum is opened with the microdissection needle and the subseptal fat with its vascular pedicle is advanced over the orbital rim, beneath the elevated orbicularis oculi muscle and sutured to the undersurface of the muscle with 5–0 rapid-absorbing plain catgut sutures (Fig. 15). Sometimes, the lateral fat pad is too full and is lightly reduced. If there is insufficient fat available such as in patients who have previously undergone a lower-eyelid blepharoplasty with fat removal, I usually can find fat in the upper lid (typically medially) to use as a free-fat graft. Careful aspiration of fat from elsewhere and placement of the fat deep to the orbicularis oculi muscle is a valuable option. The area of dissection is sprayed with dilute triamcinolone and 0.25% Marcaine with epinephrine solution. I next perform a tarsal tuck (lateral canthopexy). The next step is to develop a medially based orbicularis oculi muscle flap that is dissected off the skin from lateral to medial. Because I have released the origin of the orbicularis oculi muscle from the medial aspect of the inferior orbital rim, I can transmit a more effective force to the upper midface as the flap is advanced. When I desire more correction of the upper midface, I use the lateral aspect of the upper-eyelid incision when performing a concomitant upper-eyelid blepharoplasty or merely incise the lateral part of the upper-eyelid skin crease to allow access to the deep temporal fascia. The flap is passed beneath the lateral raphe and sutured to the deep temporal fascia with two 5–0 Vicryl sutures. Less advancement is obtained by merely retracting the lateral aspect of the lower-eyelid incision superiorly, dissecting to the deep temporal fascia, and anchoring the muscle flap slightly above the lateral canthal angle. Release of and advancement of the muscle flap works in a

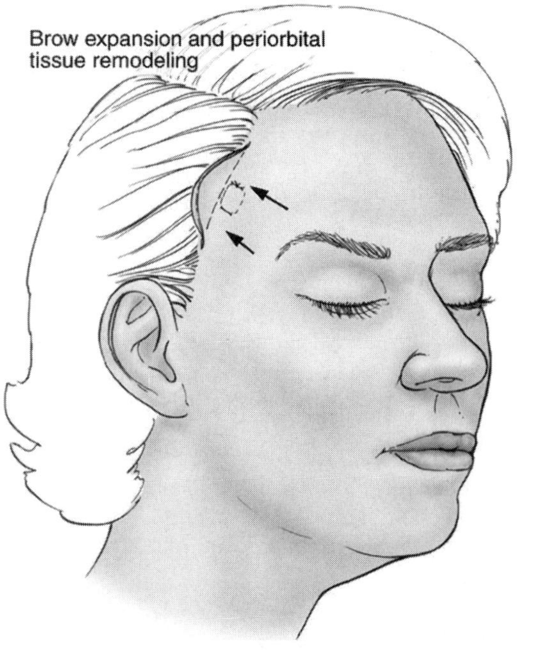

Figure 9 Redraping of temporal soft tissue.

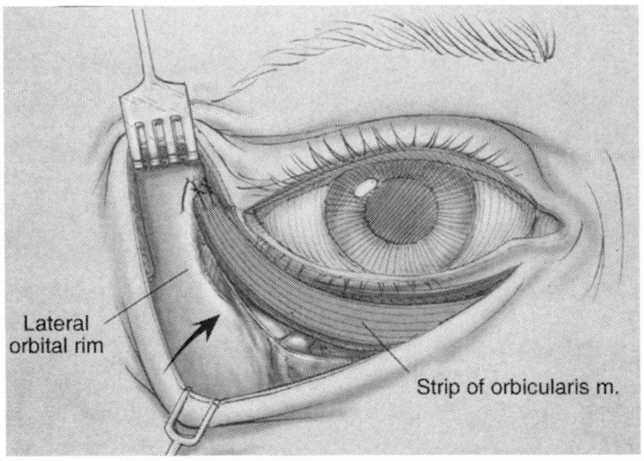

Figure 10 Muscle sling for lower eyelid support: medially based orbicularis oculi muscle flap.

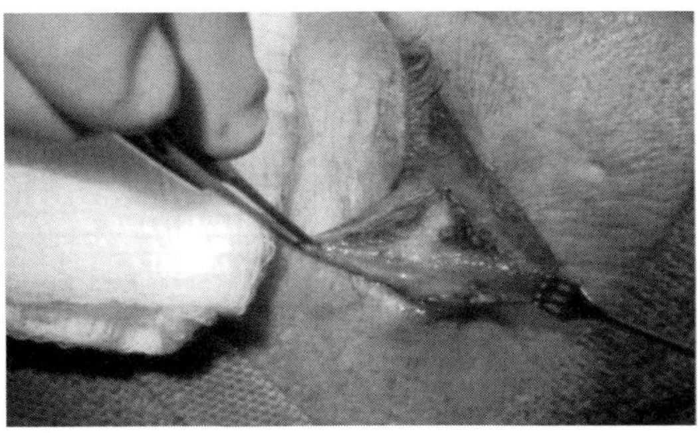

Figure 11 Muscle sling for lower eyelid support: muscle flap dissection.

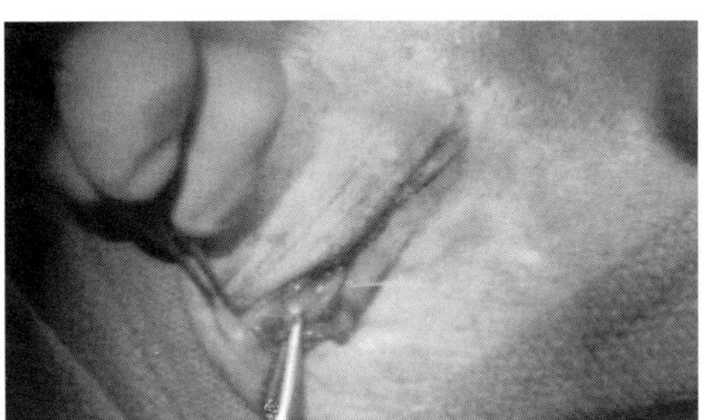

Figure 12 Muscle sling for lower eyelid support: muscle flap anchored to fascia and superior muscle.

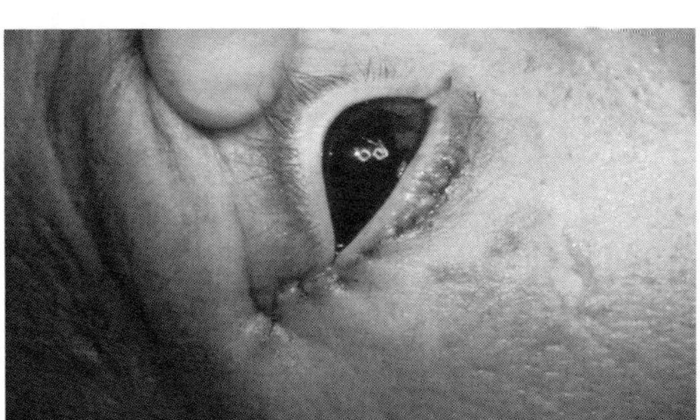

Figure 13 Muscle sling for lower eyelid support: skin closure/fast-absorbing catgut sutures.

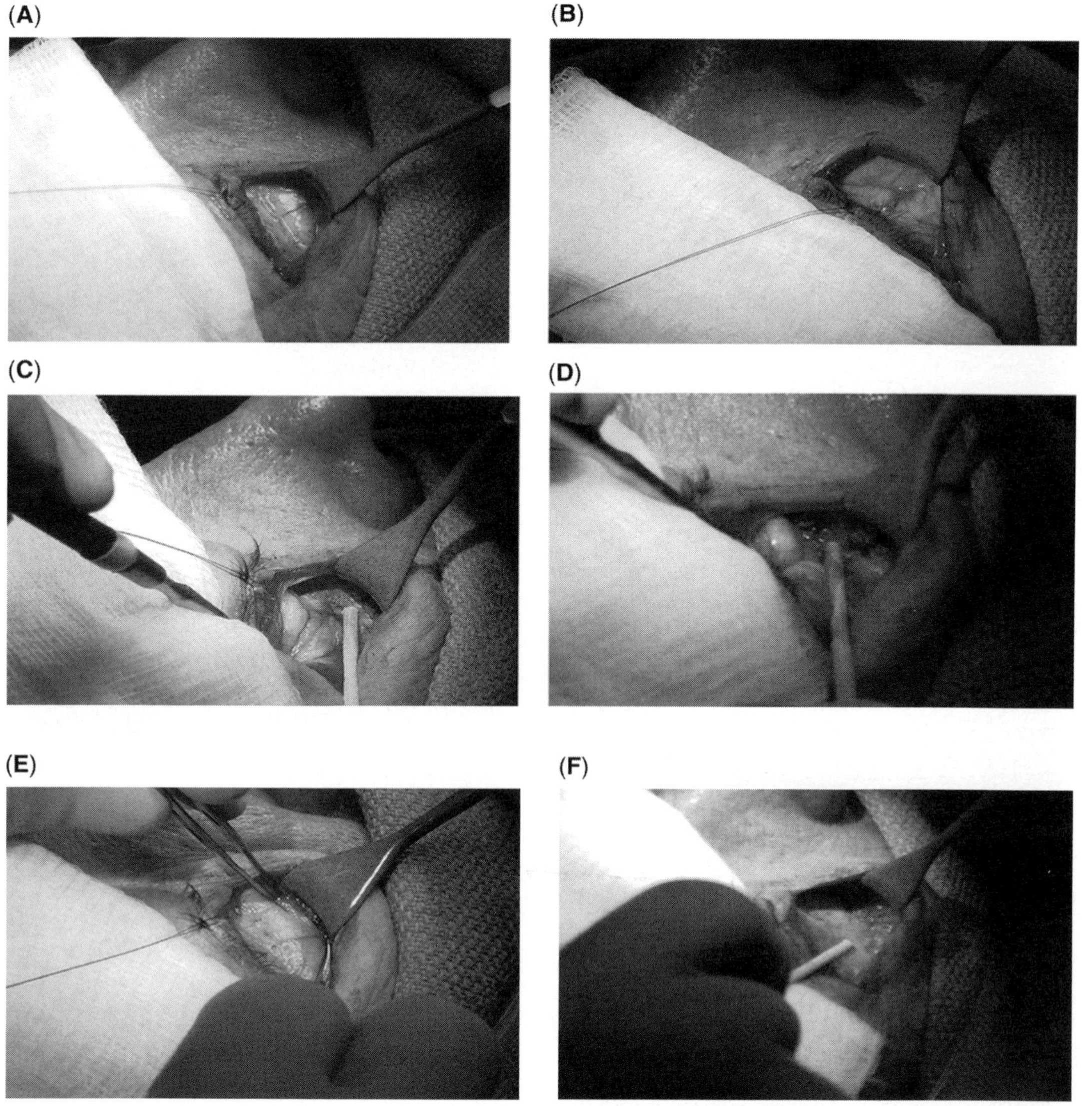

Figure 14 Septal reset: exposure.

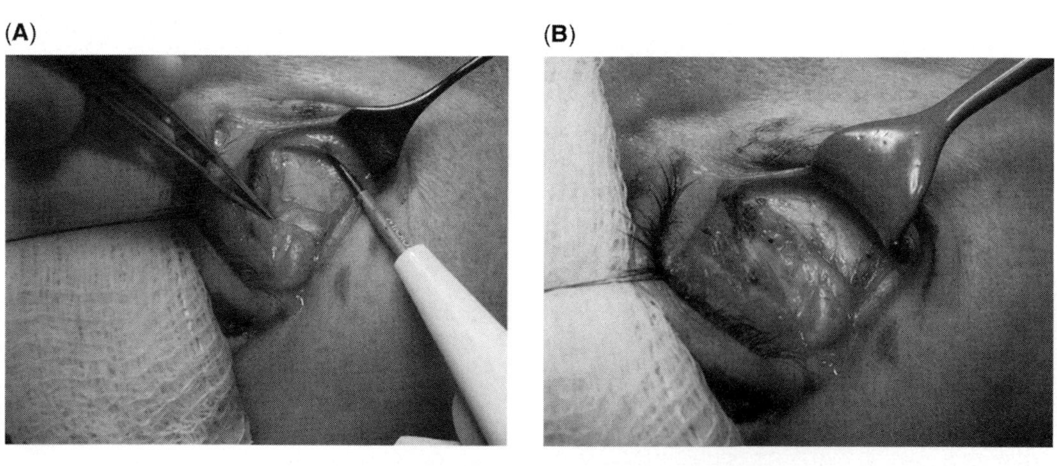

Figure 15 Complete muscle release and fat transposition: fat transposition.

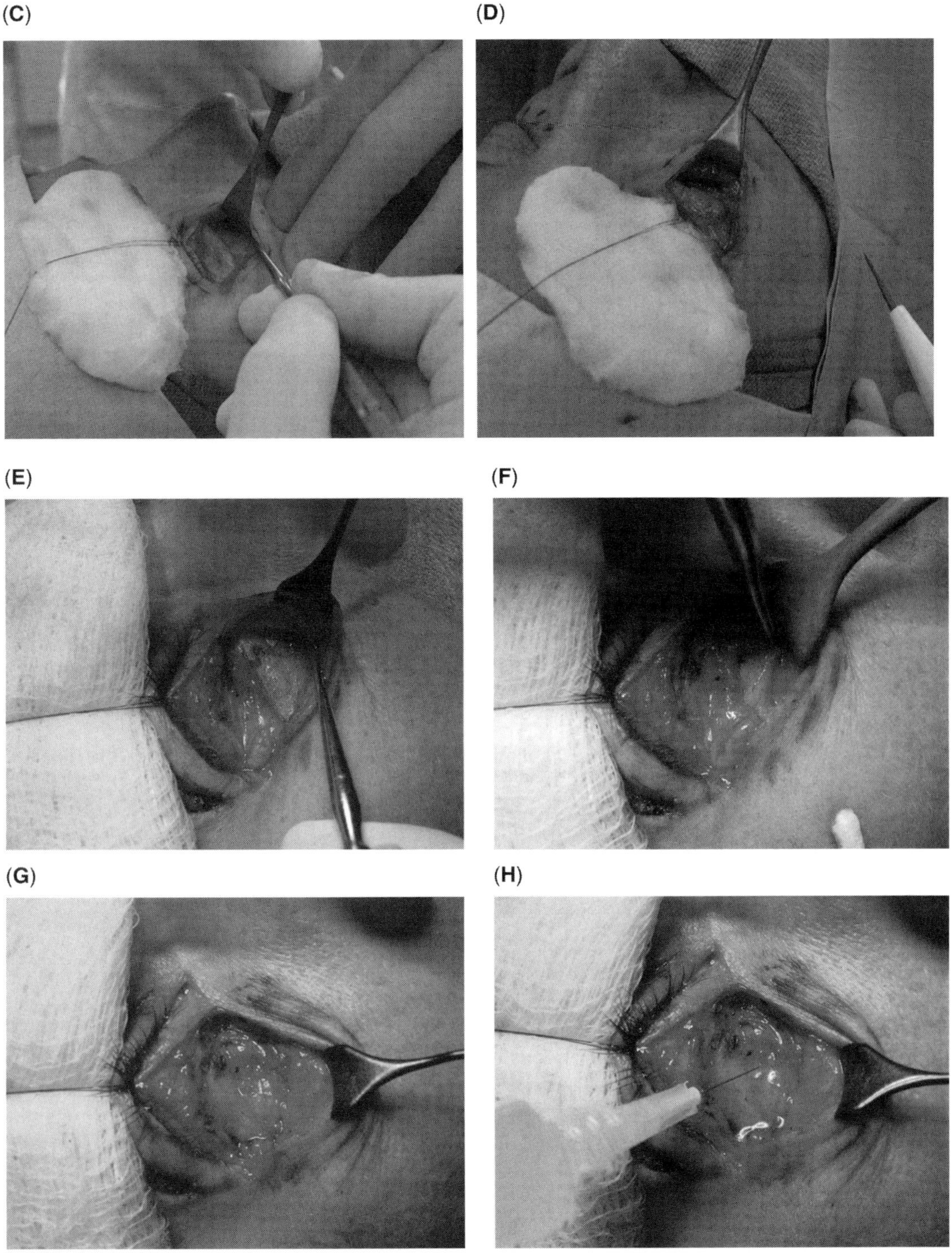

Figure 15 (*Continued*)

manner similar to utilizing the SMAS as a handle to move the medial cheek skin. This technique produces a youthful midface contour, but falls short of the profound improvement that can be obtained with the more aggressive methods presented above. I typically will not perform aggressive orbicularis oculi muscle release at the time of a subperiosteal face-lift even in patients with a prominent tear trough deformity due to concerns of cicatrical lid malposition.

Soft-tissue fillers, autogenous or allogenic, although of uncertain survivability, can nicely fill the defect without the risks associated with dissection in this area.

CONCLUSIONS

The evolution of my techniques in midface rejuvenation have provided an exciting, interesting road with obstacles that were overcome by carefully assessing the goals, understanding the risk/benefit ratio of each procedure, and meticulously working in this delicate, complex area. Midface rejuvenative procedures add enormously to the aesthetic result and truly can help return our patients to a youthful, natural appearance. When it is all said, midface rejuvenation is really about appropriate vectors and volume and the best ways to achieve both.

It is important to learn from others since you will not live long enough to make all of the mistakes yourself

—Frank McDowell
former editor, *Plastic and Reconstructive Surgery*

REFERENCES

1. Hamra ST. The deep-plane rhytidectomy. Plast Reconstr Surg 1990; 86:53.
2. Hamra ST. Composite rhytidectomy. Plast Reconstr Surg 1992; 90:1.
3. Terino EO. Alloplastic facial contouring. Surgery of the fourth plane. Aesthetic Plast Surg 1992; 16:195.
4. Owsley JQ. Lifting the malar fat pad for correction of prominent nasolabial folds. Plast Reconstr Surg 1993; 91:463.
5. Ramirez OM. Endoscopic facial rejuvenation. Perspectives Plast Surg 1995; 9:22.
6. Stuzin JM, Baker TJ, Gordon HL. Extended SMAS dissections. An approach to midface rejuvenation. Clin Plast Surg 1995; 22:295.
7. Aston SJ. Mid-facelift panel. FAME (finger assisted malar elevation). Presented at the Annual Meeting of the American Society of Plastic and Reconstructive Surgeons, Dallas, TX, 1996.
8. Hester TR, Codner MA, McCord CD. The centrofacial approach for correction of facial aging using the transblepharoplasty subperiosteal cheeklift. Aesthetic Surg Q 1996; 16:51.
9. Byrd HS, Andochick SF. The deep temporal lift: a multiplanar, lateral brow, temporal, and upper face lift. Plast Reconstr Surg 1996; 97:928.
10. Connell BF, Semlacher RA. Contemporary deep layer facial rejuvenation. Plast Reconstr Surg 1997; 100(6):1513.
11. Little JW. Three-dimensional rejuvenation of the midface: volumetric resculpture by malar imbrication. Plast Reconstr Surg 2000; 105(1):267.
12. Paul MD. An approach to correcting midfacial aging with a periosteal hinge flap. Aesthetic Surg Q 1997; 17:61.
13. Paul MD. Morphologic and gender considerations in midface rejuvenation. Aesthetic Surg J 2001; 21(4):349.

10 Autologous Volumetric Three-Dimensional Shaping of the Face

O. Onur Erol

Department of Plastic and Reconstructive Surgery, ONEP Plastic Surgery Science Institute, Istanbul Bilim University, Istanbul, Turkey

INTRODUCTION

Throughout our lives, various factors contribute to changes in the face associated with the aging process. The combinations of genetic predisposition, facial expressions, underlying bony resorption, dental deterioration, sun damage, gravity, subcutaneous tissue atrophy, and smoking are all included in the aging of the perioral and infraorbital region (1–5). Various techniques have been used in facial soft-tissue contouring, including autogenous transplants (5–52) (free fat, dermis, and dermal fat grafts), heterogeneous transplants (53–57) (bovine collagen), and alloplastic materials (silicone, methyl-methacrylate spheres, Gore-Tex, suture materials, and hyaluronic acid, as well as others). Volumetric reshaping of the face with autologous tissue injection has become a popular and reliable method (5,18–23,28,58). Since 1985, I have had extensive experience with fat injections and, in 1989, developed the "tissue cocktail injection." Since then, several modifications and improvements have made utilization of this tissue more practical and effective.

TYPE OF INJECTABLE MICROGRAFTS USED IN VOLUMETRIC SHAPING OF THE FACE

Micro-Fat Grafting

Surgical Technique

In the first group of patients to whom this technique was applied, from 1985 to 1992, a vacuum machine was used and fat was collected in a sterile interconnected bottle. In this group, the fat graft was injected without pretreatment. An 18- to 16-gauge needle was used in all patients who were overcorrected to compensate for anticipated resorption. From 1992 to 1996, fat tissue was collected utilizing a syringe and 4-mm cannula. In this group, however, the fat was treated by washing it with a Ringer's lactate solution and adding 1 g of first-generation cephalosporin for each 50 cc of specimen. Overcorrection was not done because we learned that the revascularization of a small graft is much better than a large graft. In patients who were seen after 1996, fat harvesting was similar to that of the second group. Another step was added; the fat was centrifuged to eliminate the blood and extracellular or lipid remnants. Fat is harvested with a syringe using a cannula 3 mm in diameter with the patient in a supine position. The abdominal and flank regions are preferred for harvesting; occasionally, the trochanteric regions or buttocks may be used. Harvested fat is centrifuged for three minutes at 3000 rpm; after the extracellular lipids and blood are discarded and 1 g of first-generation cephalosporin is added for each 50 cc of specimen, the fat is ready for injection and/or cryopreservation. Luer lock injectors of 1 cc are usually employed for the actual injection.

Cryopreservation

The fat or tissue cocktail to be stored is first put into sterile tubes of 10, 20, and/or 50 cc and immersed into a nitrogen tank and frozen up to −196°C, and then transferred to another freezer and maintained at −80°C for long-term storage.

Tissue Cocktail (Micro-Minigraft of Dermis, Fascia, Muscle, and Fat)

Surgical Technique

Tissue excised during other procedures such as face-lifts, forehead-lifts, and blepharoplasty is utilized to prepare the tissue cocktail after discarding the epithelial tissue. This tissue contains

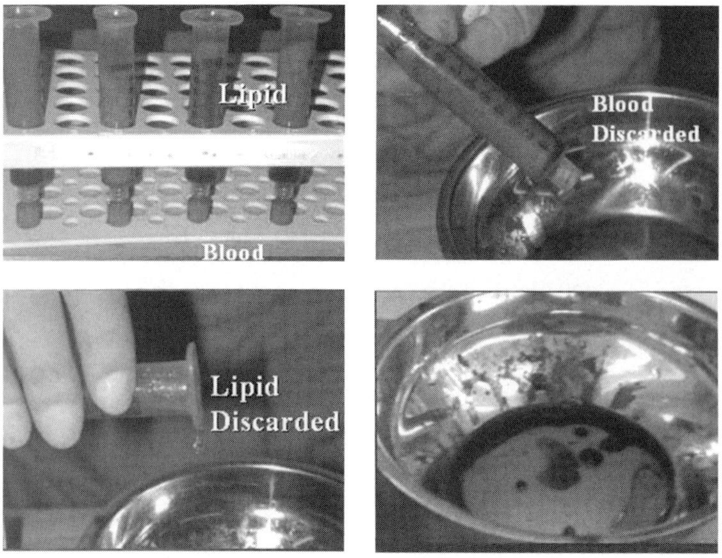

Figure 1 Harvested fat tissue centrifuged at 3000 rpm. The blood and lipid were discarded.

approximately 80% dermis and 20% fascia, fat, and muscle. Care must be taken not to include any hair follicles in the mixture. When obtaining large amounts of tissue, as from an abdominoplasty or reduction mammaplasty, the epithelial tissue and excess fat are discarded to obtain a mixture that is primarily dermal tissue (90% dermis, and 10% fascia and fat). The tissue is divided into smaller strips and then trimmed and cut until the diced tissue pieces are thin enough to pass through a 16-gauge, intravenous cannula. In doing so, mini- and micrografts of 0.5–1.0 mm are easily obtained from the mixture of tissues, creating an injectable tissue cocktail (Figs. 1–3). The required amount is used for immediate injection into different parts of the face (Figs. 4,5), and excess tissue is cryopreserved for further use. Even if a patient does not want or need facial soft-tissue rejuvenation at this time, with this technique, I preserve the tissue to utilize it in the future, depending on the needs and wishes of the patient.

Injection of Microfat or Tissue Cocktail

For fat injection, a 20- and 18-gauge Intracath disposable cannula is employed. In cases using a tissue cocktail, a 16-gauge cannula is required to ensure the passage of the semisolid liquid graft particles (Fig. 6). To inject deeper planes such as supraperiosteal areas, I use blunt metallic cannulas designed by Coleman and myself. In patients who require additional correction,

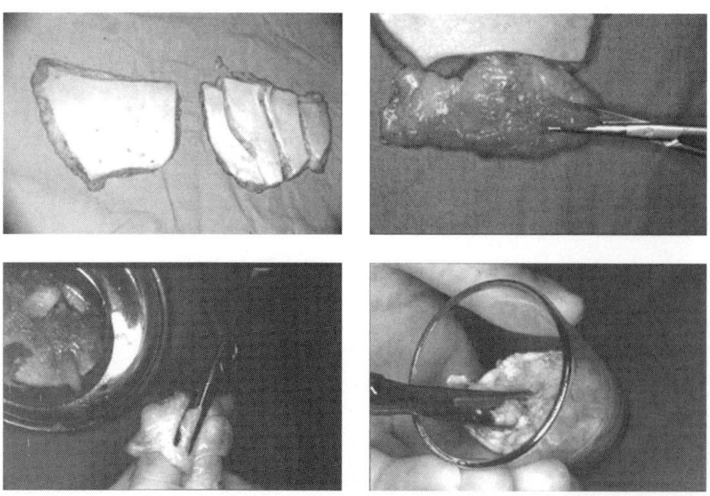

Figure 2 Excised tissue following abdominoplasty was divided into strips and the dermis was harvested.

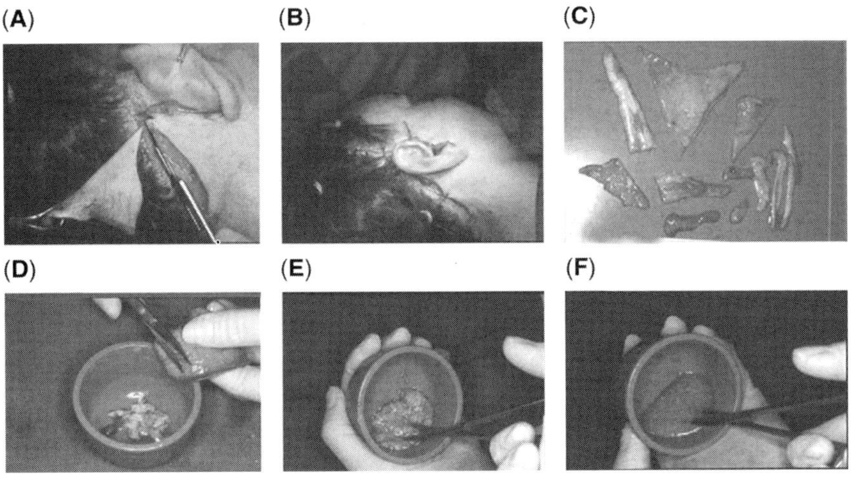

Figure 3 Following face-lift, dermis and fascia were harvested from the excised tissue and diced into small pieces of 0.5–1 mm to pass through a 16-gauge cannula.

the injection is repeated three or four times in three-month intervals for one year, with touch-up injections occasionally needed once a year thereafter. In these patients, after the first injection, cryopreserved tissue was used. The injection is performed under local or general anesthesia. Very small amounts are deposited in as many different tissue levels as practical. This maneuver maximizes the surface area of contact between newly transplanted tissue and recipient bed for revascularization and survival.

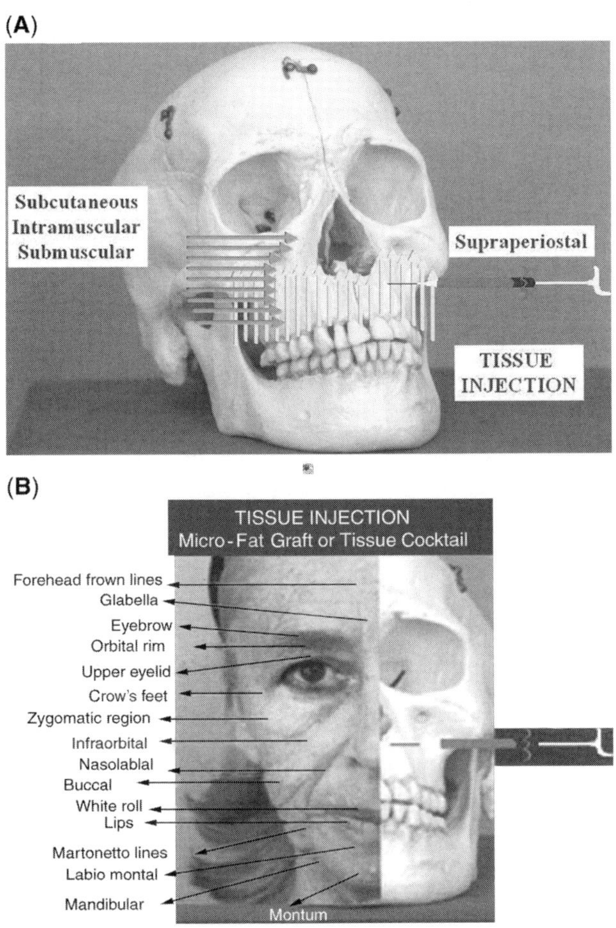

Figure 4 (**A** and **B**) The injection sites of microfat or tissue cocktail.

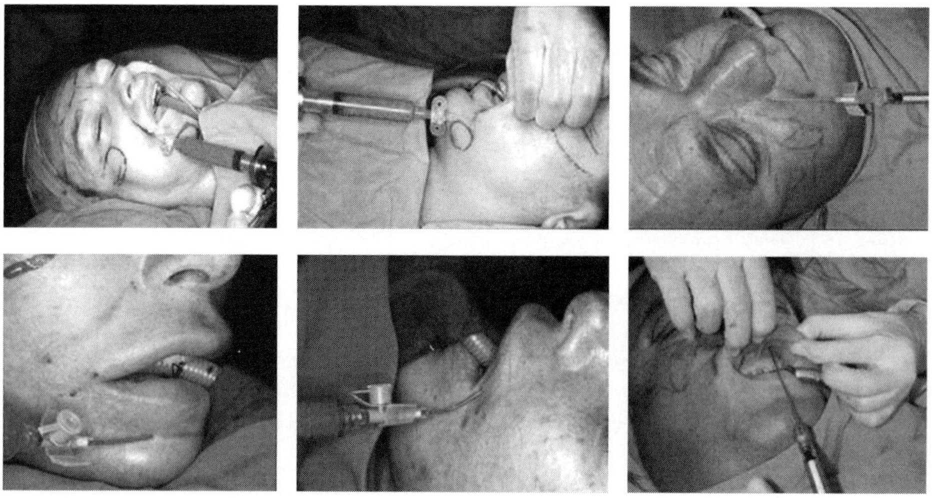

Figure 5 Intraoperative injections of microfat or tissue cocktail.

FOREHEAD REJUVENATION

Frontal and Glabellar Areas

In the frontal region, to restore convexity, it may be necessary to deposit up to 50 cc. I use a metallic cannula, and the injection is layered under and above the galea aponeurotica, close to the muscular layer. It may be useful to reduce the mobility of the frontalis muscle with a Botox injection one week before depositing the fat. If the objective is not to reshape the entire frontal area but rather to simply reduce the visibility of the frontal wrinkles, I use a 20-gauge Intracath disposable cannula for fat and a 16-gauge cannula for tissue cocktail, and inject 1 or 2 cc of tissue into every wrinkle area (Fig. 7A–C).

Temporal Area

I give a 5–10 cc injection under the deep temporal fascia and underneath the skin. Blunt cannulas should be used because many vessels will be encountered. This region is prone to develop hematoma.

Eyebrow and Upper Lid Areas

I give a 1-cc injection under and above each eyebrow. If an endo–forehead-lift is scheduled, it should be performed after the lipostructure, but the injection should be done strictly inside the soft tissues. The restructuring of this region must be performed before any palpebral skin resection because excess skin evaluation is possible only after fat grafting. The fat is deposited in the extraperiosteal plane, in the muscular plane, and in the subcutaneous plane as far

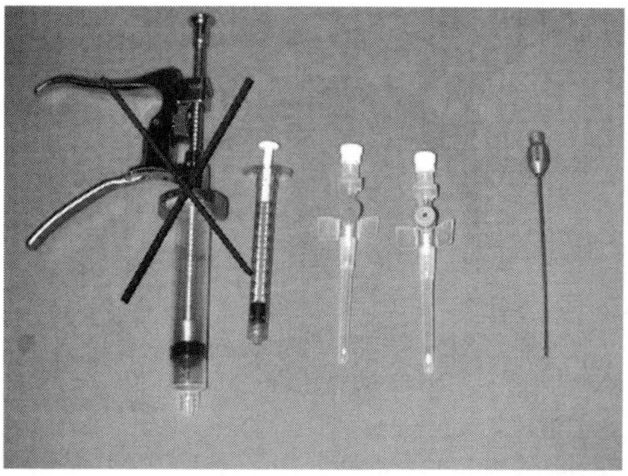

Figure 6 Tissue injection tools for facial rejuvenation.

down as the level of the upper eyelid crease. The total volume varies between 2 and 6 cc, depending on the hollowness of the eyelid to be corrected. During blepharoplasty, after the orbicularis oculi muscle is exposed, the injection of 1 cc of fat is done submuscularly under direct vision.

PERIORBITAL REJUVENATION

When a face ages, it loses its fullness because of bone resorption (maxillary and zygomatic bones). Together with bone resorption, there is also significant fat atrophy and diminution of cutaneous and subcutaneous collagen. This is particularly marked in the periorbital area, where the eyes appear sunken and a tear-trough deformity becomes visible. The muscles and fascia become loose and lose elasticity. In more advanced cases, the lower orbital rim becomes more visible and can be mistaken for a baggy eyelid. The tear-trough deformity results from reduced subcutaneous fat thickness between the baggy eyelid and the malar fat pad. After addressing the deep, excess fat, normally youthful eyelids must be restored by smoothing the transition zone to the malar area (Fig. 7C–F).

Infraorbital Area

Infraorbital hollowness gives a tired look to the patient. The lower eyelid has no support, and if the tonus of the eyelid is diminished, scleral show begins. In such patients, blepharoplasty aggravates the deformity. The infraorbital area is augmented by fat or tissue cocktail injections. As a malar support for the eyelid is recreated, the eyelid is also pushed upward, slightly modifying its slant. In moderate cases, only subcutaneous and muscular injections are done. In severe cases, I use a sublabial approach and injection is done supraperiosteally. The amount is 10 to 25 cc and covers the entire zygomatic, maxillary region up to the infraorbital rim. Then I continue with subcutaneous injections of 3–7 cc in multiple paths.

Lower Eyelid

I use only micro–fat grafts placed deeply into the supraperiosteal area, in the suborbicularis oculi fat and into the muscle. Between 1 and 3 cc of fat are deposited in the lower eyelid region using a 20-gauge Intracath cannula and/or special cannulas designed to deposit a very thin layer of fat. In the past, I had complications by using tissue cocktail in this region, where microparticles showed up for months in the dermis and I had to remove them with several stab incisions. Now in this area, I use tissue cocktail only deeply into the supraperiosteal area. After volumetric shaping of the face is performed, a blepharoplasty and face-lift is done.

I prefer a subcutaneous approach for blepharoplasty. I occasionally remove some fat, but usually only tighten the septum orbitale and orbicularis oculi muscle using bipolar cautery. In most cases, it is not necessary to remove skin from the lower eyelids because eyelid augmentation reduces the apparent excess. If fine wrinkles exist, I prefer CO_2 laser peeling.

MIDFACE REJUVENATION AND AUGMENTATION

Midface hollowness may cause a very tired look on the face. The etiology may be congenital or acquired with aging due to bone resorption and soft-tissue atrophy. The cheek region partly loses its thickness and the Bichat fat pad volume decreases. The parotid region, once convex, appears concave from a frontal viewpoint. The easiest remedy is to augment this area by tissue injection (fat or tissue cocktail). In severe cases, I augment the zygomaxillary region through the upper labial sulcus. Injections are done supraperiosteally submuscularly, deep subcutaneously in different layers (Fig. 7C–F). The injected volume varies from 10 to 25 cc for each site. If a patient has excisional skin available from an abdominoplasty or mammaplasty, I prefer to use a tissue cocktail at the same time. On the contrary situations, I use micro–fat grafting (Figs. 3A–C, 7C–F).

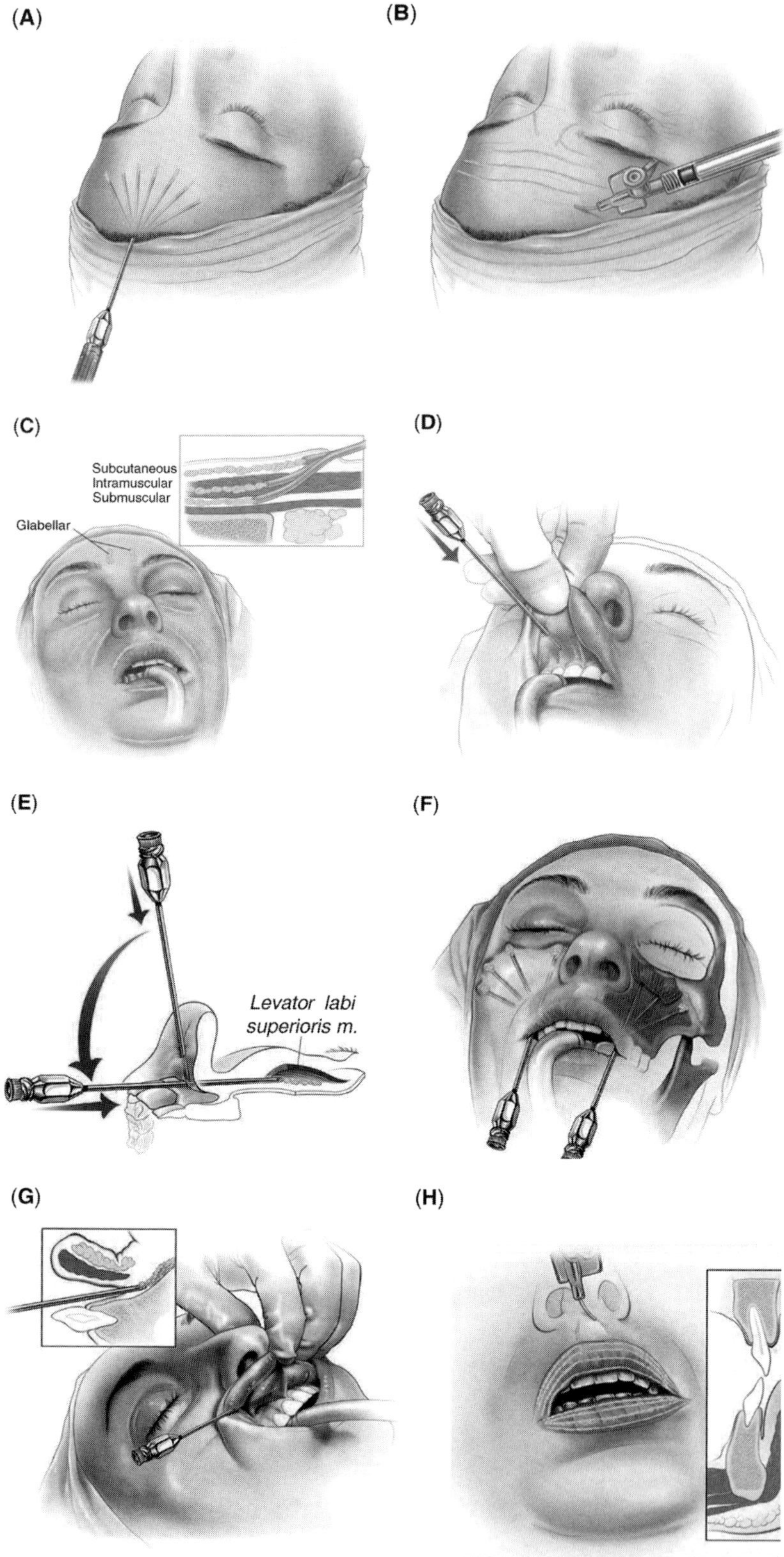

Figure 7 (*Caption on facing page*)

(I)

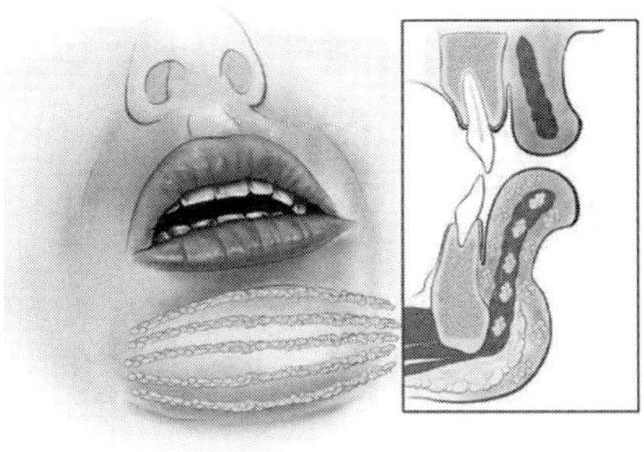

Figure 7 (*Figure starts on facing page*) (**A**) Augmentation of forehead with supraperiostal injection utilizing cannula. (**B**) Subcutaneous and intradermal injection to the wrinkles utilizing intracath disposable cannula. (**C**) Injection planes on the faces. (**D**) Vertical insertion of the cannula via upper sculcus. (**E**) Rotation of the cannula downward to start supraperiostal injection. (**F**) Supraperiostal injection on midface, intraorbital area, and check region. (**G**) Prealveolar injection utilizing cannula. (**H**) Lip injection utilizing intracath disposable cannula. (**I**) Chin augmentation by injection of microfat or tissue cocktail injection to different layers.

Cartilage Grafting

There are some instances when tissue injection is not available or the required amount is insufficient. In those cases, to augment the midface I use diced costal cartilage wrapped with Surgicel® (oxidize cellulose). The grafts are inserted supraperiosteally, through the upper labial sulcus and pushed upward to fill the entire maxillozygomatic area up to the infraorbital rim. The grafts are shaped internally and externally using fingers. There is no need for fixation. In combination I also inject some tissues subcutaneously and intramuscularly to improve the shape. Using this technique, I can obtain successful augmentation of the midface and infraorbital region with long-lasting results and with no late show of cartilage, as seen after carved cartilage is used. This approach is also very rewarding in patients with hollow lower lids and pseudo-exophthalmia caused by a retro position of the orbital rim.

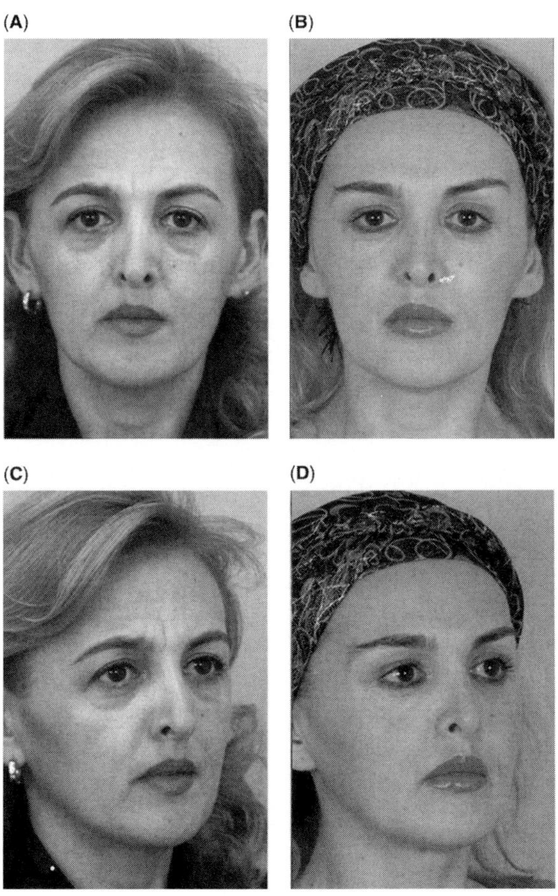

Figure 8 (**A**) Preoperative frontal view. (**B**) Postoperative frontal view two years after brow suspension and fat injection into forehead, midface, and periorbital regions. (**C**) Preoperative right oblique view. (**D**) Postoperative right oblique view two years after brow suspension and fat injection into forehead, midface, and periorbital regions. Note the improvement obtained on forehead, midface, and periorbital regions.

(A) (B) (C) (D)

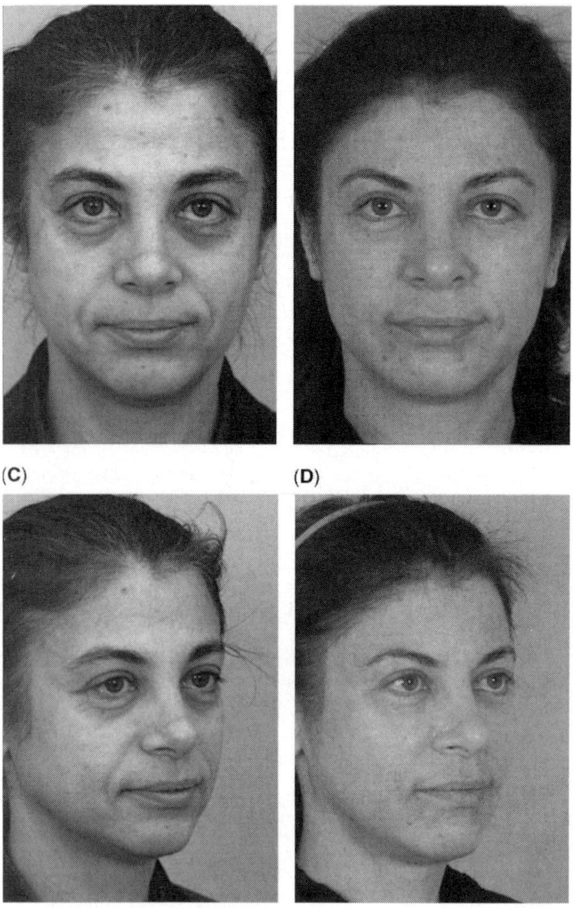

Figure 9 (**A**) Preoperative frontal view. (**B**) Postoperative frontal view two years after blepharoplasty and fat injection into midface, periorbital, and perioral regions. Note the improvement obtained on midface, periorbital, and perioral regions. (**C**) Preoperative right oblique view. (**D**) Postoperative right oblique view two years after blepharoplasty and fat injection into midface, periorbital, and perioral regions. Note the improvement obtained on midface, periorbital, and perioral regions.

PERIORAL REJUVENATION (FIGS. 4, 5, AND 7C, G, H)

Nasolabial sulcus: At different levels, 2–6 cc of tissue are injected, depending upon the depth of the sulcus. Marionette lines: Usually 0.5–1 cc of tissue is injected. White line of the vermilion: About 1–2 cc can be injected, which gives a nice contour to the upper and lower lips, and helps to improve fine skin wrinkles and the Cupid's bow curve of the upper lip. Philtral

(A) (B)

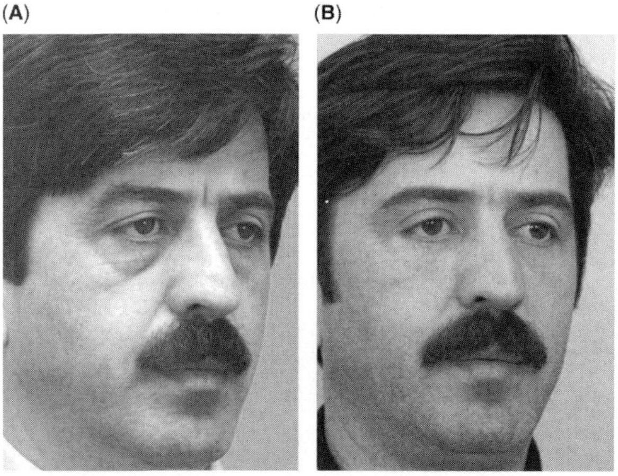

Figure 10 (**A**) Preoperative right oblique view. (**B**) Postoperative right oblique view one year after blepharoplasty and fat injection into periorbital region. Note the improvement obtained on periorbital region.

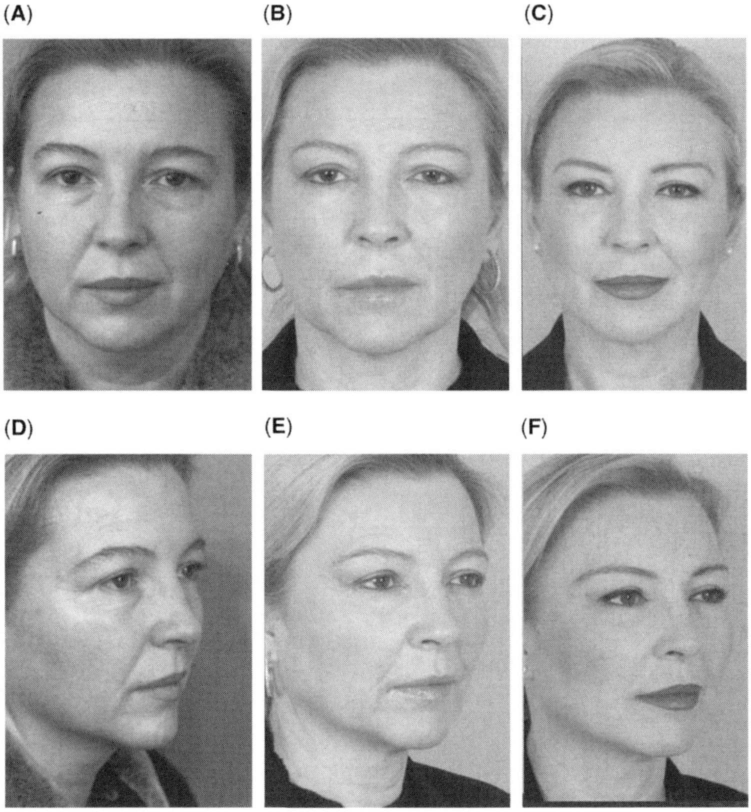

Figure 11 (**A**) Preoperative frontal view. (**B**) Postoperative frontal view six years after laser resurfacing, brow suspension, and fat injection into perioral and periorbital regions. (**C**) Postoperative frontal view two months after second session of fat injection into perioral and periorbital regions. Note the improvement obtained on perioral and periorbital regions. (**D**) Preoperative right oblique view. (**E**) Postoperative right oblique view six years after laser resurfacing, brow suspension, and fat injection into perioral and periorbital regions. (**F**) Postoperative right oblique view two months after second session of fat injection into perioral and periorbital regions. Note the improvement obtained on perioral and periorbital regions.

columns: Three-tenths to 0.5 cc is injected to heighten the philtrum on each side. Upper and lower lips: To enlarge the lips, 2–5 cc of tissue is injected at different levels, primarily intramuscular. The central tubercle can be restored. To augment the premaxillary region prealveolar region 4–12 cc may be used for each side. The injection is made subcutaneously, intra- and submuscularly, and supraperiosteally. Augmentation of this area also improves the lip shape and the nasolabial folds. Representative cases employing both fat grafts and/or the tissue cocktail, with and without ancillary procedures, are seen in (Figs. 13–18). Obviously, in addition to volumetric perioral rejuvenation there are several adjuvant procedures, which include skin resurfacing, skin excisions, lip-lifts, chin augmentations, and cosmetic dentistry, all of which contribute to our efforts in this area.

AUGMENTATION MENTOPLASTY (FIGS. 7I, 19E, F)

Mentoplasty is often a complementary procedure to rhinoplasty and face-lifting. During face-lifting, a hypoplastic chin has to be augmented to obtain a nice shape to the neck. Augmentation mentoplasty using alloplastic implants such as silicone, rubber, or other materials provides a simple approach to the treatment of the hypoplastic chin. For nine years, I have been using fat or tissue cocktail injection for augmentation mentoplasty. I use 12–16 cc for augmentation, and repeat the injection two or three times, with an interval of three months, using cryopreserved tissue.

(*Text continues on page 182.*)

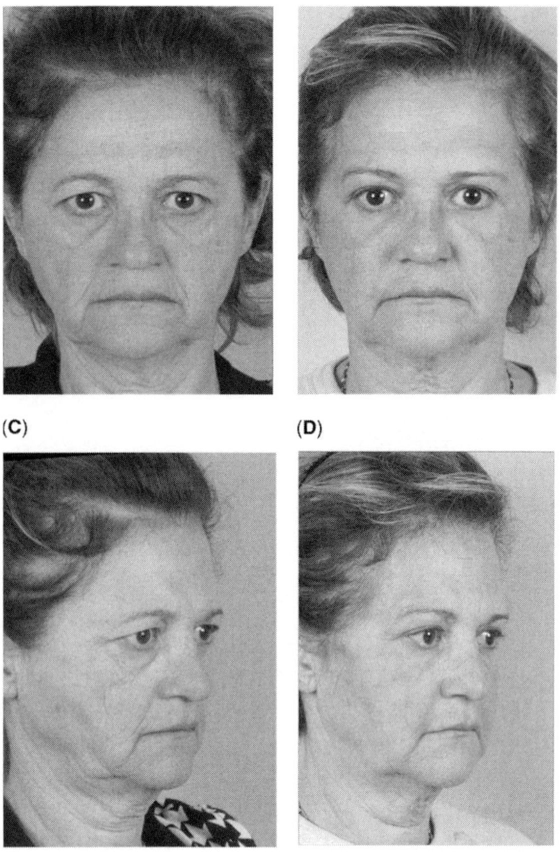

Figure 12 (**A**) Preoperative frontal view. (**B**) Postoperative frontal view six months after upper blepharoplasty; brow, cheek, neck suspension; and fat injection into midface, periorbital, and perioral regions. (**C**) Preoperative right oblique view. (**D**) Postoperative right oblique view six months after upper blepharoplasty; brow, cheek, neck suspension; and fat injection into midface, periorbital, and perioral regions. Note the improvement obtained on midface, periorbital, and perioral regions.

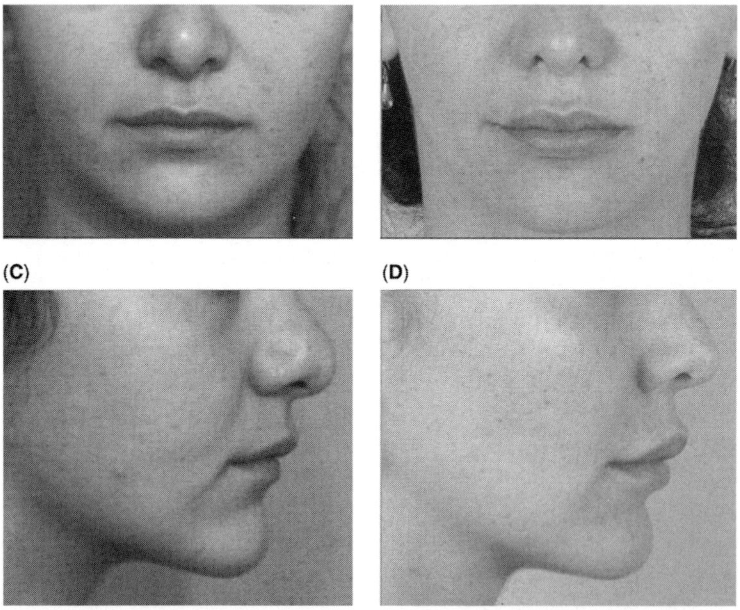

Figure 13 (**A**) Preoperative frontal view of perioral region. (**B**) Postoperative frontal view seven years after lip suspension, perioral rejuvenation, augmentation mentoplasty, and fat injection into perioral region. Note the improvement obtained on perioral region. (**C**) Preoperative lateral view. (**D**) Postoperative lateral view seven years after lip suspension, perioral rejuvenation, augmentation mentoplasty, and fat injection into perioral region. Note the improvement obtained on perioral region.

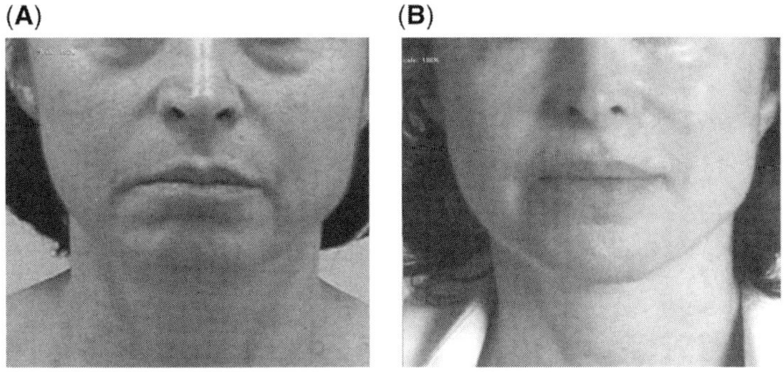

Figure 14 (**A**) Preoperative frontal view of perioral region. (**B**) Postoperative frontal view three years after lip suspension, perioral rejuvenation, augmentation mentoplasty, and fat injection into midface and perioral regions. Note the improvement obtained on midface and perioral regions.

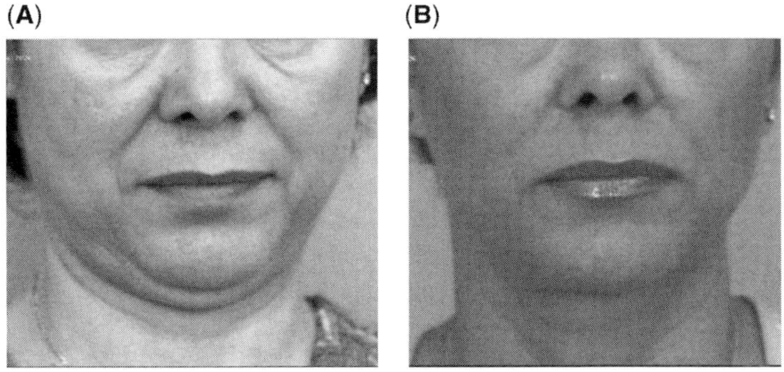

Figure 15 (**A**) Preoperative frontal view of perioral region. (**B**) Postoperative frontal view five years after lip suspension, perioral rejuvenation, augmentation mentoplasty, and fat injection into midface and perioral regions. Note the improvement obtained on midface and perioral regions.

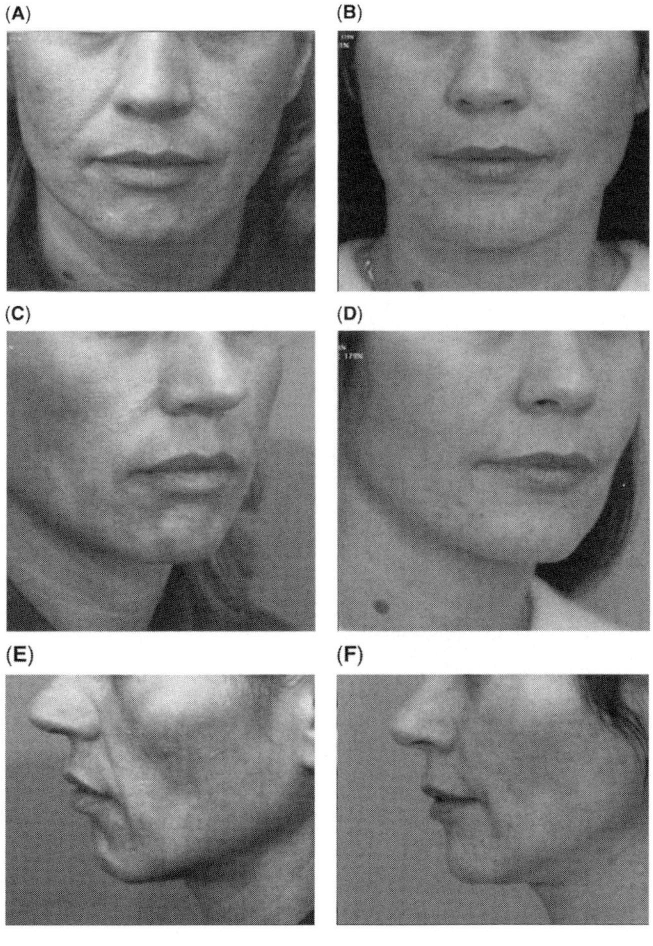

Figure 16 (**A**) Preoperative frontal view of perioral region. (**B**) Postoperative frontal view six years after fat injection into midface, perioral, and periorbital regions. Note the improvement obtained on midface, periorbital, and perioral regions. (**C**) Preoperative right oblique view. (**D**) Postoperative right oblique view six years after fat injection into midface, perioral, and periorbital regions. Note the improvement obtained on midface, periorbital, and perioral regions. (**E**) Preoperative left lateral view. (**F**) Postoperative left lateral view six years after fat injection into midface, perioral, and periorbital regions. Note the improvement obtained on midface, periorbital, and perioral regions.

(A) (B)

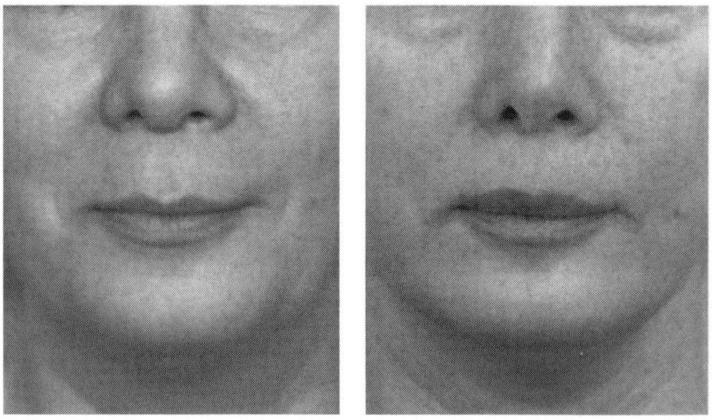

Figure 17 (**A**) Preoperative frontal view of perioral region. (**B**) Postoperative frontal view two years after face-lift and fat injection into midface and perioral regions. Note the improvement obtained on midface, perioral regions, and lips.

During the aging process, the chin area loses bulk, which might partly explain why it drops (witch's chin). This effect is further increased by a loss of thickness in the anterior part of the submental region, highlighting the looseness of the anterior cervical skin. To correct this deformity, I usually deposit 5–7 cc into the chin region, and 4–6 cc into the anterior part of the submental area before undermining the face-lift flap.

(A) (B) (C)

(D) (E) (F)

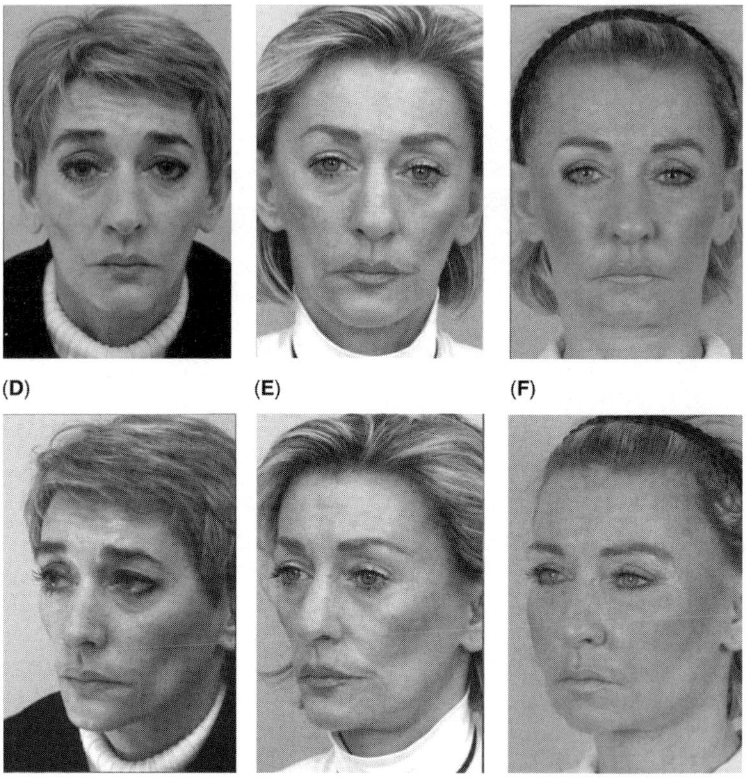

Figure 18 (**A**) Preoperative frontal view. (**B**) Postoperative frontal view four years after blepharoplasty, face-lift, brow suspension, and fat injection into forehead and midface regions. Note the improvement obtained on forehead and midface regions. (**C**) Postoperative frontal view four years after the second brow suspension and tissue cocktail injection to the face. (**D**) Preoperative left oblique view. (**E**) Postoperative left oblique view four years after blepharoplasty, face-lift, brow suspension, and fat injection into forehead and midface regions. Note the improvement obtained on forehead and midface regions. (**F**) Postoperative left oblique view four years after the second brow suspension and tissue cocktail injection to the face.

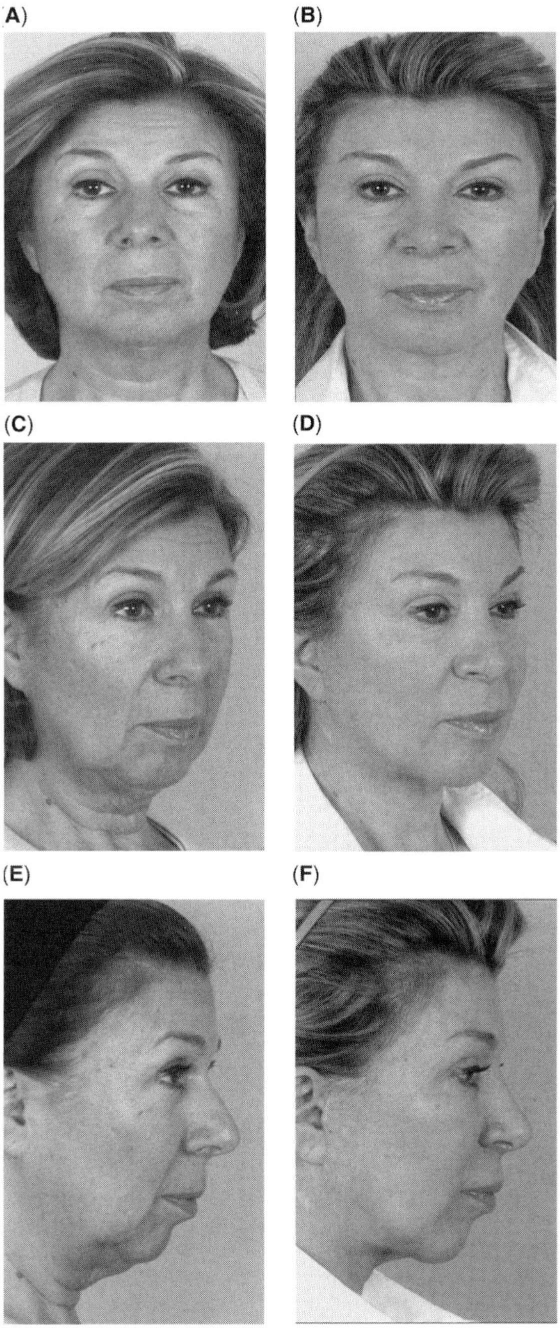

Figure 19 (**A**) Preoperative frontal view. (**B**) Postoperative frontal view one year after face-lift, septorhinoplasty, and fat injection into forehead, midface, perioral, and periorbital regions. Note the improvement obtained on forehead, midface, periorbital, and perioral regions. (**C**) Preoperative right oblique view. (**D**) Postoperative right oblique view one year after face-lift, septorhinoplasty, and fat injection into forehead, midface, periorbital, and perioral regions. Note the improvement obtained on forehead, midface, periorbital and perioral regions, and chin. (**E**) Preoperative lateral view. (**F**) Postoperative lateral view one year after face-lift, septorhinoplasty, and fat injection into forehead, midface, periorbital, and perioral regions. Note the improvement obtained on forehead, midface, periorbital, and perioral regions. Chin was augmented with microfat injection.

VOLUMETRIC FACE-LIFTING

During the past 10 years, all face-lift techniques have aimed to tighten, reposition, or redistribute facial soft tissues (59–72). Nevertheless, even in the most experienced and talented hands, the appearance of some patients cannot be improved by such techniques; these patients are not truly rejuvenated, just face-lifted (4,73–76). Since 1989, I have been using volumetric shaping with a tissue cocktail or microfat injection during all my face-lift procedures. The essentials of the technique involve reshaping rather than simply tightening (5). The area to be augmented is marked preoperatively, with the patient in the sitting position. Dr. Little made a great contribution by his work in stressing the importance of volumetric shaping. In the face-lifts that I perform, I use his technique of imbrication of the submuscular aponeurotic system to obtain a nice shape, and therefore, I need less tissue injection in the zygomatic area. I used to inject the tissue at the end of a face-lift. However, for five years, I changed this approach and I do the lipostructure before the face-lift. My technique of facial rejuvenation for 15 years involves redraping the superficial adipocutaneous system over a reshaped face as Trepsat recently described (76). A lipostructure is done during the same operative session as the face-lift but before the undermining. Of course, the undermining should not interfere with the fatty deposits, the depth of fat grafting should be planned in advance, and the undermining should be adapted to the lipostructure as Trepsat has reported (76). During the follow-up of my face-lift patients, I have found that retightening of the face in most of my patients is not necessary for more than 10 years. In these patients, in different intervals I do lipostructure to reshape their faces. In select patients, this can be combined with laser resurfacing, with satisfactory results. Sometimes, I add brow suspension and cheek suspension (no dissecting techniques) to keep the face with a fresh look. The clinical results of the patients with fat and tissue cocktail injections alone or with combined procedures are presented in Figures 8–19.

DISCUSSION

In my 20 years' experience, I have noticed that after contouring the face, the request for a face-lift has been postponed for several years. Volumetric shaping of the face utilizing micro–fat graft and/or a tissue cocktail micrograft is a key approach for rejuvenation. Not only facial contour is improved, but also with the addition of new live cells, the texture of the skin changes. The skin becomes shinier and fresh looking. The dry skin is improved, and this reality is articulated by patients. I wonder if these tissue grafts are acting as stem cells. In my opinion, the procedure of micro–tissue injection has to be accepted as a preventive medicine for skin and soft-tissue aging.

REFERENCES

1. Peer LA. Loss of weight and volume in human fat grafts. Plast Reconstr Surg 1950; 5:217.
2. Balin AK, Allen RG. Mechanisms of biologic aging. Dermatol Clin 1986; 4:347.
3. Lavker RM, Zheng P, Dong G. Morphology of aged skin. Dermatol Clin 1986; 4:379.
4. Little JW. Volumetric perceptions in midfacial aging with altered priorities for rejuvenation. Plast Reconstr Surg 2000; 105:252.
5. Erol OO. Facial autologous soft-tissue contouring by adjunction of tissue cocktail injection (micrograft and minigraft mixture of dermis, fascia, and fat). Plast Reconstr Surg 2000; 106:1375.
6. Illouz YG. Present results of fat injection. Aesthetic Plast Surg 1988; 12:175.
7. Amar RE. Micro infiltration adipocytaire dans la face ou restructuration par grefffes de tissus graisseux. Ann Chir Plast Esthet 1999; 44:593.
8. Asaadi M, Haramis HT. Successful autologous fat injection at 5-year follow-up. Plast Reconstr Surg 1993; 91:755.
9. Brandow K, Newman J. Facial multilayered micro lipo augmentation. Int J Aesthetic Restorat Surg 1996; 4:95.
10. Carraway JH, Mellow CG. Syringe aspiration and fat concentration: a simple technique for autologous fat injection. Ann Plast Surg 1990; 24:293.
11. Chajchir A, Benzaquen I, Wexler E, Arellano A. Fat injection. Aesthetic Plast Surg 1990; 14:127.
12. Coleman SR. Structural fat grafting. Plastic Reconstr Surg 2005; 11–5(6):1777–1778.
13. Coleman SR. Structural fat grafts: the ideal filler. Clin Plast Surg 2001; 28:111–119.
14. Coleman SR. Facial recontouring with lipostructure. Clin Plast Surg 1997; 24:347.
15. Coleman SR. Long-term survival of fat transplants: controlled demonstrations. Aesthetic Plast Surg 1995; 19:421.
16. Coleman WP III. Fat transplantation. Dermatol Clin 1999; 17:891.
17. Colic MM. Lip and perioral enhancement by direct intramuscular fat autografting. Aesth Plast Surg 1999; 23:36–40.
18. Erol OO. Facial rejuvenation using a different approach. Presented at the RAPS III International Symposium, Sao Paulo, Brazil, March 14–15, 1992.
19. Erol OO. Face rejuvenation: combined technique with adjunction of tissue cocktail injection. Presented at the XIII Congress of ISAPS, New York, New York, September 29–October 1, 1995.
20. Erol OO. Facial rejuvenation by adjunction of tissue cocktail injection. Presented at the EURAPS Seventh Annual Meeting, Innsbruck, Austria, May 16–18, 1996.
21. Erol OO. Face rejuvenation. Presented at the 8th Congress of the European Section of IPRAS, Lisbon, Portugal, June 22–25, 1997.

22. Erol OO. Facial rejuvenation with combined techniques. Presented at the X Anniversary International Symposium of Plastic and Aesthetic Surgery, Nice, France, April 11–12, 1997.
23. Erol OO. Temporal lift: 1-Open, 2-Endoscopic, 3-Non-endoscopic and non-invasive techniques in combination with other rejuvenation techniques. Presented at the International Society of Aesthetic Plastic Surgery XIV International Congress, São Paulo, Brazil, May 31–June3, 1997.
24. Fournier PF. Facial recontouring with fat grafting. Dermatol Clin 1990; 8:523.
25. Demir Z, Velidedeoglu H, Onur MA, Atilla E, Cakar N. Viability and mass effect of chopped fascia graft and comparison with block fascia graft (experimental study), 1996. Presented at the 19th National Congress of the Turkish Society of Plastic Surgeons, Bursa, Turkey, 1997.
26. Drommer RB, Mende U. Free fat transplantation in the face. J Craniomaxillofac Surg 1995; 23:228.
27. Eremia S, Newman N. Long-term follow-up after autologous fat grafting: analysis of results from 116 patients followed at least 12 months after receiving the last of a minimum two treatments. Dermatol Surg 2000; 26:1150–1158.
28. Erol O. Perioral Rejuvenation with Injectable Autologous Tissue, Seminars in Plastic Surgery. Vol. 17. May 2003, Number 2:173–180.
29. Guerrerosantos J. Temporoparietal free fascia grafts in rhinoplasty. Plast Reconstr Surg 1984; 74:465.
30. Guerrerosantos J, Gonzales-Mendoza A, Masmela Y, et al. Long-term survival of free fat grafts in muscle: an experimental study in rats. Aesthetic Plast Surg 1996; 20:403.
31. Hernandez-Perez E. Bi-level lipoinjection for facial wrinkles. Am J Cosmetic Surg 1992; 4:73.
32. Hernandez-Perez E. Practice perspectives: fat injection in different parts of the body. Dermatol Nurs 1998; 10:135.
33. Hernandez-Perez E. Resorcinol peel as a part of a facial rejuvenation program. Am J Cosmetic Surg 1997; 14:35.
34. Ho LC. Rejuvenative facial lipomorphoplasty. Aesthetic Plast Surg 2000; 24:22.
35. Jauffret JL. Utilisation de la Graisse Autologue en Chimrgie Plastique et Esthétique: La Technique. De Cowman SR, ed. Marseille: Thèse, 1998.
36. Kaufinan A, Mulholland S. Microfat grafting: the nurse's role. Plast Surg Nurs 2000; 229(4):216–217.
37. Kempf KK, Seyfer AE. Facial defect augmentation with a dermal-fat graft. Oral Surg Oral Med Oral Paihol 1985; 59:340.
38. Kurtay A, Velidedeouglu H, Onur MA, Atilla E, Cakar N. Viability and mass effect of chopped dermis graft and comparison with block dermis graft (experimental study), 1996. Presented at the l9th National Congress of the Turkish Society of Plastic Surgeons, Bursa, Turkey, 1997.
39. Little JW. Applications of the classic dermal fat graft in primary and secondary facial rejuvenation. Plast Reconstr Surg 2002; 109(2):788–804.
40. Loeb R. Nasolabial fold undermining and fat grafting based on histological study. Aesthetic Plast Surg 1991; 15:61.
41. Mikus JL, Koufman JA, Kilpatrick SE. Fat of liposuctioned and purified autologous fat injections in the canine vocal fold. Laryngoscope 1995; 105:17.
42. Miller TA. Temporalis fascial grafts. Plast Reconstr Surg 1980; 65:236.
43. Nicolle FV, Matti BA, Scamp T. Dermal and fascial autografts in facial aesthetic surgery. Aesthetic Plast Surg 1992; 16:219.
44. Niechajev I, Sevcuk O. Long-term results of fat transplantation: clinical and histologic studies. Plast Recohstr Surg 1994; 94:496.
45. Peer LA. Transplantation of fat. In: Transplantation of Tissue. Baltimore: Williams & Wilkins, 1969:165–244.
46. Rees TD. The application of dermis grafts in deformities of the nose (discussion). Plast Reconstr Surg 1983; 71:782.
47. Reich J. The application of dermis grafts in deformities of the nose. Plast Reconstr Surg 1983; 71:772.
48. Roddi R, Riggio E, Gilbert PM, Vaandrager JM, van der Meulen JCH. The value of microfat injection lipofilling in the treatment of soft tissue deformities of the face in Parry-Romberg syndrome. Eur J Plast Surg 1994; 17:79.
49. Saunders MG, Keller JT, Dunsker SB, Mayfield FH. Survival of autologous fat grafts in humans and in mice. Connect Tissue Res 1981; 8:85.
50. Scarborough D, Schuen W, Bisaccia E. Fat transfer for aging skin: technique for rhytids. J Dermatol Surg Oncol 1990; 16:651.
51. Toledo LS. Syringe liposculpture: a two-year experience. Aesthetic Plast Surg 1991; 15:321.
52. Bircoll M. A nine-year experience with autologous fat transplantation. Am J Cosmetic Surg 1992; 9:55.
53. Ellis DA, Makdessian AS, Brown DJ. Survey of future injectables. Fac Plast Surg Clin North Am 2001; 9:405–41.
54. Sclafani AP, Rlomo T III. Injectable fillers for soft tissue enhancement. Fac Plast Surg 2000; 16:29–34.
55. Terino EO. Alloplastic facial contouring: surgery of the fourth plane. Aesthetic Plast Surg 1992; 16:195.
56. Terino EO, Flowers RS, eds. The Art of Alloplastic Facial Contouring. St. Louis: Mosby, 2000.
57. Maas CS, Papel ID, Greene D, Stoker DA. Complications of injectable synthetic polymers in facial augmentation. Dermatol Surg 1997; 23:871–877.
58. Erol OO. Combined techniques in face rejuvenation. Presented at the First International European Appointed XX National Congress of the Turkish Society of Plastic Surgeons, Istanbul, Turkey, September 3–6, 1998.

59. Connell BF. Surgical technique of cervical lift and facial lipectomy. Aesthetic Plast Surg 1981; 5:43.
60. Delmar H. Anatomy of the superficial parts of the face and neck. Ann Chir Plast Esthet 1994; 39:527.
61. Furnas DW. The retaining ligaments of the cheek. Plast Reconstr Surg 1989; 83:11.
62. Hamra ST. Composite rhytidectomy. Plast Reconstr Surg 1992; 90:1.
63. Hoefilin SM. The extended supraplatysmal plane (ESP) face-lift. Plast Reconstr Surg 1998; 101:494.
64. Jost G, Levet Y. Parotid fascia and face lifting: a critical evaluation of the SMAS concept. Plast Reconstr Surg 1984; 74:42.
65. Mitz V, Peyronie M. The superficial musculo-aponeurotic system (SMAS) in the parotid and cheek area. Plast Reconstr Surg 1976; 58:80.
66. Mitz V, Leblanc P, Maladry D, Aboudaram T. Results of biplane face lifts with maximal skin undermining and vertical SMAS flap. Ann Chir Plast Esthet 1996; 41:603.
67. Owsley JQ, Fiala TG. Update: lifting the malar fat pad for correction of prominent nasolabial folds. Plast Reconstr Surg 1997; 100:715.
68. Ramirez OM. Full face rejuvenation in three dimensions: a "face-lifting" for the newmillennium. Aestli Plast Surg 2001; 25:152–164.
69. Tessier P, Finiiin F, Le Pesteur J, et al. Le système musculoaponéurotique de la face et ses applications diirurgicales. Presented at the Congrés National de la Société Franchise de Chirurgie Plastique Esthétique, Paris, 1974.
70. Trepsat F. Face lifts of the malar, jugal and nasolabial area. Ann Chir Plast Esthet 1994; 39:597.
71. Trepsat F. Pathogenesis and treatment of the nasolabial fat pad: nasolabial dermolipopexy. Ann Chir Plast Esthet 1996; 41:613.
72. Little JW. Hiding the posteriors scar in rhytidectomy: the omega incision. Plast Reconstr Surg 1999; 104:259.
73. Little JW. Three-dimensional rejuvenation of the midface: volumetric resculpture by malar imbrication. Plast Reconstr Surg 2000; 105:267.
74. Guerrerosantos J. Simultaneous rhytidoplasty and lipoinjection: a comprehensive aesthetic surgical strategy. Plast Reconstr Surg 1998; 102:191.
75. Stuzin JM, Baker TJ, Baker TM. Refinements in face lifting: enhanced facial contour using Vicryl mesh incorporated into SMAS fixation. Plast Reconstr Surg 2000; 105:290.
76. Trepsat F. Volumetric face lifting. Plast Reconstr Surg 2001; 108:1358.

11 Face-Lift and Facial Rejuvenation

Abel Chajchir
Department of Plastic Surgery, Barrancas Medical Center, Buenos Aires, Argentina

INTRODUCTION

A contribution to such an important topic is a great challenge to a surgeon. After so many years of a surgical career, there are different techniques to achieve. Usually after a face-lift the patient expects a total rejuvenation. After the surgery, the weaves are in their place, but the rejuvenation is completed with the correct treatement of the skin. There is a personal approach for each surgeon.

The most important topic this chapter explains is the face volume augmentation with fat grafting, boosted with growth factors (GFs). Moreover, GF has a highly positive influence in rejuvenation of the integument, in addition to any laser effect.

I direct my technique to the deficient zone I am about to treat, although this does not mean that another surgeon may not choose a different technique for the same patient.

For patients between 50 and 65 years of age presenting photoaging, facial ptosis (jowl redundancy), platysma bands, crow's-feet, and senile orbits, I suggest the following surgical plan:

1. Endoscopic brow-lift with malar suspension.
2. Blepharoplasty. Orbicular myectomy in a triangle for the crow's-feet.
3. Midface-lift, smasectomy, and suturing.
4. Neck-lift, bands myectomy.
5. Fat graft with GF, cheeks, folds, rhytids, and lips.
6. CO_2 laser one-pass, double-pass in folds and perioral rhytids, panfacial.
7. In some patients with very thin lips, submascular aponeurotic system (SMAS) strip with GF (Figs. 1–4).

According to this pattern, we discuss with our patient the steps to follow. In case the patient does not accept the CO_2 laser application, I suggest intense pulsed light combined with dermatologic skin care.

There is a lot of published literature about endoscopic technique, SMAS treatment, and platysma plications, and how to choose and adapt these techniques to each patient. The same is true for blepharoplasty. Principally, we will focus on tissue augmentation with fat grafts in the face, malar zones, cheeks, folds, rhytids, and lips (Figs. 5 and 6).

FAT GRAFTING

We use a small cannula (author's design) with a very fine tip (5 mm) to remove the fat globules. It is connected to a polyethylene tube, which in turn is attached to a receptacle of sterile glass connected to a low vacuum motor. We also use a syringe with rings and a trocar for injecting (1 mm or less).

We use local or combined anesthesia. The donor area may be chosen from the following: abdomen, trochanter, thigh, and knee. The fat tissue is removed using the usual liposuction method from an aseptic area.

The tissue must be treated carefully to cause no injury to the delicate cells and to avoid lysis of the adiposites. The fat obtained from a liposuction by low vacuum is never washed to better preserve the tissue. The transplant will not graft when the material is crushed. This aspirate is put into the syringe and injected into the deficient zone. We combine this technique with GF, mixing them with the fat before injecting them in the same syringe, to improve nasolabial folds, malar area, cheek depressions, and chin augmentation.

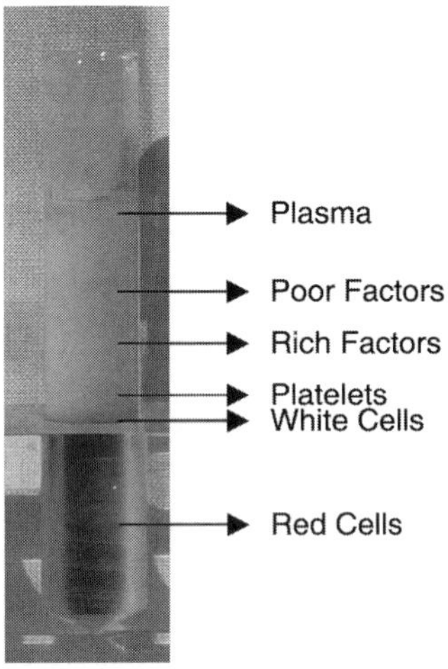

Figure 1 Separation of cells by molecular weight.

GROWTH FACTORS

The active substances that intervene in the restoration of damaged tissues are known as GF (fundamentally of the platelets), cytokines, chemokines and interleukins, tissue necrosis factor, etc. The intervening cells are the platelets, monocytes, lymphocytes (T-helper), neutrophils, and astrocytes.

The blood obtained prior to the surgical procedure is taken by an intravenous (IV) puncture, and depending on the magnitude, 20 to 60 cc or even more is needed.

Citrate 3.8%-based anticoagulants are used in the vial, we centrifuge for approximately five minutes, obtaining the separation of cells, red cells, and plasma (Fig. 1). Other authors mix the superficial part of the plasma above the platelets, called supraplasma, with calcium chloride solution (10%) and topical bovine thrombin, producing a gel for use in the surgical procedure.

We modified this technique by using, after centrifugation, the GF situated in the supraplasma. Approximately 2 cm of plasma is above the cells and is rich in GF. Another portion, 1.5 cm, has less potential and is considered to be the poorer part of the plasm. I recommend to the readers some of my literature to introduce them to the technology of GF. We start with the Anitua modified technique.

This procedure consists of the following:

1. Blood harvester.
2. Collection in a tube with sodium citrate 3.8%.
3. Centrifugation for seven minutes at 280G (Anitua procedure)—12 minutes at 300G (other authors)—We centrifuge five minutes at 350G.
4. Extraction of GF: 4.5 more minutes to collect in a sterile syringe the GF from the vacutainer.

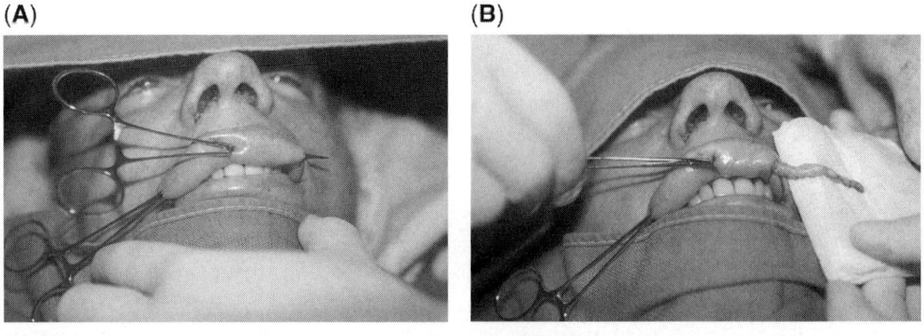

Figure 2 (**A** and **B**) Submascular aponeurotic system strip grafted into the lip.

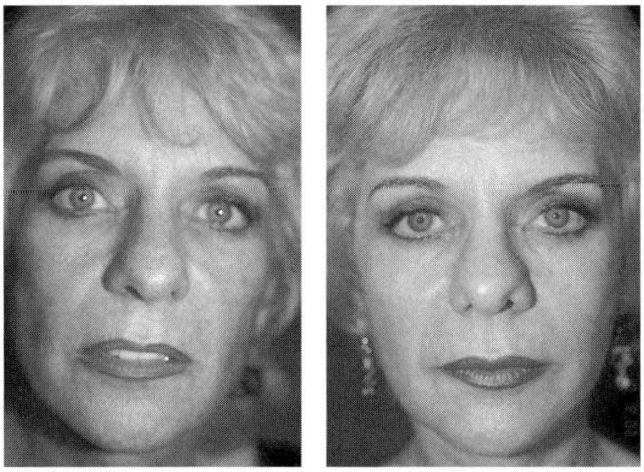

Figure 3 Preoperative and postoperative views for facial rejuvenation, with endoscopic brow-lift, blepharoplasty, one-pass CO_2 laser, and submascular aponeurotic system strip grafted in the upper lip.

5. Anitua et al. add 0.05 cc of calcium chloride (10%) for each 10 cc of GF, producing a gel mass. We do not use calcium.
6. Other authors use bovine thrombin or human thrombin. We avoid using thrombin because it can produce antibodies.
7. We use GF in a liquid form, to mix with fat graft, and introduce it by a syringe in the wounds, skin graft, or flaps.
8. Normally, we spray with a syringe on the wound surface in a face-lift in order to give better hemostasis. It prevents hematomas.

THE LASER TECHNIQUE

Long sun exposure, in addition to ozone layer damage, produces structural damage to normal skin. Injury to the dermal collagen and elastic fiber results in facial wrinkles. We have treated a large number of patients with CO_2 laser to improve their aged skin. Very few have undergone only a single procedure, and the majority have combined it with aesthetic plastic surgery and other surgical interventions.

THE HISTOPATHOLOGY

Staining with hematoxylin-eosin, periodic acid Schiff (PAS technique), orcein for elastic fibers, Mason's trichromic, and Van Gieson stain were used.

The study of the preoperative skin with hematoxylin-eosin shows an epidermis with laminar hyperkeratosis and other significant alterations. Six months later (postoperatively), the same staining procedure shows increased collagen fibers that are thin in the superficial (Fig. 7).

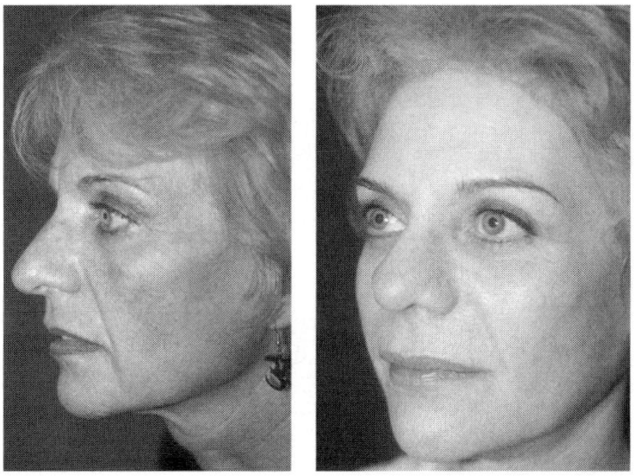

Figure 4 Same patient as in Figure 3, alternate views.

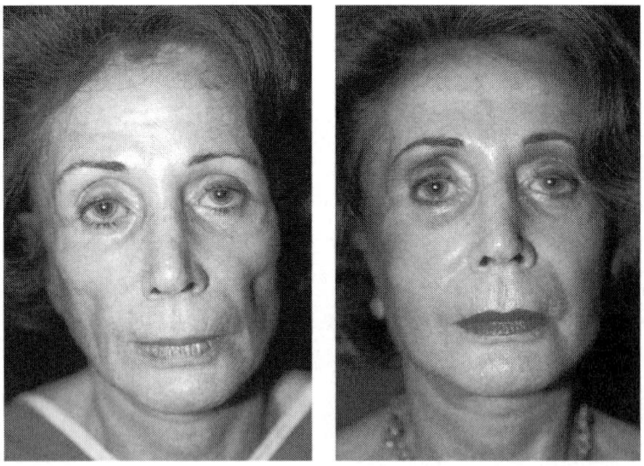

Figure 5 Preoperative and postoperative views. Face-lift, neck-lift, fat graft, and one-pass CO_2 laser.

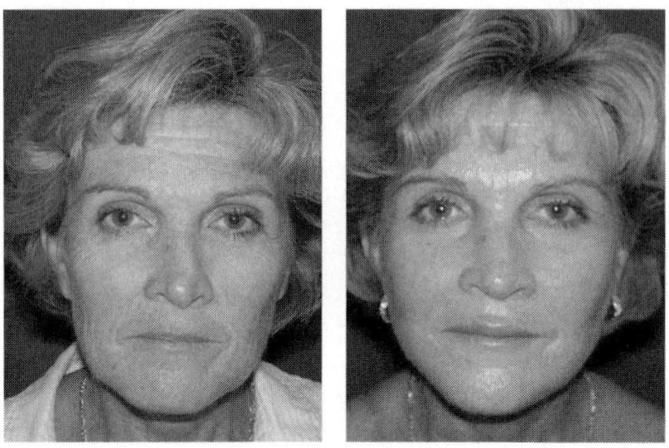

Figure 6 Preoperative and postoperative views. Endoscopic brow-lift, upper and lower blepharoplasty, reconstructive rhinoplasty, and upper lip improvement by submascular aponeurotic system strip.

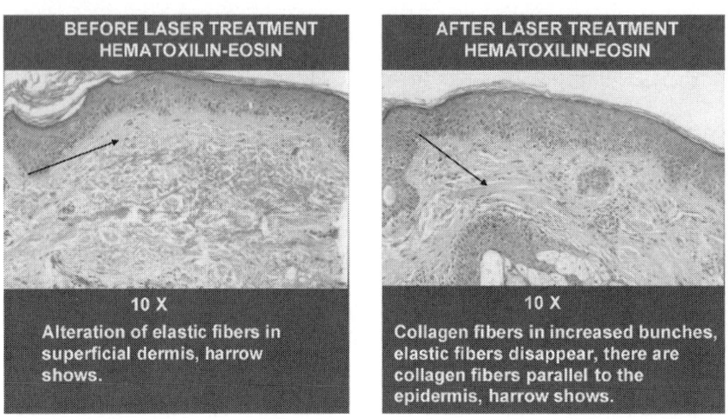

Figure 7 Histological views, before and after the treatment with CO_2 laser.

1. Panfacial treatment.
2. According to the type of skin we select intensities ranging from 18 to 26 W.
3. In the first application, shots are made through a 15 sq mm geometric pattern generator.
4. For thinner eyelid skin, only one-pass, less intensity, and a 3 to 5 sq mm geometric pattern is used.
5. For cheek folds and border of the lips, the same geometric pattern, more intensity, and a double-pass is applied.
6. The procedure takes place after face surgery, from the top of the head down to the chin. Less intensity is applied near the undermined skin. We never pass the laser on the flap.
7. A single-pass is applied and the remains of the thermal lesion are not removed. In no case are the areas wiped with wet gauze.

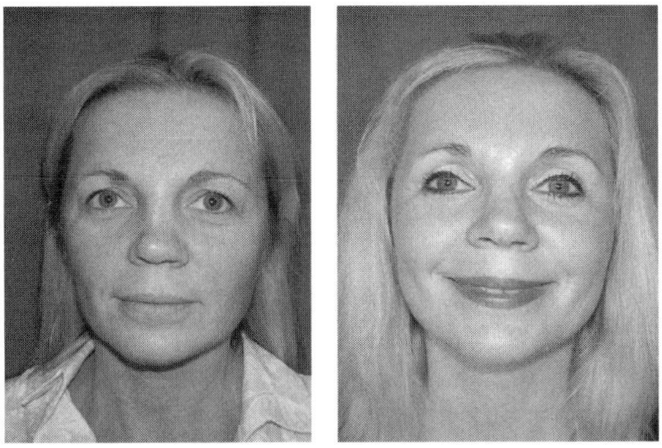

Figure 8 Preoperative and postoperative views. Endoscopic brow-lift, upper and lower blepharoplasty, repetitive reconstructive rhinoplasty, and one-pass CO_2 laser.

After analyzing patients in their preoperative period, we have observed that most of them visit us for the deep, moderate, or fine wrinkles in the perioral and periorbital regions. After laser application, we notice an evident reduction in wrinkles, which in some cases almost disappear. The skin acquires a much better aspect as dermal stains and pigmentation decrease. There is also increased skin thickness manifested in patients by a brighter and healthier looking skin.

The postoperative period is short. There have been few complaints, and they have been easily managed. Long-term results show a reduction in wrinkles in the perioral and periorbital region. This reduction is maintained for three to five years.

This procedure does not intend to totally remove wrinkles and folds, but only to improve the skin by the use of a CO_2 laser. We are in a position to assert that the CO_2 laser is one of the best methods for skin rejuvenation.

This has been proven by papers published by different authors. The single-pass of CO_2 laser produces the following:

1. Skin vaporization.
2. Collagen shrinkage and little skin tightening.
3. New collagen formation in a certain amount of time, confirmed by histopathology.
4. Less deep vaporization of the dermis.

With a photoprotection treatment for four months, we can prevent pigment disorders. In some cases of skin type Fitzpatrick IV, we suggest an earlier treatment with sunblocks. This epidermal debris in all cases is left intact as a biologic dressing. The single-pass procedure, when used as mentioned above and combined with dermatological therapy, is safe and decreases the risk of side effects. It can also allow better management in the postlaser period by improving patient comfort and accelerating recovery with satisfactory effects for both patient and surgeon. dermis (Figs. 8 and 9).

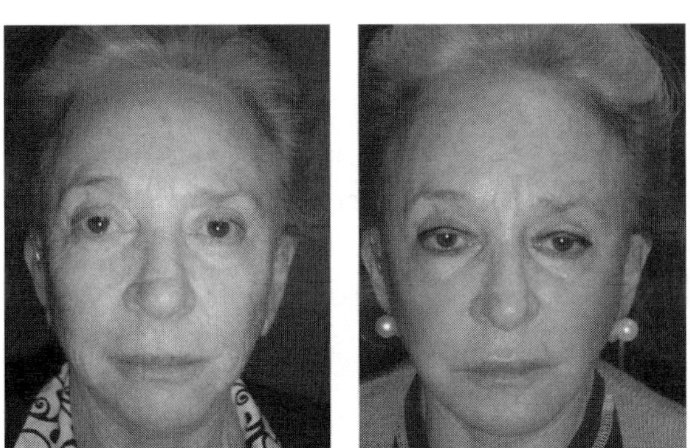

Figure 9 Preoperative and postoperative views. Face and neck-lift; fat graft with growth factor in malar zone, cheek, chin, and lips; and one-pass CO_2 laser.

BIBLIOGRAPHY

Alster TS, Apfelberg DB. Cosmetic Laser Surgery. U.S.A.: Wiley-liss, 1996.
Barton F. The "high Smass" face lift technique. Aesthet Surg J 2002; 22(5):481–487.
Bernard R. The anterior vertical Smass lift. Aesthet Surg J 2003; 23(6):486–494.
Bhanot S, Alex JC. Advances in Facial Plastic Surgery. Yale University School of Medicine, November 1, 2002.
Brown GL, Nanney LB, Griffin J, et al. Enhancement of wound healing by topical treatment with epidermal growth factor. N Engl J Med 1989; 321:76–79.
Canney PA, Dean S. Transforming growth factor beta: a promoter of late connective tissue injury following radiotherapy. Br J Radiol 1990; 63:620–623.
Chajchir A, Benzaquen I. Liposuction fat graft in face wrinkles and hemifacial atrophy. Aesthet Plast Surg 1986; 10:115–117.
Chajchir A. Fat injection: long-term follow-up. Plast Reconstr Surg 1996; 20:291–296.
Collawn SS. Re-epithelialization of the skin following CO_2 laser resurfacing. J Cosmet Laser Ther 2001; 3(3):123–127.
de Castro CC. Neck lift. Aesthet Surg J 2003; 23(3):165–169.
Eppley BL, Sadove AM. A physicochemical approach to improving free fat graft survival. Aesth Plast Surg 1991; 15:215–218.
Fisher JC. Basic biophysical principles of resurfacing of human skin by means of the carbon dioxide laser. J Clin Laser Med Surg 1996; 14(4):193–210.
Graf R. Vertical vectors in smasectomy to reshape the aging face. Aesthet Surg J 2003; 23(3):198–199.
Grossman AR, Majidian AM, Grossman PH. Thermal injuries as a result of CO_2 laser resurfacing. Plast Reconstr Surg 1998; 102(4):1247–1252.
Harding KG, Morris HL, Patel GK. Healing chronic wounds. BMJ 2002; 324:19 (www.bmj.com).
Koch RJ. Laser resurfacing of the periorbital region. Facial Plast Surg 1999; 15(3):263–270.
Lent WM, David LM. Laser resurfacing: a safe and predictable method of skin resurfacing. J Cutan Laser Ther 1999; 1(2):87–94.
Pittelkow MR. Regulation of the hair cycle and growth factor. J Cutan Aging Cosmet Dermatol 1990; 1:211–226.
Poveda M. www.diariomedico.com/cientifica. Diciembre 17, 2001.
Raines EW, Bowen-Pope DF, Ross R. Platelet-derived growth factor. In: Sporn MB, Roberts AB, eds. Peptide Growth factors and Their Receptors. New York: Springer–Verlag, 1990:173–261.
Ross EV, Miller C, Meehan K, et al. One-pass CO_2 versus multiple-pass Er:YAG laser resurfacing in the treatment of rhytides: a comparison side-by-side study of pulsed CO_2 and Er:YAG lasers. Dermatol Surg 2001; 27(8):709–715.
Shipley GD, Keeble WW, Hendrickson JE, et al. Growth and normal human fibroblasts and prokeratinocytes in serum-free medium is simulated by acids and basic fibroblast growth factors. J Cell Physiol 1989; 138:511–518.
Stuzin JM, Backer DC. Cervical contouring in face lift. Aesthet Surg J 2002; 22(6):541–548.
Tanzi EL, Alster TS. Single-pass carbon dioxide versus multiple-pass Er:YAG laser skin resurfacing: a comparison of postoperative wound healing and side-effect rates. Dermatol Surg 2003; 29(1):80–83.
Tope WD, Kageyama N. New methods in cutaneous resurfacing. Adv Dermatol 2001; 17:301–323 (Review).

12 Aesthetic Facial Contour Improvement with Microlipoinjection in Reconstructive and Aesthetic Cases

José Guerrerosantos, Fernando Guerrerosantos, and Silvia Gonzalez
Jalisco Plastic Surgery Institute and Mexico Graduate School, University Center of Health Sciences, and University of Guadalajara, Jalisco, Mexico

INTRODUCTION

Plastic surgeons can improve contour and volume of the facial soft tissues and also can augment areas of the face where the bones are not sufficiently prominent utilizing autologous fat grafts.

In our routine work of the augmentation of facial contour and volume, we utilize autologous fat grafts. In selected cases, we combine implants with autologous grafts. In this article, we will discuss mainly the utilization of autologous grafts. The tissues that we have used are fat fascia and cartilage grafts. In the last 21 years, we have operated on 3568 patients utilizing fat grafts either for reconstructive surgery or aesthetic surgery.

In 1983, we began to use fat grafts after listening to Dr. Chajchir from Argentina present his early experience as a visiting professor of the Jalisco Plastic Surgery Institute. After that we immediately began to use the procedure. Initially in the first two years we treated reconstructive surgery patients only. After we observed the success of aesthetically increasing contour and volume in these patients and also performing a research study in rats (1), we decided to start to use this procedure in aesthetic surgery cases.

The reconstructive surgery group includes patients with sequels of Parry Romberg disease, craniofacial microsomia, postsurgical and posttraumatic depressions, sequels of facial paralysis, and patients with cleft lip and palate.

Aesthetic surgery patients include facial rejuvenation, and patients who want to augment and project certain anatomical areas such as the chin, mandibular border, melolabial sulcus, and malar region. The fundamental purpose of this type of treatment has been to augment the thinned soft facial tissues.

DEMONSTRATIVE CASES

Parry Rombergs Disease and Sequels of Facial Paralysis Cases

Classification and Treatment

Before the description of each case, it is helpful to mention that in our service we classified patients with facial soft tissue atrophy into four types. Patients with mild or thinned depression are Type I and patients with moderate damage are classified as Type II. These two types are patients with damage only in soft facial tissues. Patients with damage also on the facial bones are classified Type III and are very noticeable. Severe deformities are Type IV.

We treated patients with Types I and II only with lipoinjection. Patients with Types III and IV are treated with combined procedures that include galeal flaps, dermis-fat grafts, fascia grafts, cartilage and bone grafts, and lipoinjection.

The lipoinjection procedure is very well known now by the majority of plastic surgeons, and we do several sessions of this technique in all reconstructive problems.

For the treatment of Types III and IV, we utilize galeal flaps with only fascia or with fascia and muscle, dermis-fat grafts generally harvested from the inguinal region, along with sessions of lipoinjection. In some selected cases, we utilize autologous fragmented free fascia grafts. The procedure of the galeal flap has been described by Juarez and Psillakis (2). A big flap is utilized, which is obtained on the same side as the location of the depression in Type III and IV cases. The approach consists of planning incisions on the face as follows: a preauricular one, the same as a face-lift, and on the scalp continuing the same preauricular incision and performing adequate cutting to open a wide area to design and obtain a galeal flap from the temporal, parietal, and, in some cases, occipital area (Fig. 1A). We utilize the T-inverted-shape incision on the scalp in the majority of the patients.

Undermining is performed through these incisions. The cheek or the depressed area is undermined through the preauricular incision. The procedure is exactly as we perform during a face-lift (Fig. 1E). On the scalp, incisions and undermining are carefully planned in order to get a direct view of a wide area of the galea. We calculate the exact length and thickness of the flap. When we need revascularization, we include on the flap a layer of fascia, but if we need to augment the contour and volume of the depressed area, it is important to include muscle in the galeal flap. After we perform the incisions, the scalp is undermined very carefully. We do superficial dissection to avoid damage to the superficial temporal artery and vein and to preserve vascularity of the galeal flap. At the same time, we avoid damage to the hair follicles to prevent postoperative alopecia. Galeal flaps should be planned with a shape, thickness, and length to enable rotation of the flap without tension and to improve the area and give it new vascularity (Fig. 1B).

Another surgical team should obtain a de-epithelialized dermis-fat graft from the inguinal region. With a careful suture, this graft is place over the depressed area with the fat

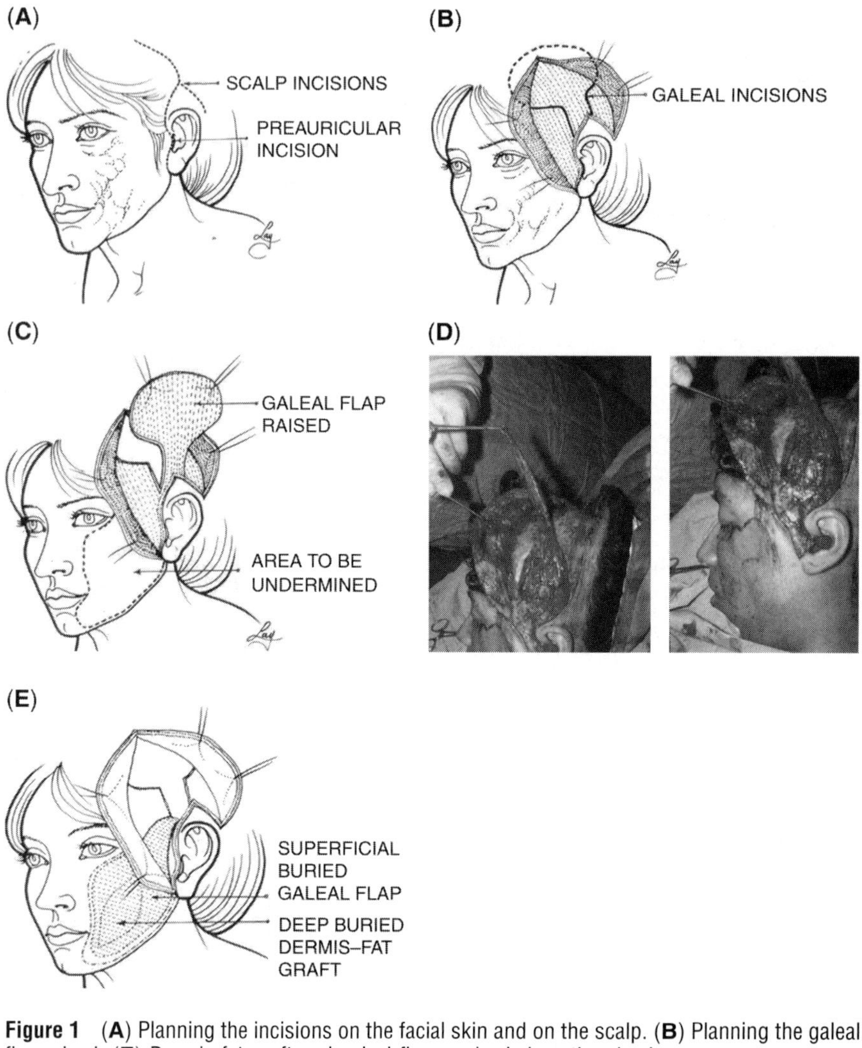

Figure 1 (**A**) Planning the incisions on the facial skin and on the scalp. (**B**) Planning the galeal flap. (**C** and **D**) Galeal flap raised. (**E**) Dermis-fat graft and galeal flap are buried on the cheek.

surface facing the SMAS (Fig. 1F). Then the galeal flap is raised (Fig. 1C–E), and introduced and placed over the denuded dermis surface of the dermis-fat grafts (Fig. 1E). Both flaps give volume and new contour to the depressed area. To fix the galeal flap appropriately, a moderate bit of muscle and fascia is taken at the distal borders of some areas of the galeal flap. The ends of each suture emerge through the skin of the cheek and mandibular area with some pulling sutures applied and tied over gauze boli (Fig. 1G). Since these sutures pull the galeal flap

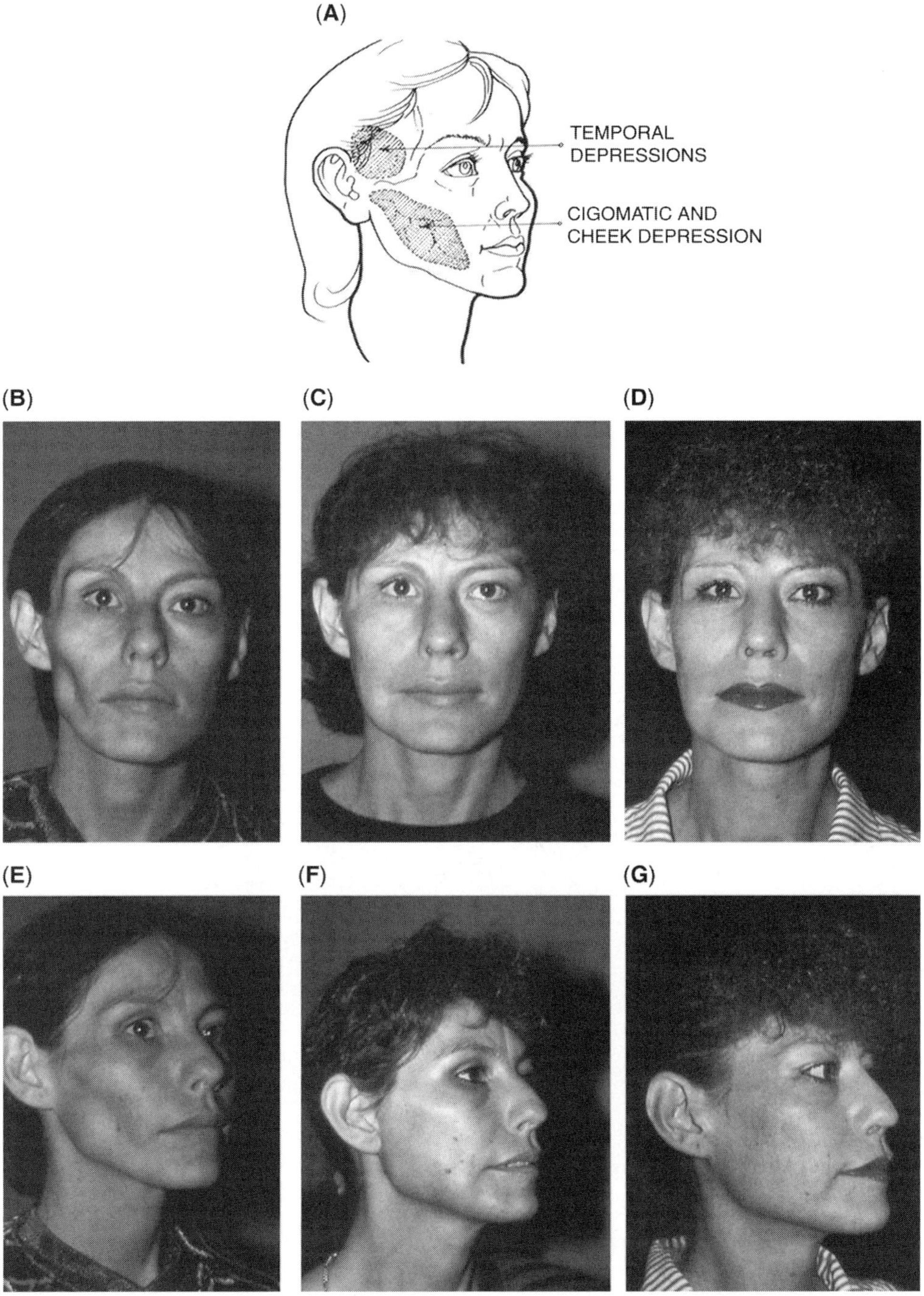

Figure 2 (**A**) Drawing showing temporal and cheek depressions. Case 1—(**B** and **E**) Patient before treatment. (**C** and **F**) Two years after the first lipoinjection and six months after the second lipoinjection. (**D** and **G**) Six years after the first lipoinjection and one year after the second one.

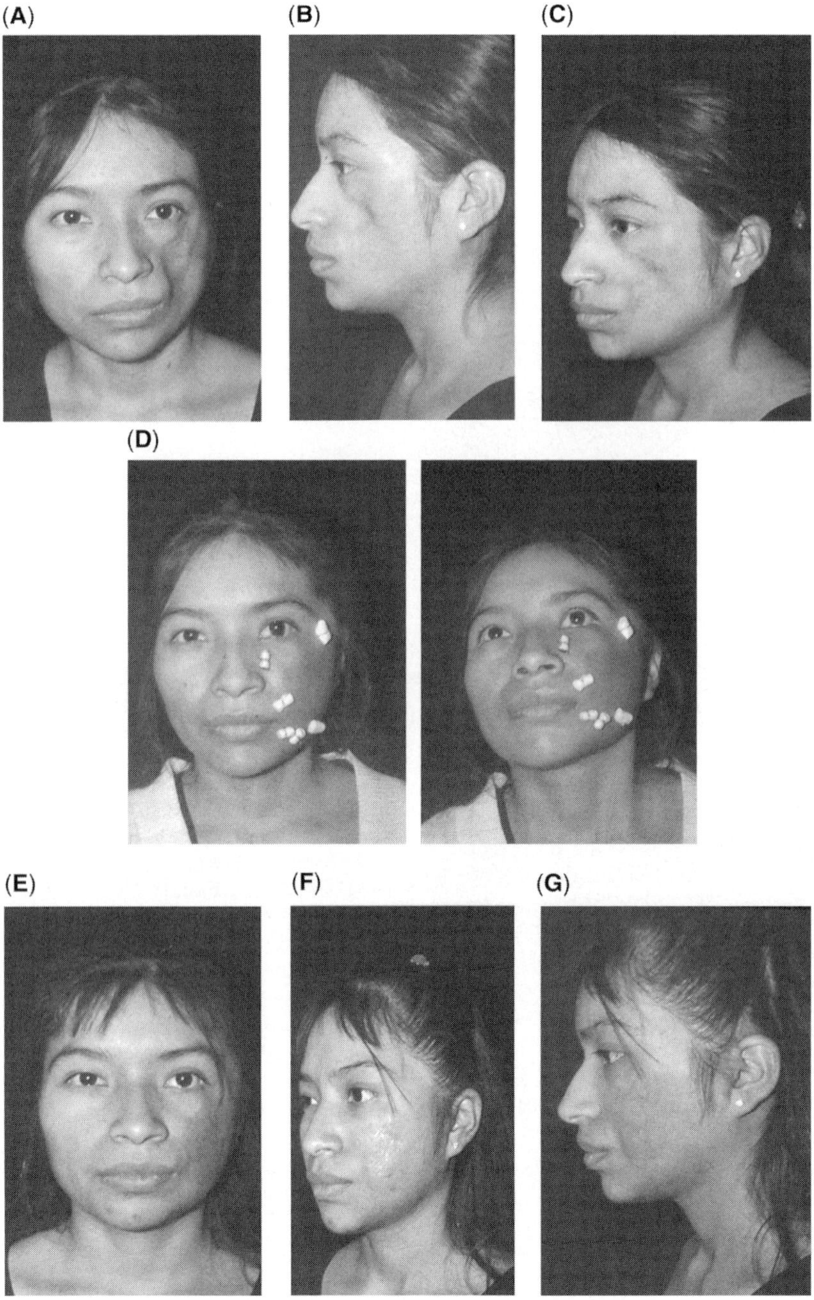

Figure 3 *Case 2*—Type III depression in Parry Romberg's Disease before treatment (**A**, **B**, **C**). (**D**) Face with pull-out Sutures fixing the galeal flap. Two years after combined treatment with great contour and volume improvement (**E**, **F**, **G**).

laterally, avoid retraction of the flap, with the purpose of preventing the formation of palpable and visible steps around the galeal flap. Lipoinjection is applied on the galeal flap and on deep soft tissues. We observe the patient periodically, and, if necessary, additional lipoinjections are performed at least every six months.

Case 1—A 27-year-old female patient with Type II soft-tissue depressions in right temporal and cheek regions (Fig. 2B and E). She developed old Parry Romberg disease at the age of 14. Consequently, atrophy of the soft tissues developed. She underwent previous treatment elsewhere without success. After an

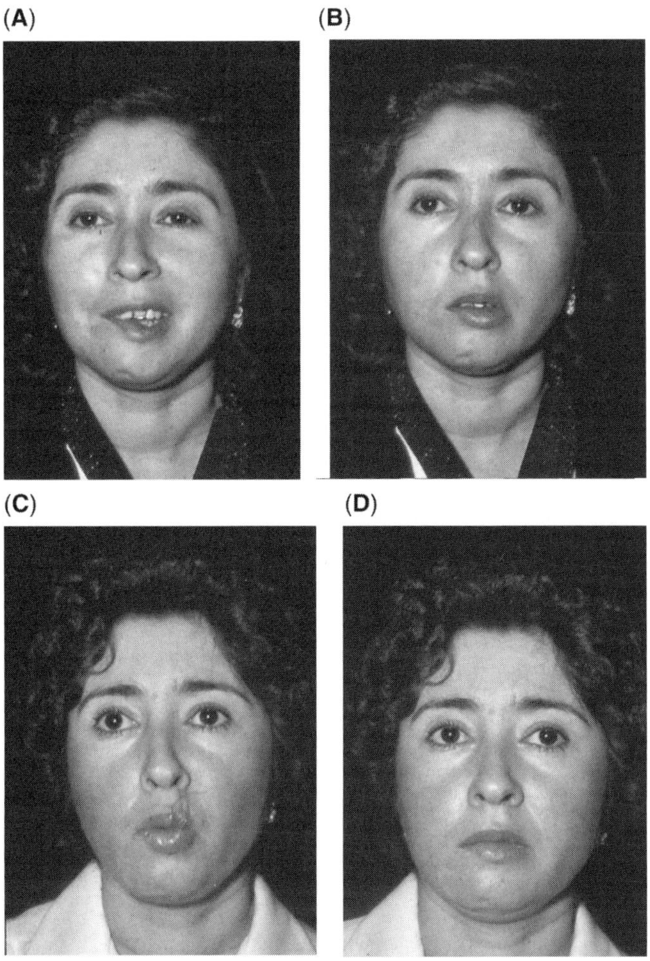

Figure 4 *Case 3*—Patient with sequels of facial paralysis including labial and facial deviation and soft tissues thinned, before surgery (**A**, **B**). Same patient two years after treatment (**C**, **D**).

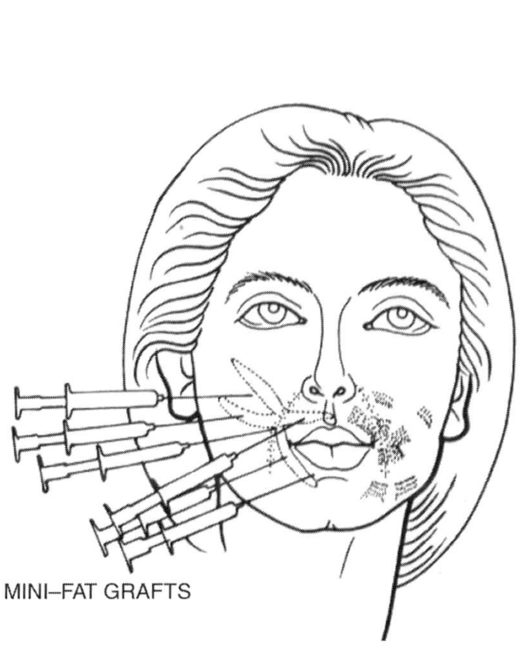

Figure 5 *Case 3*—Drawings of the combined treatment includes microlipoinjecton, removal of muscle pieces, and denuded buried facial flaps.

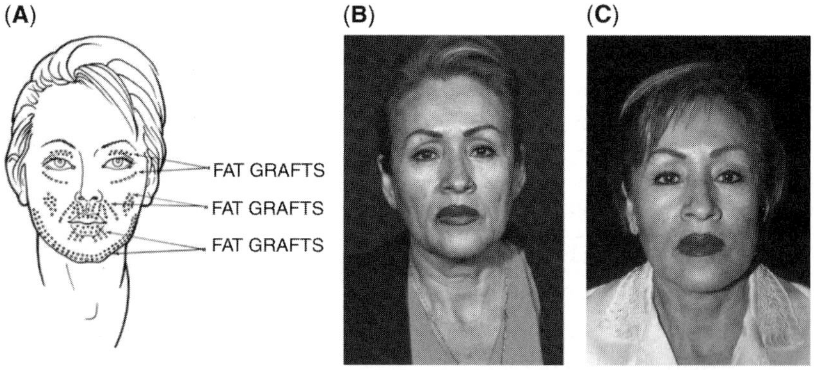

Figure 6 *Case 4*—Drawing showing areas submitted to microlipoinjection in addition to rhytidoplasty (**A**), patient before rhytidoplasty and microlipoinjection (**B**), and results at one-and-a-half years postoperative (observe the eyelid improvement) (**C**).

in-depth study of her case, we decided to perform three lipoinjection sessions. In the first one, we infiltrated 25 mL sub-SMAS in each depressed area. The second infiltration of 10 mL in each area was performed one year later. Follow-up of the patient two years after the first infiltration, and one year after the second one (Fig. 2C and F), demonstrated a very significant improvement. We performed the third infiltration with only 5 mL in each area and when examining her six years after the first infiltration, and one year after the third infiltration, the improvement was highly satisfactory (Fig. 2D and G).

Case 2—A 31-year-old female patient, presented with a severe Type III depression on the left cheek as a sequel of Parry Romberg disease (Fig. 3A, B, and C). We performed a combined surgical treatment, utilizing a well-planned galeal flap with fascia and muscle (Fig. 1), a de-epithelialized dermis-fat graft, and lipoinfiltration in two sessions, one every six months. When seeing the patient two years after the

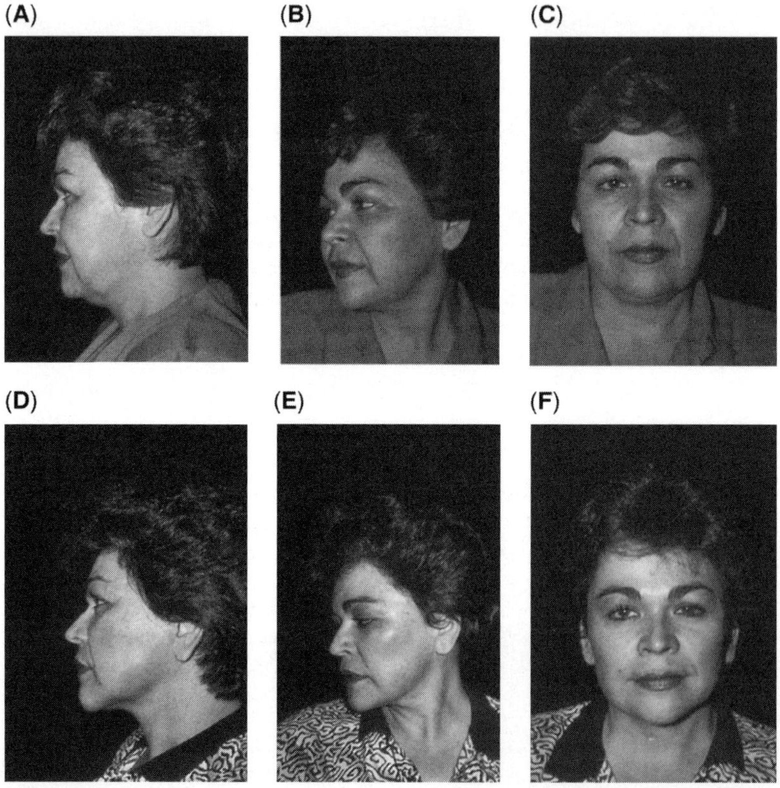

Figure 7 *Case 5*—Lateral, three-quarter, and front views of the patient before surgery (**A**, **B**, **C**). Result is shown after combined treatment two years later (**D**, **E**, **F**).

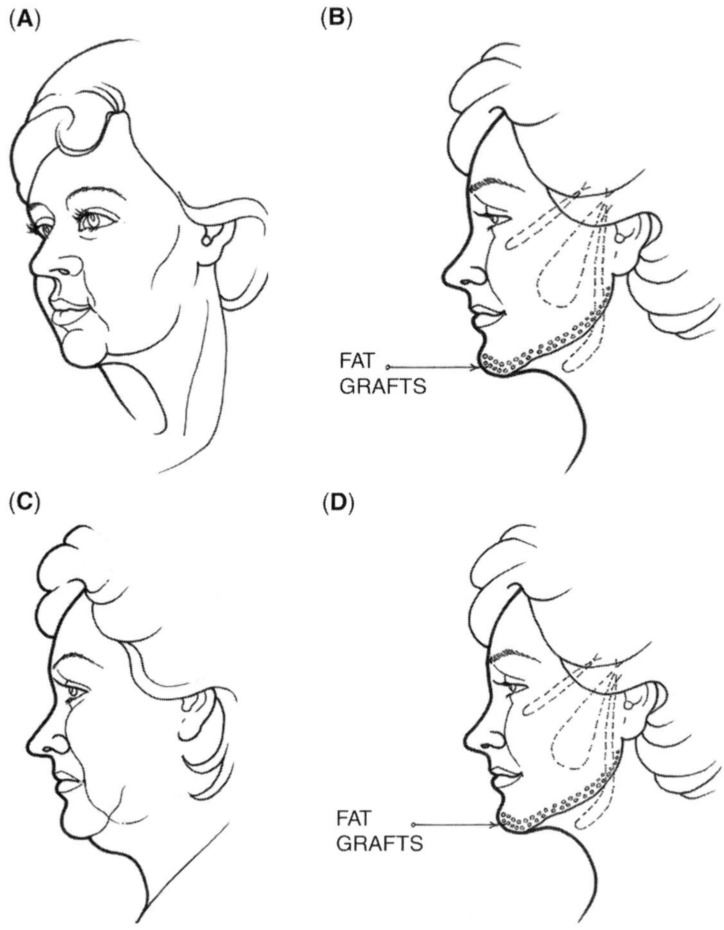

Figure 8 *Case 5*—Drawings showing rhytidoplasty, microlipoinjection, and plication suspension sutures (**A**–**D**).

treatment, we could observe a great improvement in volume, in contour, and also in the revascularization of her skin on the cheek of the affected side (Fig. 3D, E and F).

Case 3—A 33-year-old female patient with Type II tissue atrophy on the right side of her face as a sequel to facial paralysis (Fig. 4A and B). Treatment included infiltration of 40 mL of sub-SMAS fat in the depressed areas, resection of portions of 1 cm in length of normal facial muscles with movement of the left healthy side of her face, and the use of four denuded flaps raised from the right melolabial sulcus and buried in the right cheek and the right side of the upper and lower lips (Fig. 5). The patient showed great improvement aesthetically and functionally two years after treatment (Fig. 4C and D).

AESTHETIC SURGERY CASES

As previously mentioned, after being successful with the aesthetic improvement in cases with sequels of Parry Romberg disease, craniofacial microsomia, and facial paralysis, and by observing the long-term survival of infiltrated fat when it is correctly infiltrating 3-mm-wide rolls after placing the fat in well-vascularized tissue layers such as muscle, we decided in 1985 to use it in cases of aesthetic surgery after observing that increasing volume and contour of soft tissues greatly improved the patient's appearance. We will show now some demonstrative cases:

Case 4—A 57-year-old female patient who presented flaccidity and thinned facial tissues, especially sunken eyelids (Fig. 6B). We performed rhytidoplasty and microlipoinfiltration in some areas of the face and in the

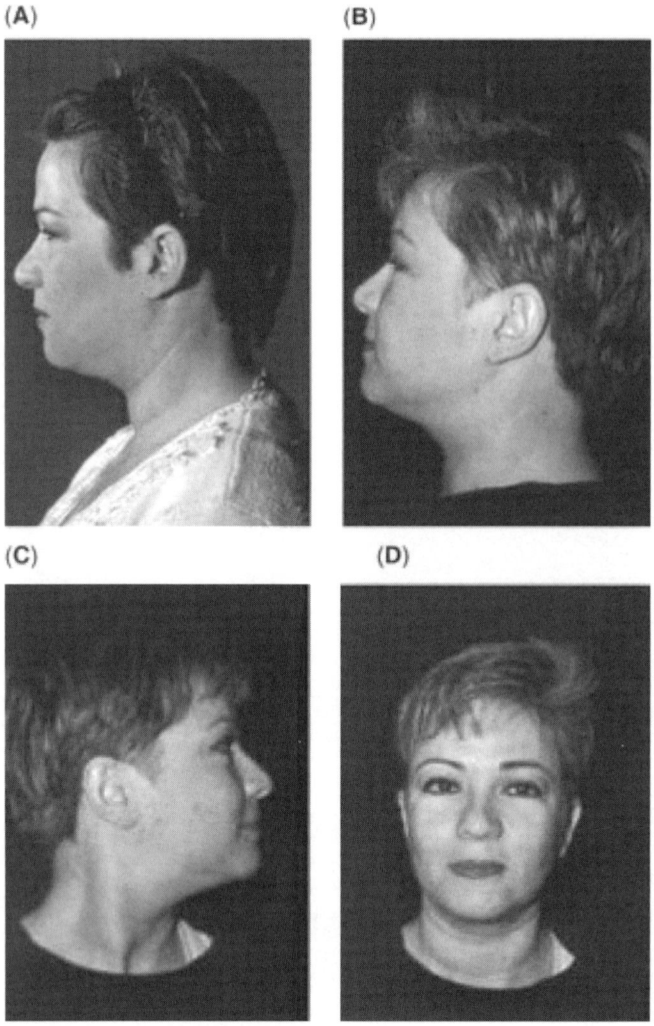

Figure 9 *Case 6*—Young female patient with submental and submandibular adiposis, poor definition of the jawline, and "low neck fat roll," before treatment (**A**, **B**, **C**, **D**). Patient one year after (**E**, **F**, **G**) and four years after treatment (**H**, **I**, **J**).

eyelids (Fig. 6A). We could observe a very favorable facial aesthetic result with correction of the face and lids, two years later (Fig. 6C).

Case 5—A 52-year-old female patient presented cervicofacial flaccidity, noticeable melolabial sulcus, lack of definition of the mandibular border, mild chin retraction, and bulky cheeks (Fig. 7A, B, and C). We performed the following procedures: cervicofacial rhytidoplasty with plication sutures, partial removal of the buccal fat pad, liposuction of the neck, and microlipoinfiltration of the melolabial sulcus, chin, and mandibular border (Fig. 8A–D). The photos show the patient before and two years later, in which we can observe the improvement of her facial features and the rejuvenation achieved (Fig. 7D, E, and F).

Case 6—A 23-year-old female patient presenting several aesthetic problems such as submental and submandibular adiposis, "low neck fat roll" with poor definition of the jawline (Fig. 9A, B, C, and D). Surgical treatment consisted of liposuction of the submental, submandibular, and low neck, and lipoinjection in the jawline (Fig. 10). When examining the patient operated on in 1996, one (Fig. 9E, F, and G) and four years later (Fig. 9H, I, and J), we could observe a very favorable aesthetic result.

(E) (F) (G)

(H) (I) (J)

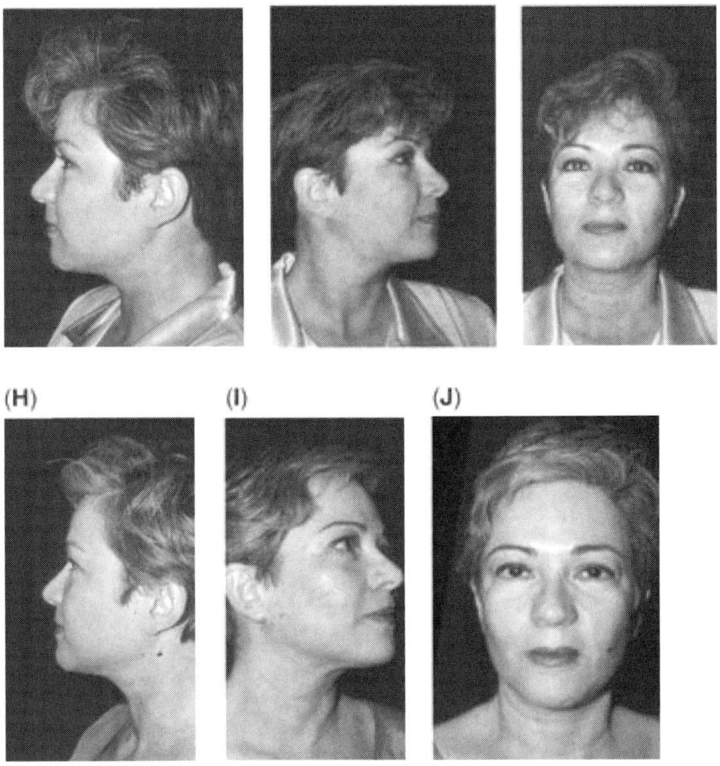

Figure 9 (*Continued*)

Case 7—A 31-year-old female patient presenting extremely deep melolabial sulcus, bulky and drooping cheek fat pad, deep "marionette groove," poor definition of the jawline, and hollow cheeks (Fig. 11A and D). As treatment, we performed surgical cheek fat pad–lifting with plication sutures (Fig. 12), and microlipoinjection of the upper lip, mandibular border, marionette groove, zygoma, and buccal fat pad compartment. The result has been excellent one (Fig. 11B and E) and two years after surgery (Fig. 11C and F).

PREBONE CONTOUR AUGMENTATION WITH MICROLIPOFILLING

Enhancing the contour and shape of the face is possible with fat autografting; we can restore, rejuvenate, and enhance facial features by thickening soft tissues adjacent to bones (3). Anatomical areas to be augmented could be chin, mandible, malar, zygoma, and paranasal area.

Clinical Cases: *Case 8*—A 31-year-old female patient with a poorly defined nose, acute nasolabial angle, retrusion of the paranasal area, and chin retraction (Fig. 13A, B, and C). Treatment consisted of performing liposuction of the neck, rhinoplasty with cartilage and fascia graft on the nasal dorsum (4), and nasal tip cartilage graft, cartilage, and fascia graft in paranasal areas (5). In the chin and the jawline, we used microlipofilling (Fig. 14A and B). When examining the patient one year later, we saw a nice improvement, especially in the chin, nose, and facial contour (Fig. 13D, E, and F).

Case 9—A 33-year-old male patient with noticeable cervical adiposity, chin retrusion, and lack of definition of the mandibular border (Fig. 15A, B, and C). We performed cervical liposuction, microlipofilling in the chin and mandibular border (Fig. 16A and B). Six months later, the patient showed an improved and different aesthetic contour (Fig. 15D, E, and F).

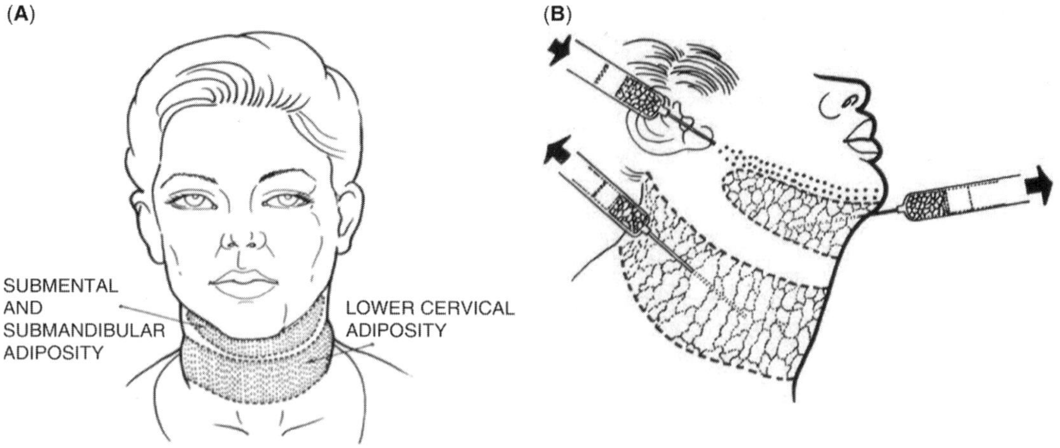

Figure 10 *Case 6*—Drawing showing the treatment of this case including liposuction of the submental and submandibular areas and "the low neck fat roll" (**A**) and microlipoinjection of the jawline (**B**).

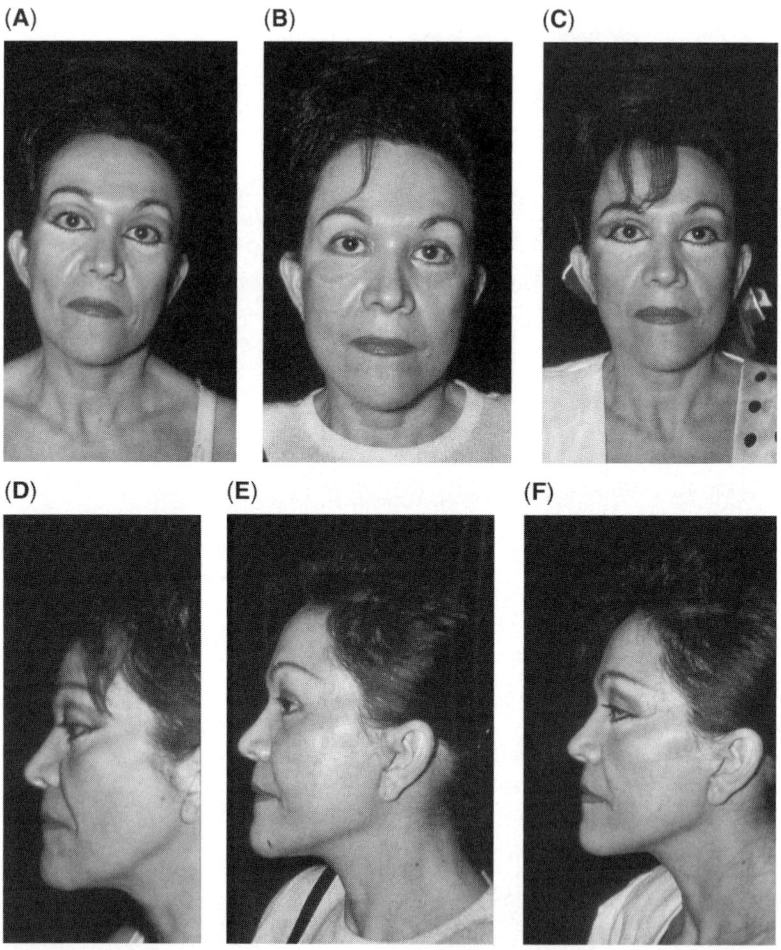

Figure 11 *Case 7*—Patient before surgery with deep melolabial sulcus, bulky and drooping cheek fat pad, noticeable "marionette grove," poor definition of the jawline, and hollow cheeks (**A**, **D**). Patient one year after surgical treatment (**B**, **E**), and two years later (**C**, **F**).

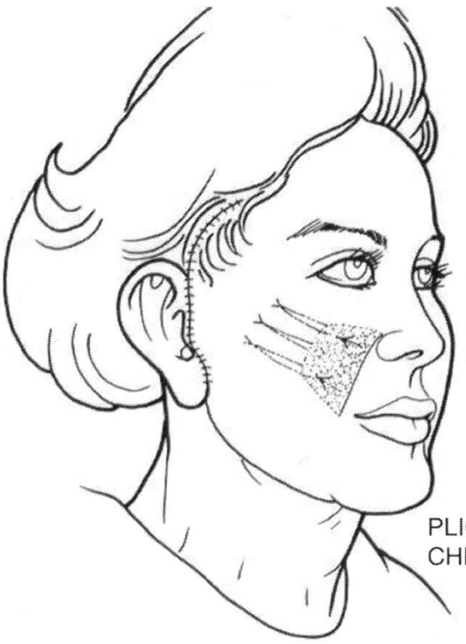

Figure 12 *Case 7*—Drawing showing the procedure utilizing cheek fat pad–lifting with plication sutures.

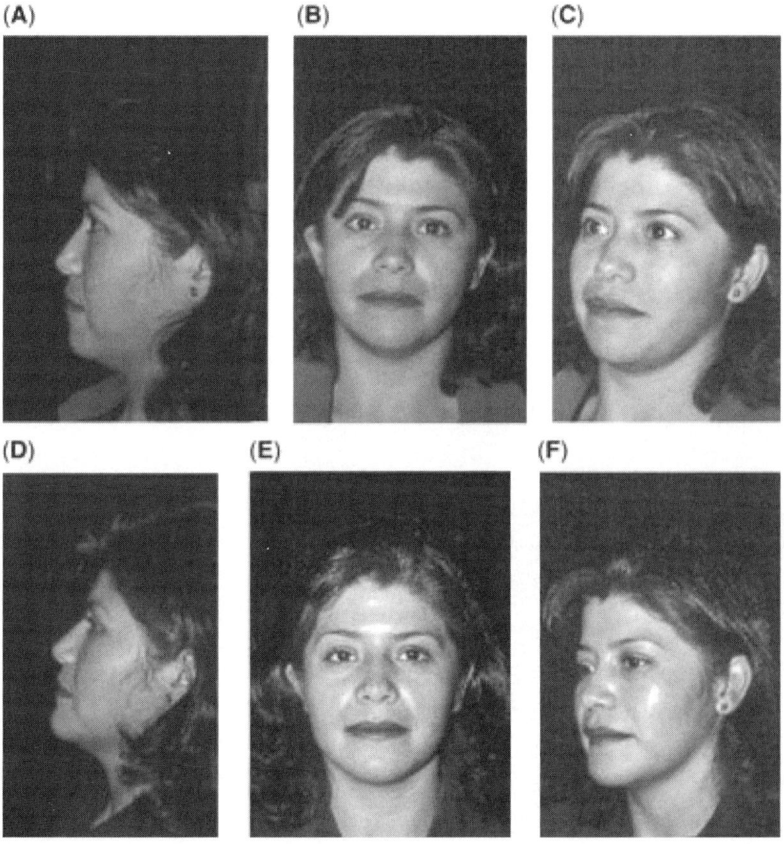

Figure 13 *Case 8*—Patient with nose with poor definition, acute nasolabial angle, retrusion of paranasal area, chin retraction, and poor definition of the jawline, before surgery (**A**, **B**, **C**). Patient one year after surgical improvement (**D**, **E**, **F**).

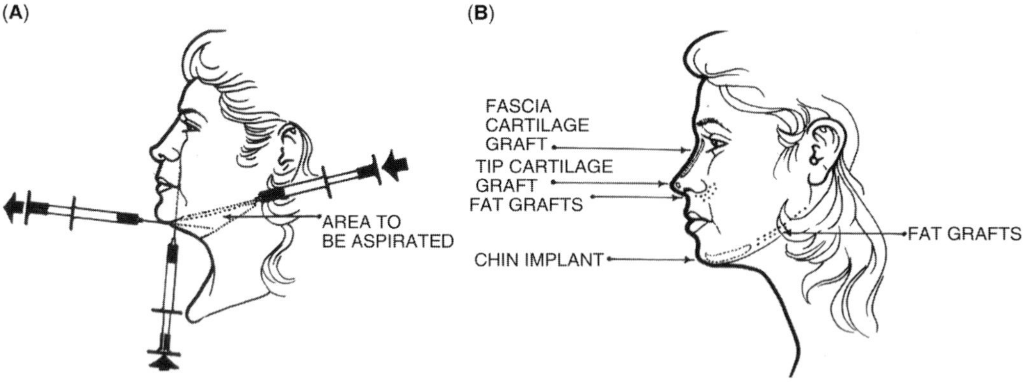

Figure 14 *Case 8*—Drawings showing neck liposuction (**A**), augmentation rhinoplasty with combined cartilage and fascia grafts, tip cartilage graft, cartilage and fascia augmentation of the paranasal area, and chin and jawline micro-lipoinjection (**B**).

Case 10—A 21-year-old female patient with flat and depressed nasal dorsum, bulky cheeks, chin retrusion, and cervical adiposity (Fig. 17A, B, and C). We performed buccal fat pad removal (10), cervical liposuction, and microlipofilling in the paranasal area, chin, and mandibular border (Fig. 18A and B). The result is shown one year later, with a significant aesthetic improvement (Fig. 17D, E, and F).

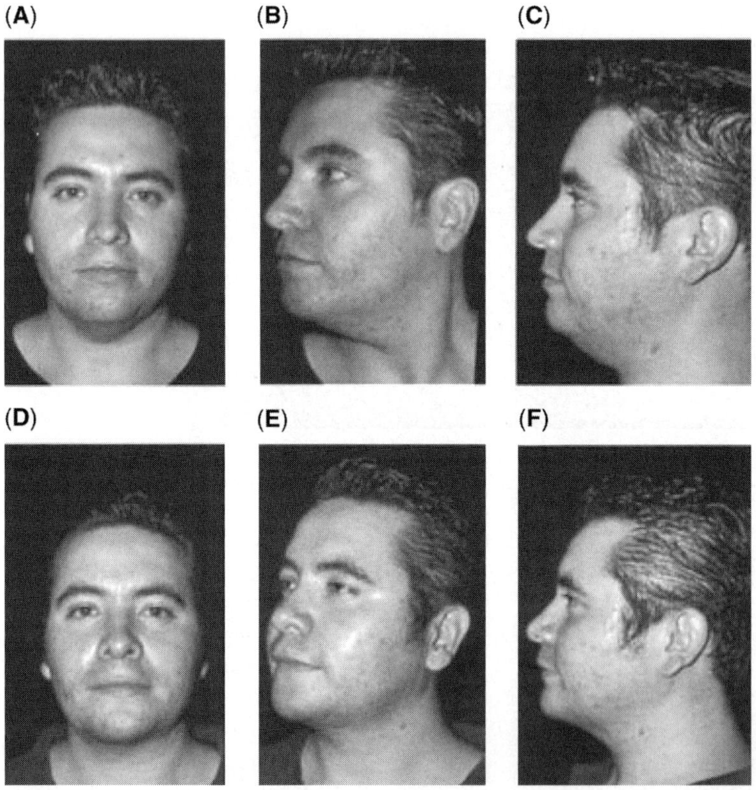

Figure 15 *Case 9*—Male patient with neck adiposity, chin retraction, and poor definition of the mandibular line (**A**, **B**, **C**). Patient six months after surgical treatment showing nice aesthetic result with new chin and mandible line definition (**D**, **E**, **F**).

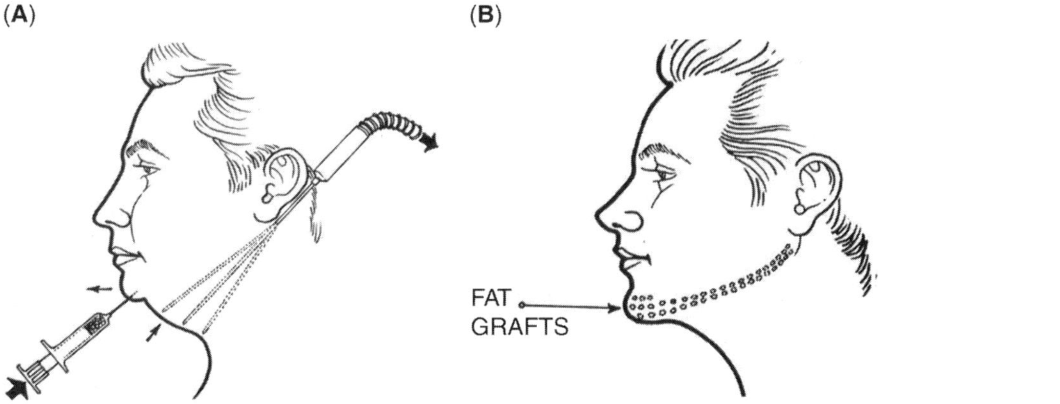

Figure 16 *Case 9*—Drawings showing the preoperative condition (**A**) and treatment utilized, including neck liposuction and chin and mandible microlipoinjection (**B**).

COMMENTS

Fat autografting has proven to be a very good technique to obtain aesthetic improvement in both aesthetic and reconstructive cases in our routine work. We have cases infiltrated with fat grafts for more than 17 years with long-lasting survival (6–9). The key to success in this procedure is to apply the fat grafts in a well-vascularized tissue and also in thin rolls in order

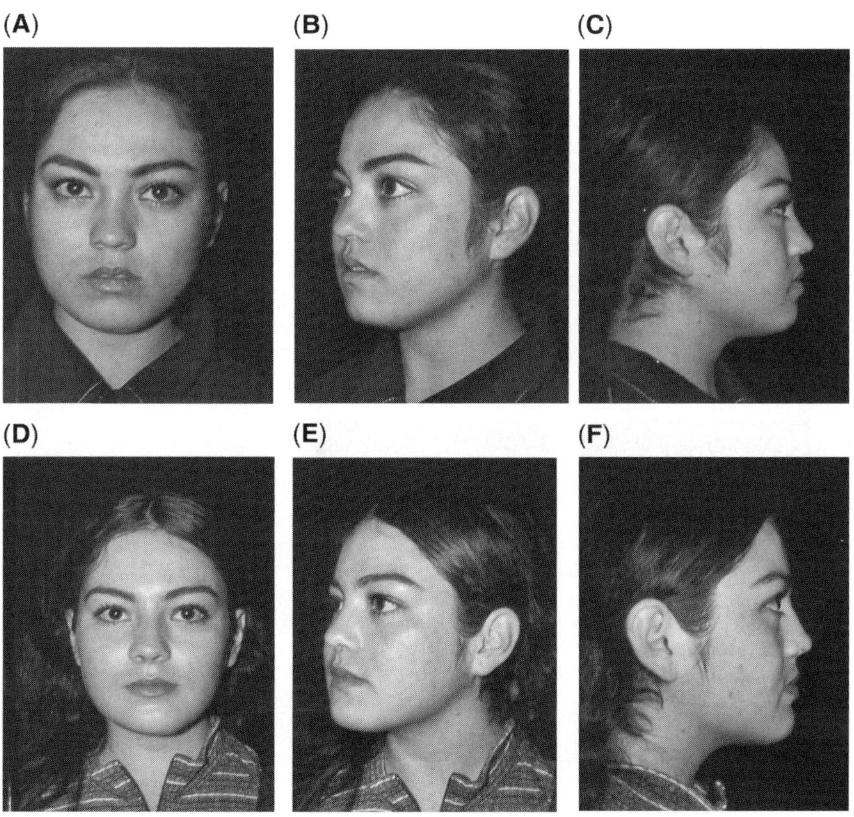

Figure 17 *Case 10*—Patient before treatment (**A**, **B**, **C**). Result is shown one year later (**D**, **E**, **F**).

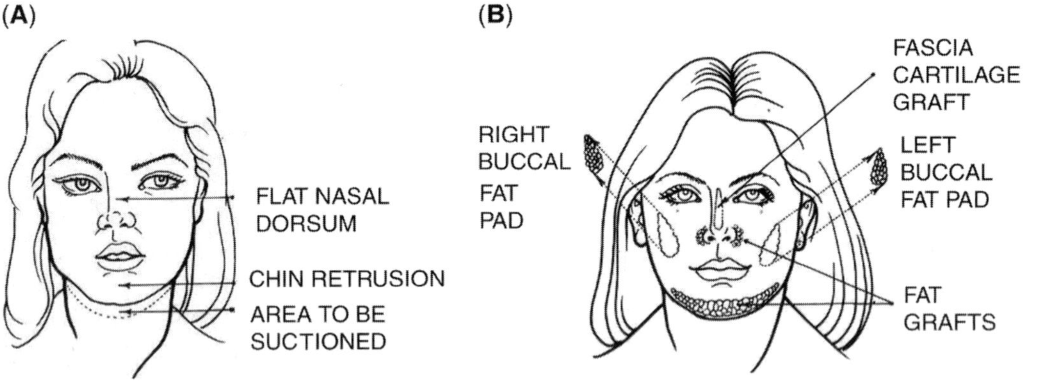

Figure 18 *Case 10*—Drawings showing flat nasal dorsum, chin retraction, chubby cheeks, and moderate neck adiposity (**A**). Treatment includes nasal dorsum augmentation with cartilage graft, bilateral buccal fat pad removal, and microlipoinjection of the paranasal areas, chin, and mandible (**B**).

to get the best revascularization. Simple instruments give similar results to those obtained with sophisticated equipment. There are many reports of various authors utilizing fat autografting with success (11–20).

REFERENCES

1. Guerrerosantos J, González-Mendoza A, Masmela Y, et al. Long-term result survival of free fat grafts in muscle: an experimental study in rats. Aesth Plast Surg 1996; 20:403.
2. Juarez JM, Psillakis JM. The use of galeal flaps in craniofacial deformities. Ann Plast Surg 1981; 6:464.
3. Guerrerosantos J, Balza I. Facial contour Aesthetic improvement with microlipoinjection. Oper Tech Plast Reconstr Surg 2002; 8:151.
4. Guerrerosantos J. Temporoparietal free fascia graft in rhinoplasty. Plast Reconstr Surg 1984; 74:465.
5. Guerrerosantos J. Nose and paranasal augmentation: autogenous, fascia and cartilage. Clin Plast Surg 1991; 18:65.
6. Guerrerosantos J, Flores M, De-Leon O. Free fat autografting cervicofacial augmentation: a 5-year study. Plast Surg Forum 1988; 11:216.
7. Guerrerosantos J. Autologous fat grafting for body contouring. Cli Plast Surg 1966; 23:619.
8. Guerrerosantos J. Simultaneous rhytidoplasty and lipoinjection. A comprehensive aesthetic surgical strategy. Plast Reconstr Surg 1998; 102:191.
9. Guerrerosantos J. Long-term outcome of autologous fat transplantation in aesthetic facial recontouring: sixteen years of experience with 1936 cases. Clin Plast Surg 2000; 27:515.
10. Guerrerosantos J. Intraoral meloplasty: a new approach for rejuvenating and recontouring the cheeks. Worldplast 1996; 1:185.
11. Aboudib JHS Jr, Cardoso de Castro C, Gradel J. Hand rejuvenescense by fat filling. Ann Plast Sur 1998; 41:503.
12. Cardenas-Camarena L, Lacouture AM, Tobar-Losada A. Combined gluteoplasty: liposuction and lipoinjection. Plast Reconstr Surg 1999; 104:1524.
13. Carraway JH, Mellow CG. Syringe aspiration and fat concentration: simple technique of autologous fat injection. Ann Plast Surg 1990; 24:293.
14. Chajchir A, Benzaquen I. Liposuction fat grafts in face wrinkles and hemifacial atrophy. Aesth Plast Surg 1986; 10:115.
15. Coleman SR. The technique of periorbital lipoinfiltration. Oper Tech Plast Reconstr Surg 1994; 1:120.
16. De la Fuente A, Tavora T. Fat injection for the correction of facial lipodystrophy: a preliminary report. Aesth Plast Surg 1988; 12:39.
17. Ellenbogen R. Free autologous pearl fat grafts in the face: preliminary report: A preliminary report. Ann Plast Surg 1986; 16:179.
18. Ersek RA, Chang P, Salisbury MA. Lipo layering in autologous fat: an improved technique with promising results. Plast Reconstr Surg 1998; 101:820–26.
19. Illiouz YG. Present results of fat injection. Aesth Plast Surg 1988; 12:175.
20. Lambros V. Fat injections for aesthetic facial rejuvenation. Aesth Surg J 1997; 17:190.

13 Neck Lift

Foad Nahai and M. Keith Hanna
Paces Plastic Surgery, Atlanta, Georgia, U.S.A.

INTRODUCTION

Volume assessment and modification is an integral part of neck lifts. Volume reduction is almost always a component of neck lifts in contrast to other areas of facial rejuvenation that commonly involve volume enhancement. A critical factor in achieving good results is preoperative assessment of volume in the three planes of the neck (superficial, intermediate, and deep) and the proper intraoperative techniques necessary to modify volume in each of these planes. These areas of possible volume modification include subcutaneous fat, fat between the platysma muscles, platysma muscles, subplatysmal fat, digastric muscles, and submandibular glands. We believe that the most common error in neck recontouring is over-reduction of volume in the superficial (subcutaneous) plane in an attempt to improve or disguise volume problems in the intermediate or deep planes. The hesitancy of some surgeons to operate in the deeper layers of the neck may lead to suboptimal results.

This chapter serves to review neck anatomy pertinent to neck-lift procedures as well as systematic preoperative and intraoperative assessment to evaluate the different components of neck volume from each of the different planes of the neck. The procedures for volume modification in the neck range from simple liposuction to a full open neck lift with tangential excision of the anterior digastric muscle, partial submandibular gland excision, and platysmal plication.

PERTINENT ANATOMY

Necks vary in anatomic structure and in response to aging. Each neck should be assessed individually in order to optimize the outcome. We assess the neck in three planes—superficial, intermediate, and deep. The superficial plane is between the skin and the platysma and includes the subcutaneous fat. The intermediate plane consists of the platysma muscles and the interplatysmal fat. The deep plane beneath the platysma contains the subplatysmal fat, the digastric muscles, and the submandibular glands. The amount of fat in these three planes, as well as digastric muscle hypertrophy and submandibular gland ptosis or hypertrophy, all may affect the overall volume and appearance of the neck. Careful examination of a patient's neck, considering these planes, is performed in order to select the appropriate surgical options and to prepare a preoperative plan, which will maximize the postoperative result (Fig. 1).

Fat

All three planes of the neck contain fat. The subcutaneous fat within the superficial plane can vary in thickness with differences in a patient's anatomy and weight. There is usually more accumulation of fat in the submental area that may extend into the intermediate plane between the platysma muscles depending on the degree of platysmal decussation. This interplatysmal fat will occasionally contain a lymph node. The deep plane fat is located deep to the platysma muscle but superficial to the digastric muscles and submandibular glands. Subplatysmal fat resection should always be performed by direct excision, not suction. It can be performed safely with care taken to avoid anterior neck veins within the fat. Significant change in neck contour can be obtained by reducing the volume of fat within these three different planes. The most dramatic effect, however, results from removal of fat that is below the skin.

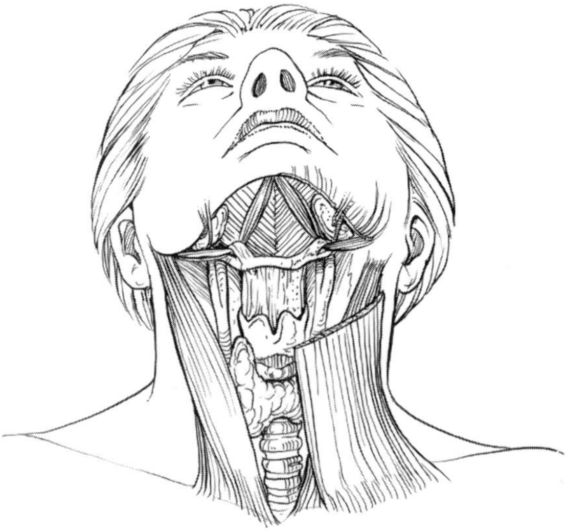

Figure 1 Planes of the neck. The superficial plane is between the skin and the platysma and includes the subcutaneous fat. The intermediate plane consists of the platysma muscles and the interplatysmal fat. The deep plane beneath the platysma contains the subplatysmal fat, the digastric muscles, and the submandibular glands.

Muscles

The platysma muscles are bilateral, thin sheets of muscles extending from the face down the neck to the clavicles, separating the planes of the neck into superficial and deep. Platysmal anatomy varies in the submental area, as classified by Cardoso de Castro into three types in relation to midline muscle decussation:

- Figure 2: Type I (75%)—decussation of the platysma muscles 1–2 cm below the mandibular symphysis.
- Figure 3: Type II (15%)—decussation of the platysma muscles from the mandible symphysis to the thyroid cartilage.
- Figure 4: Type III (10%)—no decussation.

The absence of decussation of the platysma muscles in the majority of individuals is demonstrated by visible platysmal bands. Retaining ligaments, as described by Stuzin, which hold the platysma to the deep cervical fascia, can attenuate with aging and cause platysmal descent, resulting in an oblique cervical angle. The increased obliquity of the cervical angle accentuates the appearance of increased volume in the neck. Plication of the platysma medially and laterally serves to make the cervical angle more acute and thereby decreases the apparent volume in the neck. Platysmal tightening has a significant effect on neck contouring.

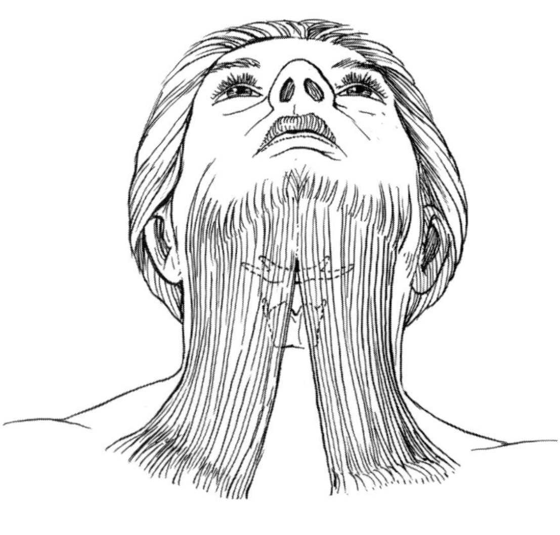

Figure 2 Platysma anatomy. Type I (75%)—decussation of the platysma muscles 1–2 cm below the mandibular symphysis.

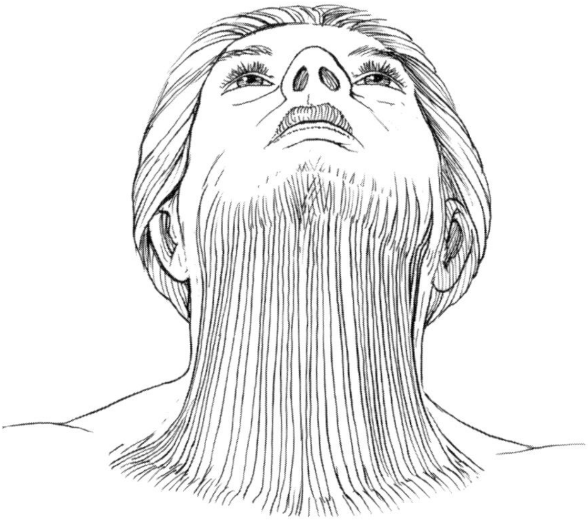

Figure 3 Platysmal anatomy. Type II (15%)—decussation of the platysma muscles from the mandible symphysis to the thyroid cartilage.

The anterior belly of the digastric muscle is occasionally modified during neck lifts. This muscle forms one side of the submental triangle that contains the submandibular gland, facial artery and vein, lingual nerve, and marginal mandibular branch of the facial nerve. The other two sides of the submental triangle are formed by the posterior belly of the digastric muscle and the ramus of the mandible. Debulking of the anterior belly of the digastric (partial digastric myectomy) is relatively safe and bloodless (Fig. 5).

SUBMANDIBULAR GLAND

Lying within the submental triangle, the submandibular gland is in close proximity to important anatomic structures that the surgeon must be aware of. The facial artery crosses superficial to the posterior portion of the gland, and the marginal mandibular branch of the facial nerve also runs superficial to the gland. As all of these structures are external to the capsule of the submandibular gland, intracapsular resection is the safest approach. Extracapsular dissection or dissection beyond the superficial lobe of the submandibular gland is more likely to result in nerve injury or vascular injury with profuse bleeding (Fig. 5).

PREOPERATIVE PLANNING AND ASSESSMENT

Detailed evaluation of the neck is essential, as is choice of appropriate procedures, to produce optimal outcomes. Volume assessment is the most crucial part of the preoperative

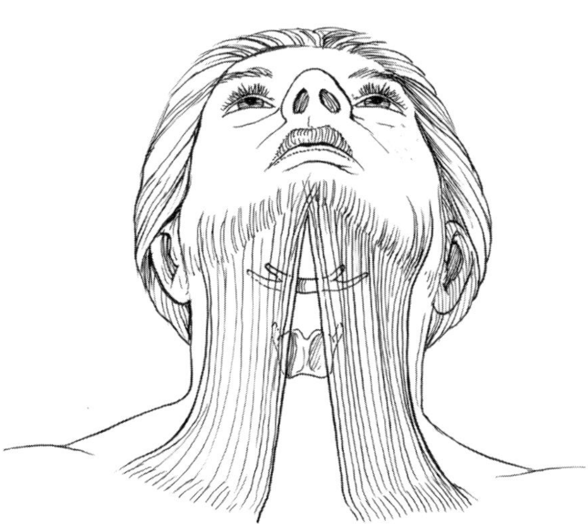

Figure 4 Platysmal anatomy. Type III (10%)—no decussation.

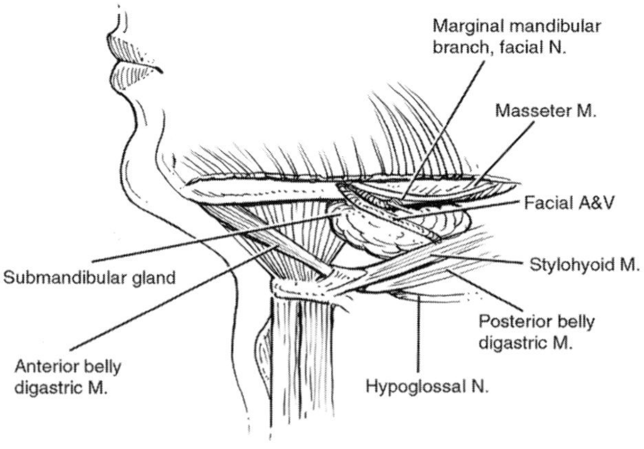

Figure 5 Submental triangle.

examination, because volume modification results in the most dramatic and lasting change in neck contour. In order of importance we evaluate the fat, the muscles, the submandibular gland, the skin, and the interface of the neck and face. The fat, muscles, and submandibular glands are the structures that contribute to volume in the neck, which will be discussed below.

Fat reduction, by far, has the most impressive and profound effect on neck recontouring. Thus, the importance of accurately determining the location of fat in the neck, whether only subcutaneous or also between and beneath the platysma muscles, cannot be overstated. Subplatysmal and subcutaneous fat can be differentiated on physical examination by pinching the submental area with the patient at rest and during platysmal contraction. If the same amount of fat is pinched at rest and during contraction, then most of the fat is in the superficial plane and subcutaneous fat removal or liposuction may be all that is needed. However, if the amount of pinchable fat diminishes with muscular contraction, then a significant portion of fat is located deep to the platysma muscle and an open procedure is indicated for direct excision of fat from this deep plane.

The platysma and digastric muscles are evaluated prior to any neck-lift procedure. The platysma is assessed at rest and during animation for banding and platysmal descent. Platysmal descent exaggerates the appearance of increased volume, and if present plication of this muscle should be planned. Evaluation of the digastric muscles may not always be possible preoperatively, particularly in thick necks. The best way to assess the digastrics is intraoperatively after subcutaneous fat removal. Partial excision of the digastric muscles may be indicated if a bulge in the neck is observed during flexion of the neck. Transcutaneous visibility of the digastric muscles is more common in secondary neck lift patients, usually due to the overresection of subcutaneous fat during the first procedure.

A bulge within the submental triangle may be observed on physical examination, indicating submandibular gland ptosis or hypertrophy. However, this may not be perceptible in the thick neck, and a plan for intraoperative assessment should be made to determine the need for submandibular gland modification.

After thorough assessment of the neck has been performed, planning of the operative approach is made. Liposuction in the superficial plane is the procedure of choice if only subcutaneous fat excision is required. The need for platysmal plication necessitates intervention in the intermediate plane. The deep plane must be addressed if modification of the subplatysmal fat, digastric muscles, or submandibular glands is needed. Frequently, intervention in all three planes is necessary.

PROCEDURES

Liposuction

Liposuction only is best for patients who have superficial excess fat localized in the submental area with normal skin tone. These patients are usually young. Liposuction in the superficial plane significantly improves neck contour but relies on healthy skin elasticity for redraping. Careful evaluation of these patients for subplatysmal fat and platysmal banding should be performed, and if present an open procedure would be required for intervention in the intermediate and deep planes of the neck.

Neck liposuction can be performed under local or general anesthesia; however, general anesthesia is preferred if multiple additional procedures are planned in conjunction with the liposuction. Positioning of the patient on the operating table is supine with full neck extension. The access incision should be placed in the submental area with the possibility of additional incision behind each earlobe. The neck is infiltrated with approximately 100 mL of wetting solution consisting of Ringer's lactate with 1 mg of epinephrine and 250 mg of lidocaine per liter of fluid. Liposuction is delayed for 12 to 15 minutes after infusion in order to allow time for the full vasoconstriction effect of the epinephrine.

Ultrasonic-assisted liposuction (UAL) and suction-assisted liposuction (SAL) are suitable for the neck. For UAL a short 2- or 3-mm-diameter solid probe is used for no longer than two to three minutes at a setting of 50% to 60% energy on the Mentor contour genesis device. Aspiration of the neck follows with a flat 2- or 2.5-mm single-hole cannula with the hole always towards the deep surface and never towards the dermis. The cannula is slowly moved by fanning out from the submental incision, taking care not to pass more than one or two times in each tunnel made by the cannula. Repeated passes in the same tunnel will result in overresection and postoperative irregularities. Separate incisions behind the earlobes are made if the lateral neck or jawline requires suctioning. Dressing includes compression of the neck with an elastic garment or foam tape; however, no drains are required.

Postoperative irregularities are avoided by leaving at least 3–5 mm of subcutaneous fat on the deep surface of the skin. If a layer of fat is not left under the skin, the dermis will adhere to the platysma and result in tethering and irregularities. Excessive liposuction in the superficial plane of the neck to camouflage deep plane volume problems is a common error and very difficult to correct. Occasionally, aggressive liposuction in the neck will reveal prominent digastric muscles or platysmal bands, which can only be addressed with an open procedure.

Case 1 is a 44-year-old patient who was evaluated to have a significant amount of excess fat superficial to the platysma. This was determined by pinching the submental area at rest and during platysmal contraction. No platysmal banding was identified and the patient had normal skin tone, therefore was felt to be a good candidate for liposuction only. UAL was performed with a short 2-mm-diameter solid probe at a setting of 50% energy, then evacuation was completed with SAL. As can be seen in the postoperative photos (two months' postop), much improvement in the cervicomental angle can be obtained with liposuction only in the appropriate patient.

Submental Neck Lift

The submental neck lift may be performed alone or in conjunction with a face-lift. It consists of a submental incision, variable neck undermining, and intervention in all three planes of the neck as needed. We prefer general anesthesia for this procedure. The patient is placed on the operating table in the supine position with the neck extended. A dilute solution of 0.5% xylocaine with epinephrine 1:200,000 is infiltrated into the neck and adequate time is allowed for the epinephrine effect. A 3- to 5-cm incision is then made just posterior to the submental crease, and dissection under the crease is performed to release it from its underlying attachments. The mandibular ligaments may be released by carrying this dissection anterior and lateral.

The next step is subcutaneous defatting, which is preferably done under direct vision rather than by liposuction. The skin, with a 3- to 5-mm layer of fat, is elevated from the underlying tissue using scissors, dissecting towards the thyroid cartilage and laterally as needed. The remaining submental fat on the superficial surface of the platysma is then resected (Fig. 6).

If intervention in the deep plane of the neck is planned, the platysma is elevated bilaterally and any amount of fat between or deep to this muscle is excised. Excellent exposure to the submental space is obtained by retraction on the medial borders of the elevated platysma muscles (Fig. 7).

At this point, the anterior belly of the digastric muscle is easily seen and can be excised partially, totally, or plicated in the midline to reduce neck volume. Partial tangential excision is accomplished by placing a hemostat halfway through the thickness of the muscle at its

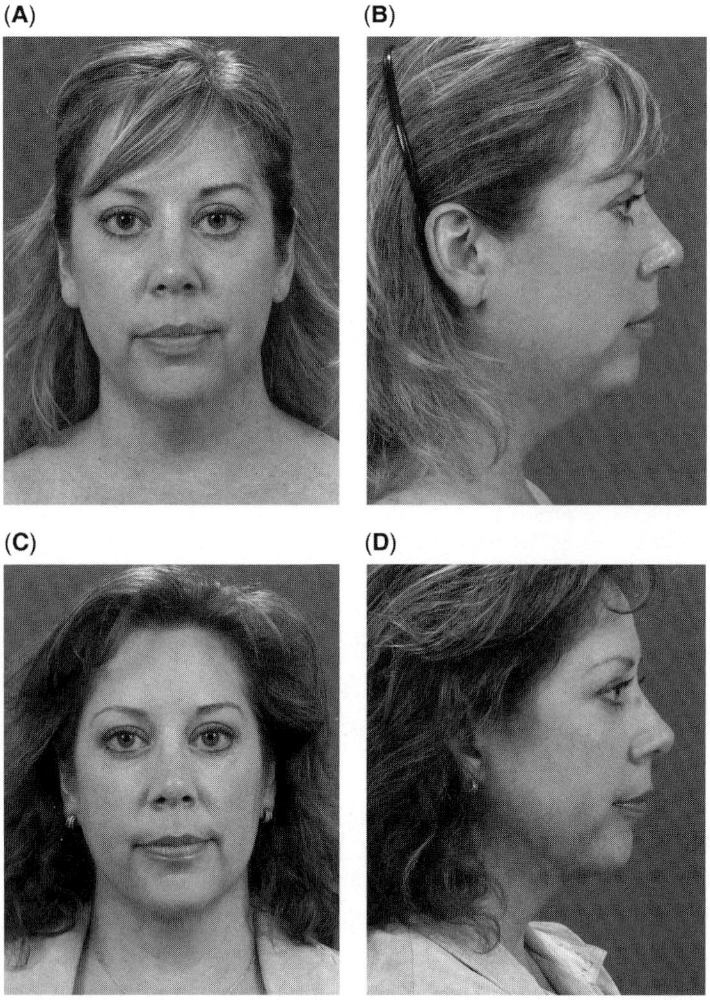

Case No. 1 Liposuction-only [preop, (**A**); preop lateral, (**B**); post-op, (**C**); and post-op lateral, (**D**)].

anterior end. The muscle is then divided with electrocautery between the tips of the hemostat, and tangential excision is performed by continuing the dissection posteriorly to the tendinous junction (Fig. 8).

With the digastric muscle being reduced, an enlarged submandibular gland may be seen. The key to safe partial resection of the submandibular gland is to incise the capsule and perform an intracapsular resection in a piecemeal fashion. This will reduce the risk of bleeding and nerve damage. An Allis clamp or 3–0 suture is used to pull the gland into view, with the needle tip cautery of the capsule is incised, and piecemeal resection is performed. The neck is flexed prior to and intermittently during the resection to assess neck contour and to avoid an unattractive depression because of overresection. Detailed knowledge of the anatomic structures associated with the submandibular gland is extremely important.

Once all of the structures contributing to the true volume in all three planes of the neck have been addressed, the platysma muscles are plicated in the midline to contour the neck further and correct banding. Anterior platysmaplasty is performed from the mentum to the superior portion of the thyroid cartilage in one to two rows of permanent suture in an interrupted fashion with the knots buried. The patient's neck should be at a 90° angle or less during this plication to reduce tension (Fig. 9).

Finally, the skin of the neck is dissected laterally until it can be effectively redraped. Contour irregularities are treated with direct fat excision or liposuction. A suction drain is placed in the neck and the skin is closed in layers and the dressings applied.

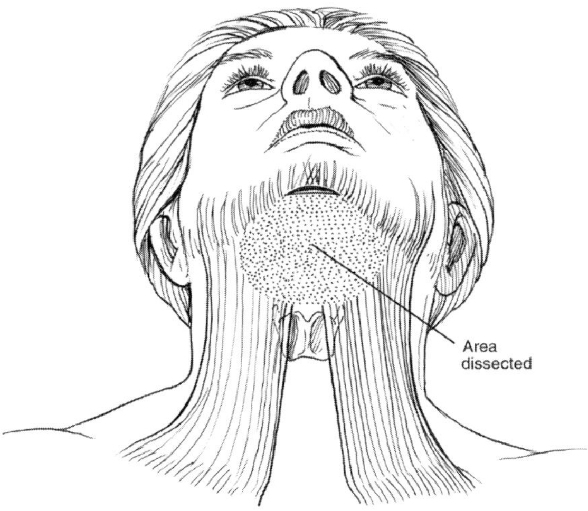

Figure 6 Area of subcutaneous fat excision.

The submental neck lift can be performed in conjunction with a short-scar face-lift or a full-scar face-lift. The short-scar face-lift is best in a patient with jowls and aging of the neck–face interface without neck skin excess. Patients with aging of the face and neck with inelastic and excessive skin of the lower and posterior neck require a full-scar face-lift, so that inelastic excess skin can be removed.

Case No. 2 is a 50-year-old patient who underwent a neck lift with submental lipectomy and platysmal plication. No subcutaneous fat was excised in this patient, only fat deep to the platysma was removed. Intraoperative evaluation of the deep layer of the neck revealed no need for modification of the digastric muscles or the submandibular gland. The postoperative photos (18 months' postop) demonstrate an improvement in the cervicomental angle. Of note, other simultaneous procedures performed included face-lift, secondary upper and lower blepharoplasties, cheek-lift, and Erbium laser resurfacing of the nose, glabella, and perioral area.

Case No. 3 is a 60-year-old patient who had a neck lift with submental lipectomy, tangential excision of the digastric muscles, and platysmal plication. Intraoperative examination of the deep layer of the neck showed enlarged bilateral digastric muscles. There was also no need for modification of the submandibular glands. Postoperative photos (two years' postop) illustrate the improvement in neck contour and volume. This patient also had an endoscopic forehead-lift, upper and lower blepharoplasties, midface-lift, face-lift, autologous fat transfer

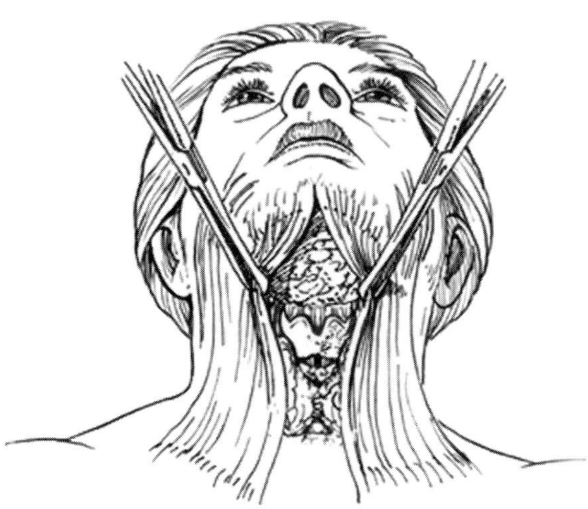

Figure 7 Elevation of the platysmal muscles bilaterally for access to the submental space.

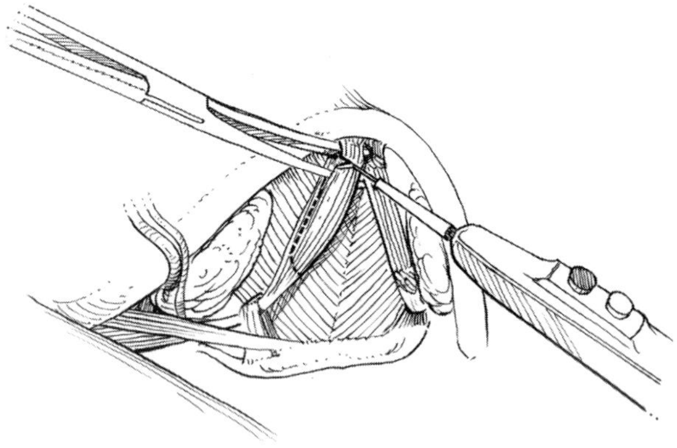

Figure 8 Partial tangential excision of the anterior belly of the digastric muscle.

to the cheeks, and Erbium laser resurfacing to the forehead, glabella, and perioral area in conjunction with the neck lift.

Case No. 4 is a 65-year-old patient who had a neck lift with submental lipectomy, partial excision of bilateral submandibular glands, and platysmal placation. Intraoperative examination revealed enlarged bilateral submandibular glands that were excised through an intracapsular incision. There was no need for modification of the digastric muscles. Postoperative photos (16 months' postop) demonstrate a significant improvement in neck contour in relation to the cervicomental angle as well as neck volume. This patient also had an endoscopic brow-lift, autologous fascia transfer to the glabella vertical frown lines, and autologous submascular aneurotic system (SMAS) transfer to the marionette lines in addition to the neck lift.

POSTOPERATIVE CARE

Patients who have only a submental neck lift are discharged on the same day after surgery; however, those who also have a face-lift are kept overnight for observation. Instructions are given to keep the head elevated but with care to avoid neck flexion, to help reduce swelling and to preserve skin adherence in the neck. The drain is removed the next day and the compression garment is worn for several days.

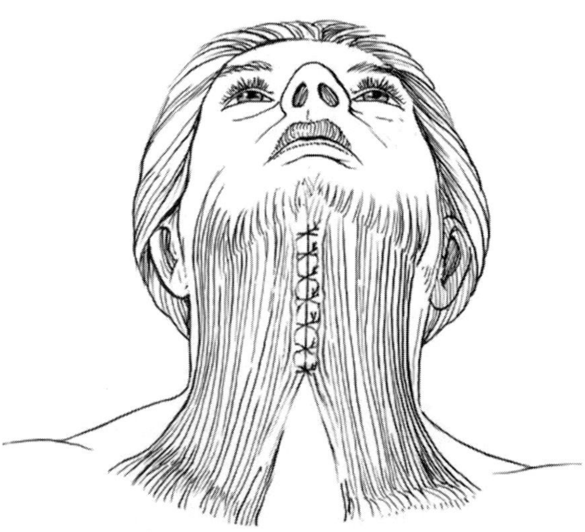

Figure 9 Platysmal plication.

(A) (B)

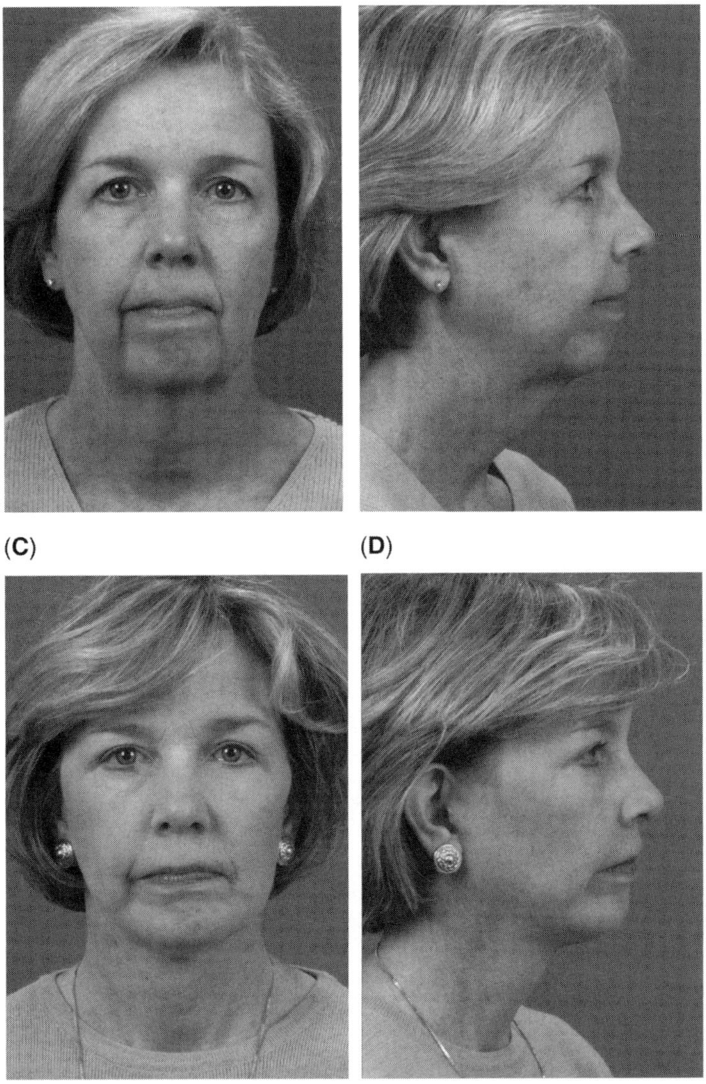

(C) (D)

Case No. 2 Neck lift with submental lipectomy and platysmal plication. No subcutaneous fat was excised, only fat deep to the platysma was removed [preop, (**A**); preop lateral, (**B**); post-op, (**C**); and post-op lateral, (**D**)].

COMPLICATIONS

The most frequent complication seen in neck recontouring is overreduction of volume in the superficial plane in an attempt to improve or conceal volume problems in the intermediate or deep planes. This problem results from a reluctance to deal with the deeper layers of the neck including the interplatysmal fat, subplatysmal fat, digastric muscle, and submandibular gland. Attempting to mask deeper volume problems, through excess removal of superficial subcutaneous fat, results in suboptimal neck contouring and adherence of the denuded dermis to the underlying platysma muscle. As a secondary procedure, the management of the subplatysmal volume problems is relatively straightforward. However, correction of adhesions between the skin and the platysma is extremely difficult. In this situation, some improvement may be obtained by complete mobilization of the skin off the platysma with subsequent redraping. Autologous fat or dermal grafts may also offer some assistance in these difficult reoperations. Excess removal of subcutaneous fat during liposuction can be avoided by the

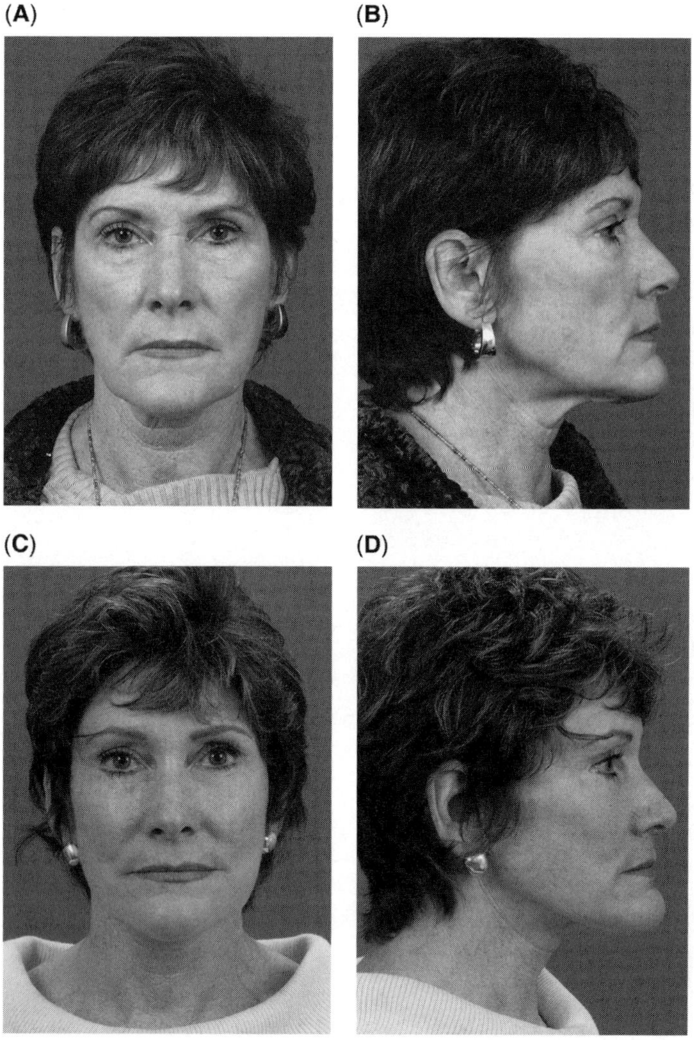

Case No. 3 Neck lift with submental lipectomy, tangential excision of the digastric muscles, and platysmal plication [preop, (**A**); preop lateral, (**B**); post-op, (**C**); and post-op lateral, (**D**)].

use of smaller cannulae with the opening away from the skin and limiting the number of passes within the same tunnel. With liposuction or the open approach, a 3- to 5-mm-thick layer of fat should remain deep to the skin.

Another complication is inadequate volume reduction most often in the deep plane, including interplatysmal or subplatysmal fat, the digastrics, or the submandibular glands. Appropriate preoperative planning and intraoperative management of each plane of the neck will minimize this, but secondary correction is relatively straightforward. A residual bulge in the submental area may represent the anterior belly of the digastric, whereas a bulge in the submental triangle corresponds to an enlarged submandibular gland. Correction of both these problems involves direct excision through a submental incision.

Just as insufficient volume reduction in the deep plane of the neck can produce suboptimal results, so can excess reduction of volume be a problem. Overcorrection of volume in the deep plane of the neck results in a hollowed-out depression in the submental area. This depression is accentuated if failure of the midline platsymal plication occurs. Constant reassessment of the effects of various interventions in the deep plane is performed to avoid these problems.

The results of procedures in all three planes of the neck have been pleasing for both the patients and the surgeons in our practice. Minimal morbidity and complications have been

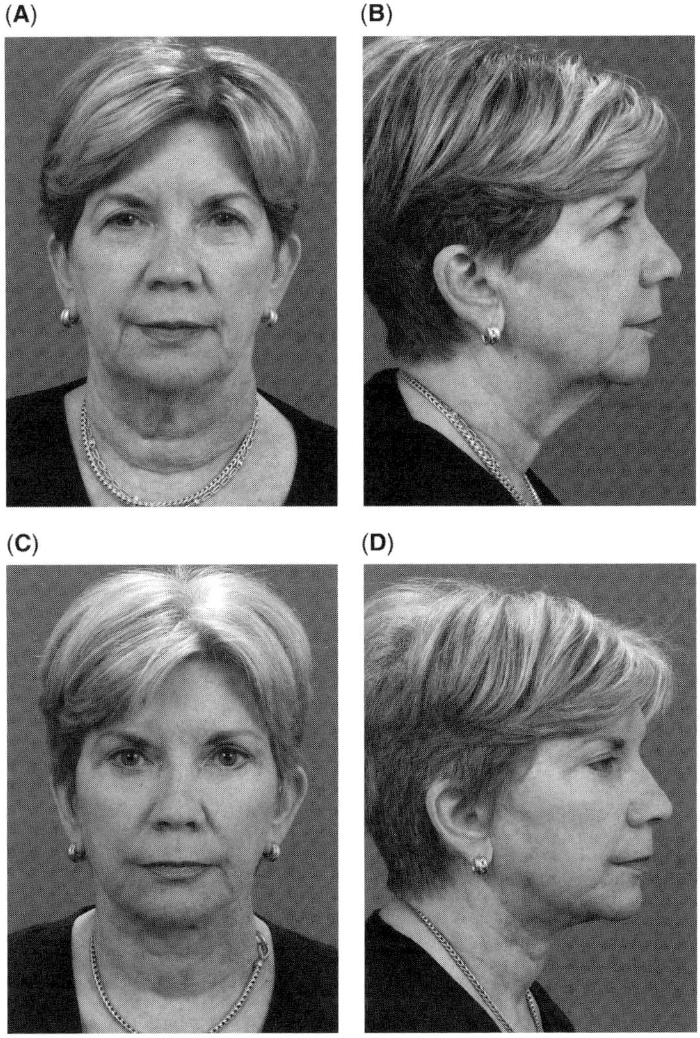

Case No. 4 Neck lift with submental lipectomy, partial excision of bilateral submandibular glands, and platysmal plication [preop, (**A**); preop lateral, (**B**); post-op, (**C**); and post-op lateral, (**D**)].

observed. To date, no hematomas, seromas, or nerve injuries have been experienced as a result of procedures in the deep plane. Therefore, in our hands, the three-plane approach to neck recontouring has proven to be safe and effective.

CONCLUSION

The layered approach to neck contouring with assessment of volume of each layer facilitates neck contouring. After the proper identification of volume, the optimal technique of volume modification must be performed in the appropriate plane to obtain a pleasing result. The most common problem in neck contouring is overexcision of fat in the superficial plane in an attempt to overcome problems in the deeper planes. Optimal outcomes result when the deeper planes are addressed through an open approach and adequate subcutaneous fat is left under the skin. Liposuction should only be performed in the subcutaneous plane with cannulae that are 2.5 mm or smaller in diameter with the hole turned away from the skin and limiting the number of passes in each cannula tunnel. A layer of fat 3–5 mm thick should be left on the skin to avoid irregularities and skin-platysma adherence. Recontouring through removal of subplatysmal fat is preferable to overresection subcutaneous fat. It is important to evaluate the digastric muscles and submandibular glands intraoperatively for possible modification.

Digastric excision is usually performed tangentially, and submandibular gland excision is done intracapsular in a piecemeal fashion. If every patient is approached with these principles of volume assessment and modification in mind, optimal results for the surgeon and the patient can be achieved.

SUGGESTED READING

Connell BF. Neck contour deformities: the art, engineering, anatomic diagnosis, architectural planning and aesthetics of surgical correction. Clin Plast Surg 1987; 14(4):683–692.

Connell BF. SMAS facelift. Semin Plast Surg 2002; 16(4):305–317.

Connell BF, Hosn W. Importance of the digastric muscle in cervical contouring: an update. Aesthetic Surg J 2000; 20:12–16.

Connell BF, Marten TJ. Submental crease: elimination of the double chin deformity at rhytidectomy. Aesthetic Surg 1990; 10:10–12.

Connell BF, Shamooun JM. The significance of digastric muscle contouring for rejuvenation of the submental area of the face. Plast Reconstr Surg 1997; 99(6):1586–1590.

de Castro CC. The anatomy of the platysma muscle. Plast Reconstr Surg 1980; 66(5):680–683.

Fisher G. Male facelift: state of the art. Semin Plast Surg 2002; 16(4):319–330.

Gradinger GP. Anterior cervicoplasty in the male patient. Plast Reconstr Surg 2000; 106(5):1146–1154.

Kesselring UK. Direct approach to the difficult anterior neck region. Aesthetic Plast Surg 1992; 16(4):277–282.

Marten TJ. Facelift: planning and technique. Clin Plast Surg 1997; 24(2):269–308.

Michalany FS. Neck rhytidectomy: aesthetic treatment variations. Aesthetic Plast Surg 1997; 21(1):32–37.

Millard DR Jr, Mullin WR, Ketch LL. Surgical correction of the fat neck. Ann Plast Surg 1983; 10(5):371–385.

Nahai F. Reconsidering neck suspension sutures. Aesthetic Surg J 2004; 24:365–367.

Stuzin JM, Baker TJ, Gordon HL. The relationship of the superficial and deep fascial fascias: relevance to rhytidectomy and aging. Plast Reconstr Surg 1992; 89(3):441–449.

14 Aesthetic Facial Osteotomies

Fernando Ortiz-Monasterio
School of Medicine, Universidad Nacional Autónoma de México, Mexico City, Mexico

INTRODUCTION

Body contour is conditioned by the skeletal structure, the muscle and ligament support, and the soft tissue coverage. The participation of each of these elements varies in different areas of the body. Subcutaneous fat is the main component of the abdomen and hips; bone is mainly responsible for the shape of the face. The craniofacial skeleton not only determines the size, the dimensions, and the contour of the face but also the relationship between its various segments.

There are three prominent areas in the face. The first is the supraorbital ridge limited on each side by the temporal crest; the second is the zygomatic malar prominence; the third is the inferior border of the mandible. The protruding zones form the limits for depressed areas located more posteriorly. These shallow areas are the temporals, the orbits, the lower midface, and the neck immediately below the mandibular margin. All these elements of the facial topography are determined by the skeletal framework. The relationship of the soft tissue cover and the subjacent solid foundation determines the angularity and the character of the face (1–4).

In order to study the face it is appropriate to start the examination with the full-face view, locating the various classic points accepted in physical anthropology: trichion, the highest point at the center of the forehead at the hairline; temporal crest; nasion, the deepest point of the frontonasal groove; zygoma, the most prominent point of the zygomatic arch; malar, the vertex of the malar prominence; alar, the lateral border of the nasal alae; subnasal, the junction of the columella with the upper lip; stomion, the contact point between the lips at the midline; chirium, the buccal commissures; gonion, the most prominent point of the mandibular angle; and menton, the most caudal point of the mandibular symphisis. As a general rule, the bitemporal–bimalar and bigonial diameters should be equal. If we divide the face into four sections with horizontal lines at the level of the chirion, the medial canthus, the subnasal, the stomion, and the menton, it is possible to establish a "golden" relationship between the upper two and the lower two segments and also the components of each segment (Fig. 1A).

In the profile view, we use the same anthropometrical references to analyze facial convexity, which is related to the prominence of the forehead, the nose, the dental arches, and the chin (Fig. 1B).

Surgical alterations of the upper third of the face by osteotomies, by remodeling, or by implants contribute to facial aesthetics, especially around the orbital rims and the malar. These procedures are discussed elsewhere in this book. The scope of this chapter is limited to the surgical procedures on the skeleton of the middle and lower third, which have a dramatic effect on the beauty of the face and which are frequently performed in combination with nasal and rejuvenation surgery.

The most common aesthetic surgical procedures on the facial skeleton include LeFort I osteotomy of the maxilla, segmental maxillary and mandibular osteotomies for the correction of dentoalveolar disharmonies, and some mandibular osteotomies to advance or retroposition the lower jaw or to alter the contour of the mandibular body. To cover all that territory is beyond the scope of this chapter, so it will be limited to the most common procedures that alter the central part of the middle and lower thirds of the face.

The middle third includes maxilla from the fronto zygomatic, the orbital floor, and the nose to the upper dental arch. To correct sagittal disharmonies it is necessary to mobilize the maxilla anteriorly or posteriorly. Vertical discrepancies require elongation or shortening of the maxilla, and in some cases maxillary advancement may be combined with retroposition of the mandible. The most frequent aesthetic procedure of the middle third is the LeFort I type osteotomy (5–9). This is a horizontal osteotomy of the maxilla above the dental roots more or less following the tracing of a fracture described by Rene LeFort in 1900. This technique was

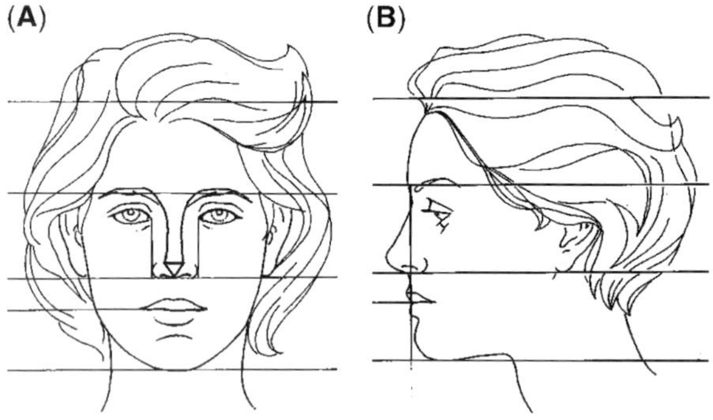

Figure 1 (**A**) To determine the proportions, the face should be examined by tracing five imaginary horizontal lines at the level of the trichion, the supraorbital, the subnasal, the stomium, and the menton. Ideally these segments should fit into the golden proportion Tr-subnasale = 1: subnasale = menton 0.618–subnasale-stomium = 0.618. Stomium-menton = 1. (**B**) Temporal bizygomalar and bigonial diameters should have the same dimension. The width of the nasal base should be equal to the intercantal distance. On the profile view, the proportions of the segments are visualized as well as facial convexity. A vertical line (perpendicular to the Frankfort plane) from the nasion to the lower lip should be slightly in front of the menton.

initially described by Dingman and Obwegeser for the correction of orthognathic problems, but it had been used by surgeons in the 19th century as an access route to reach the pterigo maxillary region. With the advent of rigid fixation and refined instrumentation, this is now a common operation to modify the shape, the position, and the dimensions of the bones with almost millimetric precision without the need for interdental fixation. This osteotomy is routinely used to advance the middle third to correct maxillary hypoplasia manifested by decreased facial convexity and flattening of the face. These patients present alterations of dental occlusion type Angle 3, and it is relatively common to see maxillary hypoplasia associated with mandibular prognathism. The same horizontal osteotomy can be used to retroposition the maxilla, combining it with bone resection in the posterior segment.

This type of surgery as well as the mandibular surgery requires orthodontic preparation. To achieve a permanent result, a stable dental occlusion is mandatory. Preoperative orthodontic treatment might be minimal in some cases or may require a prolonged process, but it is unacceptable in aesthetic surgery to have an incorrect or unstable occlusion. Orthodontic bands are also necessary during the transoperative stage to maintain the dental occlusion while rigid fixation plates are applied. During the planning process, the orthodontist simulates the osteotomies on the dental casts and prepares an occlusal plate that determines the exact position of the segments during the operation.

This surgery is always performed under general anesthesia controlled by an experienced anesthetist in a surgical center with all the necessary facilities including an intensive care unit. It is also important to have the required instruments, namely, saws, oscillatory, reciprocating, and rotatory-type burrs, drills, and a complete set for rigid fixation. We usually employ titanium miniplates, and the equipment includes plates of different shapes and dimensions, cutting and bending tools as well as titanium forceps for handling the plates, and a variety of screws of different caliber and length with appropriate screwdrivers. Microplates and monocortical screws are occasionally used.

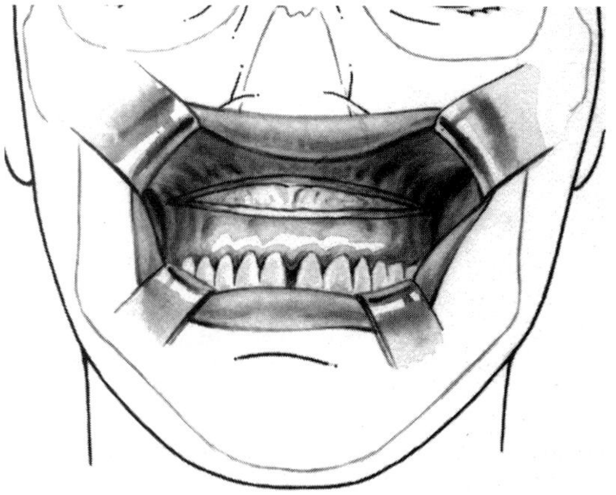

Figure 2 LeFort I osteotomy. A horizontal incision is made slightly in front of the upper vestibular sulcus extending to the first molar on each side.

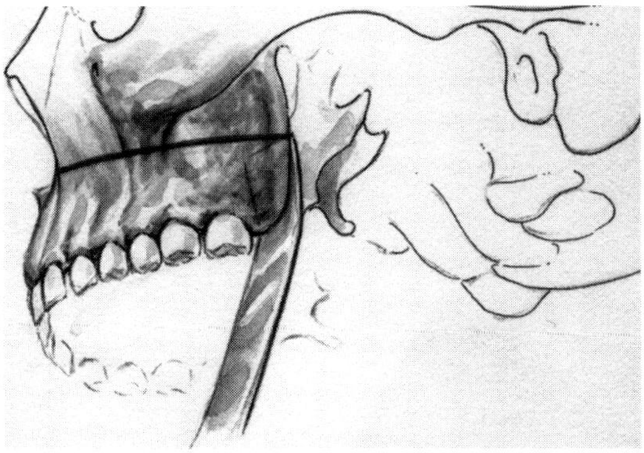

Figure 3 LeFort I osteotomy. The pterigomaxillary disjunction is done with a slightly curved osteotome introduced in a cephalad direction through the mucosa of the retromolar area immediately posterior to the tuberosity.

SURGICAL TECHNIQUE

Anesthesia should be given through a nasotracheal intubation that allows the mouth to close temporarily transoperatively. The operative field is infiltrated with a 1:10,000 adrenaline solution. A gull-wing incision is made slightly in front of the upper buccal sulcus extending to the first molar on each side (Fig. 2). The periosteum is elevated from the anterior aspect of the maxilla extending superiorly to the emergence of the infraorbital nerve and medially to the edge of the pyriform aperture. Laterally, the dissection is extended to the pterigomaxillary junction to maintain the subperiosteal plane to avoid exposing the buccal fat pad. The dissection of the nasal cavity begins on the lateral wall, introducing a periosteal elevator at the edge of the pyriform aperture and proceeding to free the lateral nasal wall all the way to the posterior edge of the maxilla. The undermining is extended inferiorly, carefully elevating the mucoperiosteal lining of the nasal floor its full length to the limit of the nasal crest. At this time, the medial nasal wall is dissected, exposing the junction of the septum with the nasal crest. The line of osteotomy on the anterior aspect of the maxilla is traced above the dental roots. Protecting the nasal mucosa with a thin malleable retractor, the osteotomy is made from medial to lateral with a fine reciprocating saw introduced into the nasal cavity. The cut is extended to the lateral maxillary wall (Fig. 3). The medial and lateral osteotomies are completed with a 7-mm chisel introduced horizontally. The junction of the septum with the nasal crest is freed with a fine osteotome. Finally the pterigomaxillary disjunction is performed. This can be done either with a curved chisel introduced laterally through a vestibular incision or with a wider chisel introduced through the buccal cavity behind the alveolar ridge between the tuberosity and the hamulus of the pterigoid, which is easily palpable (Fig. 3). At this stage, the maxilla is totally freed and can be mobilized with Rowe forceps exerting lateral and vertical movements, and placed in the desired position (Fig. 4). Bone irregularities of the walls of the maxillary antrum interfering with the mobilization of the maxilla may be eliminated at this time with a burr.

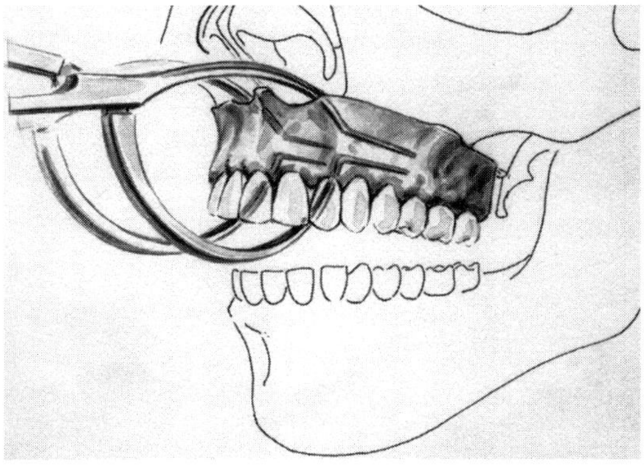

Figure 4 LeFort I osteotomy. Once the osteotomies are completed, the maxilla is mobilized with the Rowe forceps.

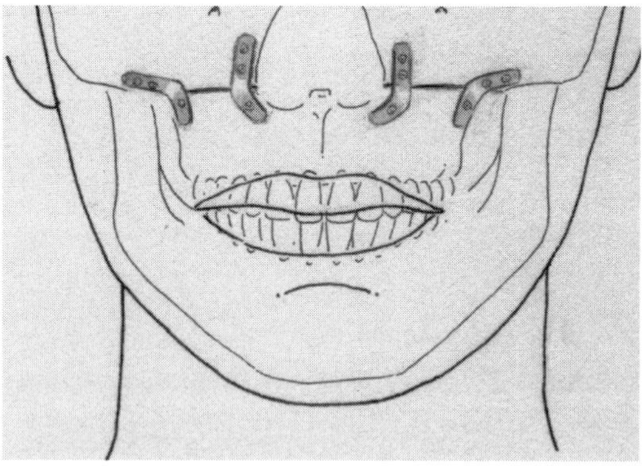

Figure 5 LeFort I osteotomy. The maxilla is fixed on its new position with titanium miniplates. Two L-shaped plates are used for the pyriform area, and two straight plates are placed on the lateral buttress.

There might be some bleeding, usually from the pterigoid plexus. The internal maxillary is located behind the tuberosity and there is no reason to endanger this vessel with correct technique. To control the bleeding, the free maxillary segment is taken between the thumb and index finger of the surgeon and displaced inferiorly, while the bleeding vessels are electrocoagulated. Generous irrigation with cold saline solution helps to visualize the origin of the bleeding and also controls the hemorrhage.

At this time the occlusal plate is placed and intermaxillary fixation is done with rubber bands or fine wire. To achieve the fixation of the maxilla in the new position we employ two L-shaped miniplates medially and two straight plates laterally. We start with the medial segment on top of the canine eminence, taking care to model the plates to achieve a snug adaptation to the osseous surface. This is critical, because if the fit is not perfect, the maxilla will be displaced when the screws are introduced, throwing off the dental occlusion. Once the L-plates are fixed, we remove the interdental fixation to confirm that the bone is in the proper position (Fig. 5). If there was some movement and the occlusion is not correct, it is necessary to remove the plates and the screws and replace them in the correct position. The two lateral miniplates are then fixed, and the intermaxillary fixation is removed. Before closing the mucosa, it is important to replace the paranasal tissues in their original position using nonabsorbable suture to prevent widening of the nasal bone (Fig. 6). The mucosa is closed with fine absorbable sutures (Fig. 7).

LONG FACE

The exaggerated vertical dimension of the maxilla produces a facial characteristic commonly called long face. Insufficient vertical development produces the short face. On frontal examination, the long face presents a disproportion between the height and the width, giving an

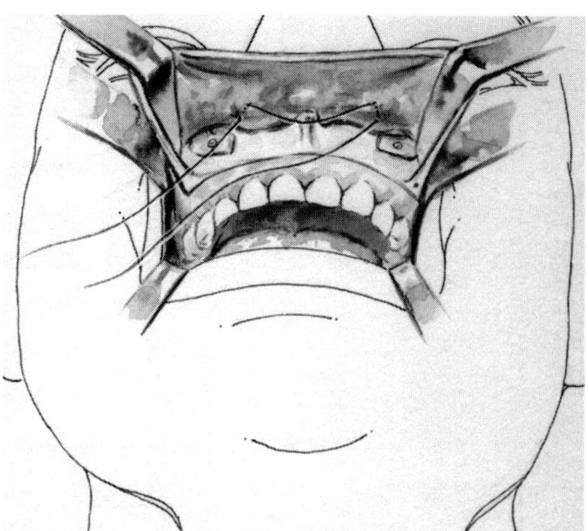

Figure 6 The muscles at the midline of the paranasal area are sutured to each other to prevent postoperative widening of the nasal base.

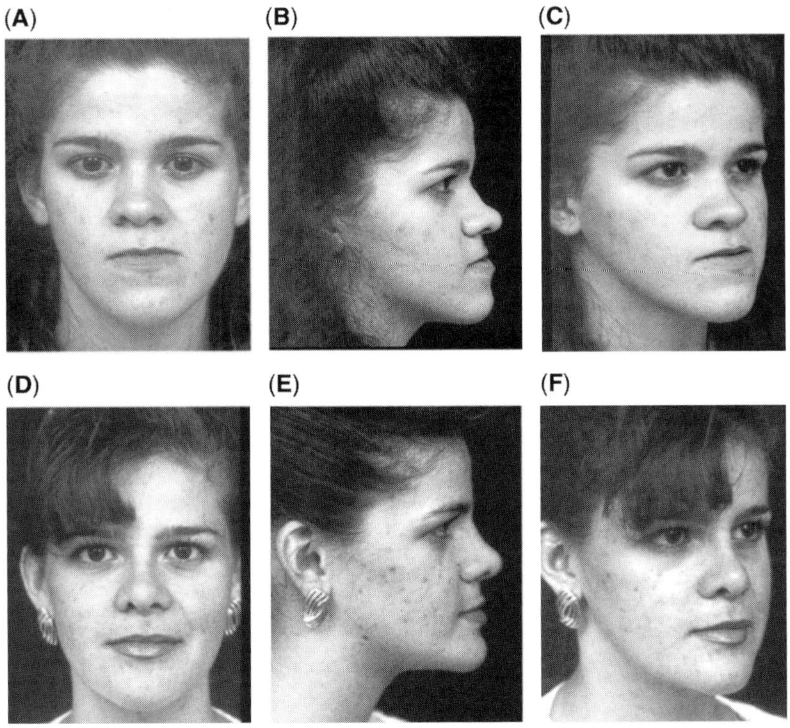

Figure 7 (**A–C**) Preoperative views of a 19-year-old female with mandibular prognathism, maxillary hypoplasia, and nasal deformity. Inadequate lip position is produced by the position of the mandibular alveolar ridge, which is also responsible for the absence of the sublabial groove. The nasion is caudally displaced and the nasal tip appears very prominent in relation to the dorsum. (**D–F**) Postoperative result after maxillary advancement by LeFort I osteotomy, segmental mandibular osteotomy to retroposition the alveolar ridge, and chondrocostal graft to the nasal dorsum.

impression of thinness even when the transverse diameters are normal. The nose is usually thin, and the distance between the nasion and the nasal tip may be exaggerated. With the mouth in the rest position, the upper incisors are visualized. When the mouth is completely closed, lip strain can be observed, while a smile reveals the free gingival edge excessively (Fig. 9). On the profile view, the same characteristics of vertical excess are associated with an apparent microgenia. This deficiency of the anterior projection of the chin is produced by the increase of the vertical dimension of the maxilla, limiting the mandibular rotation. The aperture of the nasolabial angle may be exaggerated as a result of the projection of the nasal spine displacing anteriorly the base of the columella. For the correction of a long face,

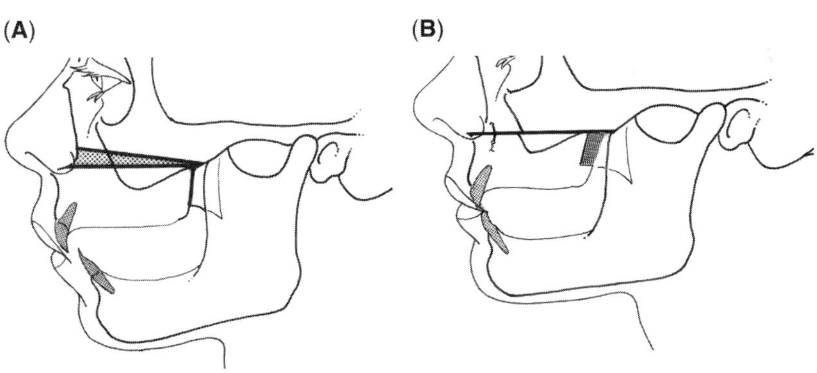

Figure 8 (**A**) To shorten the midface it is necessary to resect a wedge of the maxilla. (**B**) After shortening the maxilla, there is an increase of mandibular rotation, which projects the chin anteriorly.

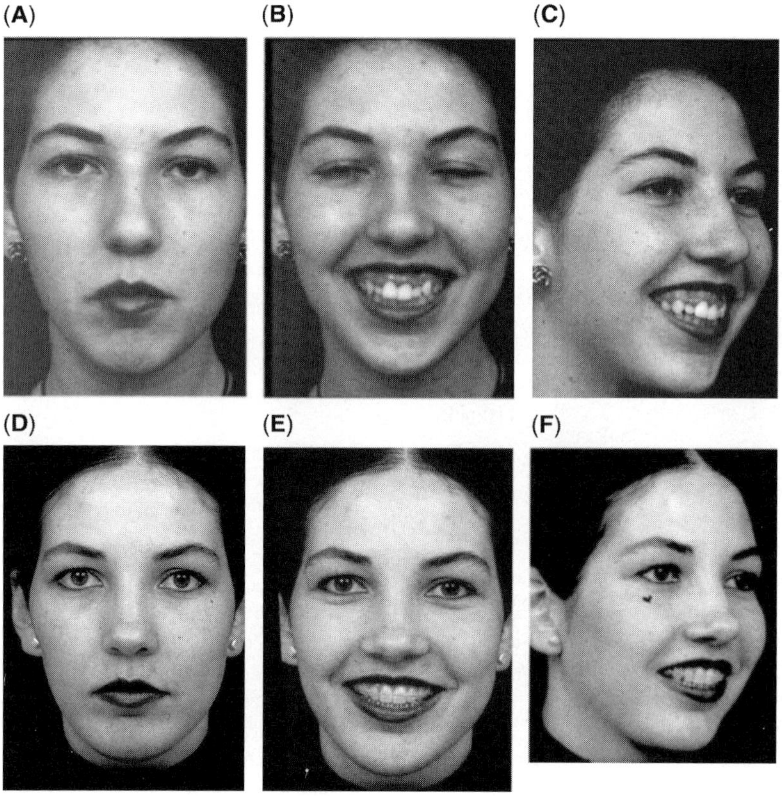

Figure 9 (**A–C**) Preoperative views of a 21-year-old female with a long face. Lip strain can be observed when the lips are closed and gingival exposure is exaggerated when smiling. (**D–F**) Postoperative results after a 7-mm shortening of the maxilla. Lip strain has disappeared as well as the gummy smile.

it is important to evaluate the soft tissues, especially the vertical dimension of the upper lip, which may be short. In the lateral cephalometry, it is possible to measure exactly the vertical excess and to determine the extent of the resection. This is important data, which should be compared with the clinical observation and the anthropometric measurements. Usually both methods give the same information, but the aesthetic judgment should prevail. In some cases preoperative orthodontic treatment may be necessary.

The operation is the same as described for the classic LeFort I except that a slice of bone should be removed to decrease the vertical dimension. For this, accurate measurements should be made, and the limits of the osteotomy should be marked on the anterior aspect of the maxilla (Fig. 10). The slice of bone to be removed should be slightly thicker anteriorly than posteriorly to maintain a good occlusion and to prevent an anterior open bite. The free maxillary segment should be easily moved without resistance to the new position while the mandible is maintained in its occlusal position. If the upper lip is short, it is possible to increase the length at the end of the operation by suturing the paranasal muscles to each other at the midline with a nonabsorbable material. The elongation may be completed, closing the mucosal incision in the shape of V-Y by performing backup cuts in the two lateral extremes of the incision (Fig. 9).

SHORT FACE

The vertical hypoplasia of the maxilla produces a typical short face. On the front view, there is disharmony between the vertical and the transverse dimensions. The face appears broad in the position of rest, i.e., when the contact between the upper and the lower lip is maintained and when complete closure is achieved the lips project anteriorly. During the smile, the free edge of the gingiva is covered as well as part of the front teeth. The nasal tip is usually displaced

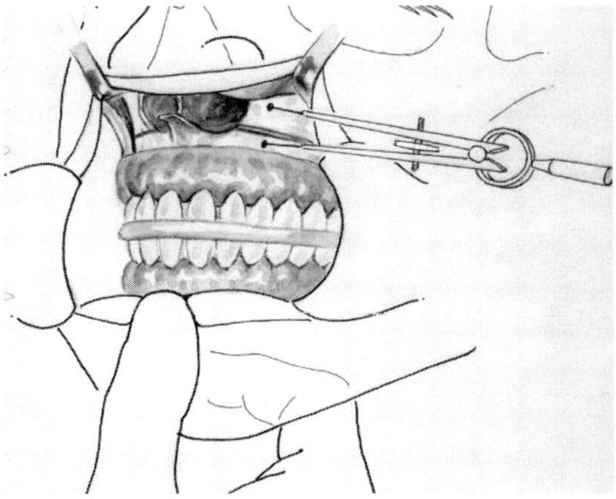

Figure 10 To shorten the midface a horizontal maxillary osteotomy is combined with a wedge resection, which must be accurately done according to the preoperative planning.

caudally with an acute nasolabial angle. On the profile view, the position of the lips protruding anteriorly when the mouth is closed is confirmed and the chin is prominent because of the exaggerated rotation of the mandible resulting from the short maxilla (Fig. 11).

The correction of the short face is made by an elongation of the maxilla. The extent of the elongation is determined by measurements in the lateral cephalometry and physical anthropology but again the aesthetic judgment should prevail. As a result of the exaggerated rotation of the mandible an edge-to-edge occlusion is frequently seen.

The aesthetic appreciation is based on direct observation of the face at rest and during the smile. A practical way to predict the final result is to ask the patient to bite a rubber block between the central incisors and then to close the mouth. The diameter of the rubber block correlates with the prospective increase of the vertical dimension of the mandible. With this simple test, it is possible to see the change between the vertical and the transverse dimensions of the face as well the position of the lips and the decrease of the chin projection. The patient may see in a mirror the expected changes (Fig. 11).

For the correction of the short face the LeFort I operation is slightly modified. If the vertical hypoplasia is associated with minor sagittal maxillo-mandibular discrepancy, it is necessary to change the direction of the osteotomy cutting obliquely in a superior and posterior direction so the free segment can be mobilized anteriorly and inferiorly, maintaining contact with the cranial section. Another method is to start the osteotomy horizontally and then make a step at the level of lateral buttress so the bone can be mobilized, maintaining contact with the cranium. Stabilization is achieved by means of the four miniplates inserted medially and laterally. It is occasionally necessary to insert a bone graft taken from the parietal area or from the ribs between the two segments at the level of the pyriform aperture. The bone graft is fixed with the L-shaped miniplate. Some authors report the successful use of hydroxyapatite instead of the bone graft, but in our experience this material is not a substitute for bone (Fig. 12).

DENTOALVEOLAR DEFORMITIES

Maxillary alveolar protrusion is a relatively common deformity affecting the aesthetics of the face and is related to abnormal movements of the tongue or associated with retromandibulism in which the sublabial fold is exaggerated. Protrusion may be present in patients with a type 1 occlusion but it is more frequently seen in type 2. It may be associated with alveolar mandibular protrusion, altering the facial profile and the relationship between the middle third and the chin. This bimaxillary protrusion, considered as a deformity in the Indo-European race, is a common characteristic in many ethnic groups in Asia as well the Amerindians and their descendents, resulting from a mixture with Europeans. Although this is a normal anatomic characteristic of this group, it does not conform to the accepted contemporary aesthetic standards, so we frequently see patients presenting biprocidence with excellent dental occlusion requesting aesthetic improvement. Some of these patients have been treated by dental extractions and long orthodontic treatments without obtaining the desired results, because orthodontics alters the position of the teeth but does not change the shape of the bone (Fig. 13).

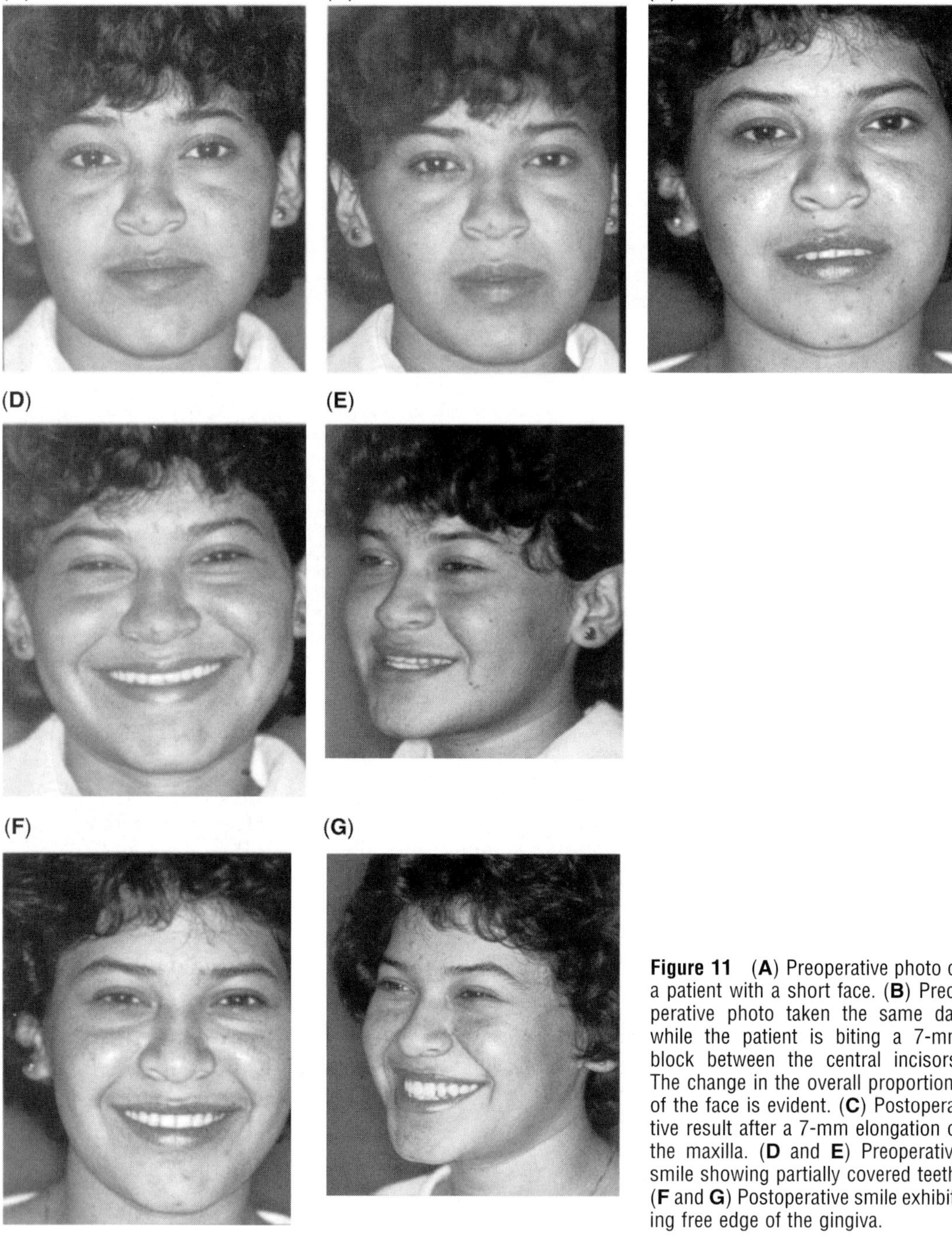

Figure 11 (**A**) Preoperative photo of a patient with a short face. (**B**) Preoperative photo taken the same day while the patient is biting a 7-mm block between the central incisors. The change in the overall proportions of the face is evident. (**C**) Postoperative result after a 7-mm elongation of the maxilla. (**D** and **E**) Preoperative smile showing partially covered teeth. (**F** and **G**) Postoperative smile exhibiting free edge of the gingiva.

Maxillary alveolar protrusion is characterized by overprojection of the upper lip that is located well in front of the lower, resulting in lip strain to achieve mouth closure. In the bimaxillary protrusion, both lips are projected anteriorly, and the gingival exhibition as well as the lip strain is exaggerated. The relationship with the chin is altered, and the sublabial sulcus is absent. Surgical treatment of the alveolar protrusion requires careful planning, and preoperative orthodontics is often necessary. An occlusal plate must be prepared to be used transoperatively after the segmental maxillary osteotomy, and two plates are necessary when maxillary and mandible protrusion are going to be corrected in one stage (Fig. 14).

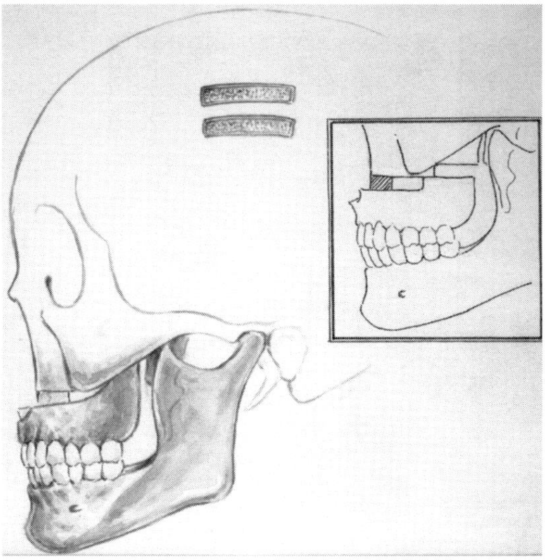

Figure 12 In order to maintain contact between the maxilla and the cranium during midface elongation, the transverse osteotomy is extended obliquely in a posterior and superior direction. A bone graft may be used anteriorly. Another option is to cut a step on the lateral aspect of the maxilla.

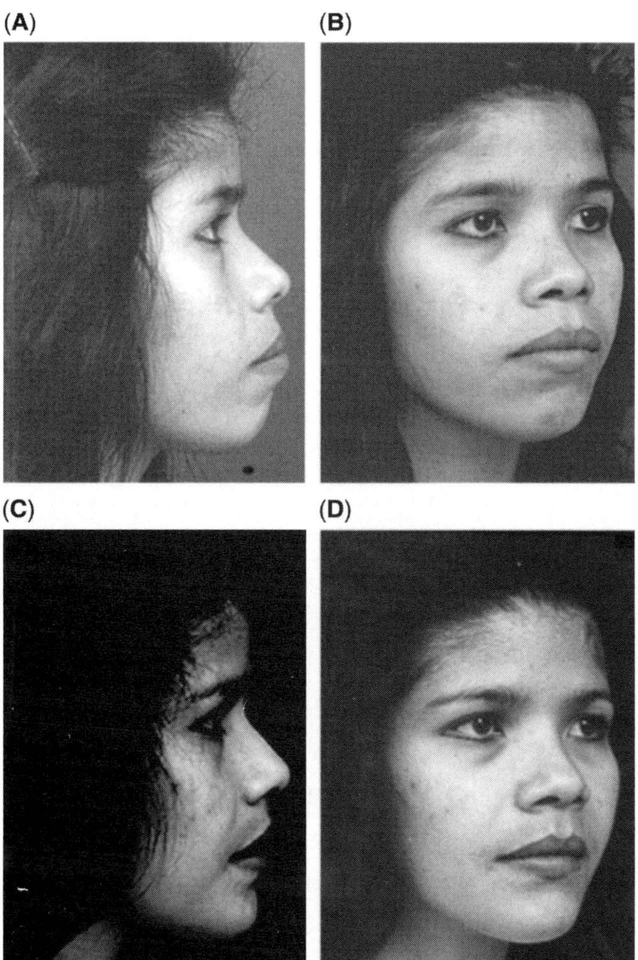

Figure 13 (*Continued on next page*) (**A** and **B**) Preoperative views of a female with an ethnically related bimaxillary alveolar protrusion. (**C** and **D**) Preoperative views of the same patient during orthodontic preparation. The first premolars have been extracted. (**E**, **F**, and **G**) Postoperative results after segmental mandibular and maxillary osteotomies.

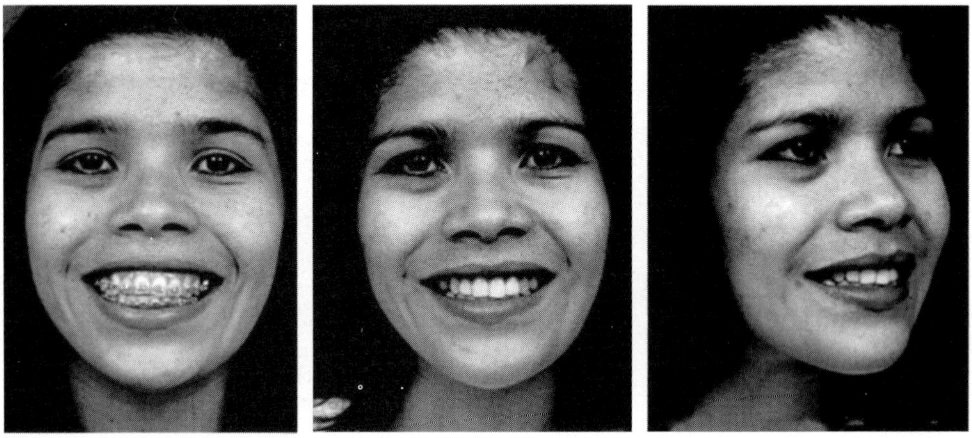

Figure 13 (*Continued from previous page*)

Segmental osteotomies proposed early in the 20th century were later discarded because of the number of complications resulting from incorrect technique and inadequate instrumentation. Surgical refinements and better understanding of the vascularity of the maxilla have made these operations safe, with predictable results and minimal morbidity (10–13). Segmental aesthetic osteotomies have several requirements (i) Provide adequate exposure for the osteotomies without injuring adjacent teeth; (ii) preserve blood supply of the mucosa and of the osseous segment; and (iii) achieve mobilization of the segments without intermaxillary postoperative fixation (14).

Surgery for Maxillary Alveolar Protrusion

The operation is performed under general anesthesia with nasotracheal intubation. The operating field is infiltrated with a small amount of 1:10,000 adrenaline solution. Usually the first molars have been previously extracted or are removed before beginning the operation. Contrary to many techniques proposed in the past using labial or palatine pedicles, we feel that the integrity of the palatine and the vestibular mucosa should be preserved. A vertical incision is made on each side from the central part of the alveolus of the first premolar directed superiorly until the cul-de-sac of the vestibulum (Fig. 15). Subperiosteal dissection on the anterior aspect of the maxilla is performed, carefully protecting the mucosa communicating both vertical incisions (Fig. 16). It may be convenient in some cases to make a 1-cm vertical incision at the midline to facilitate the subperiosteal dissection of the nasal spine and the anterior segment of the nasal floor (Fig. 17). The palatine mucosa is elevated with a thin periosteal elevator

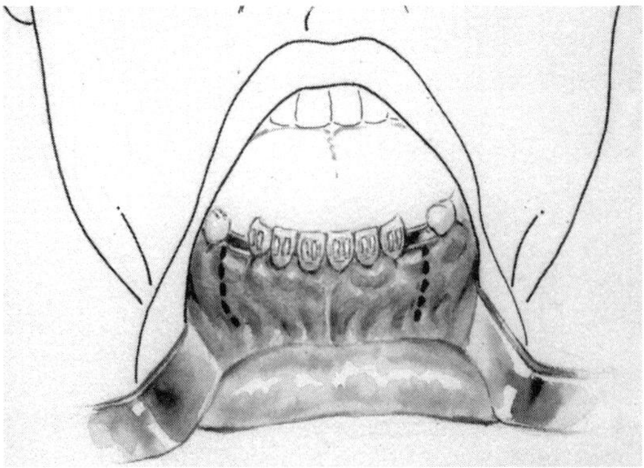

Figure 14 Segmental mandibular osteotomy. First premolars are extracted on both sides, and a vertical incision is made on the vestibular mucosa.

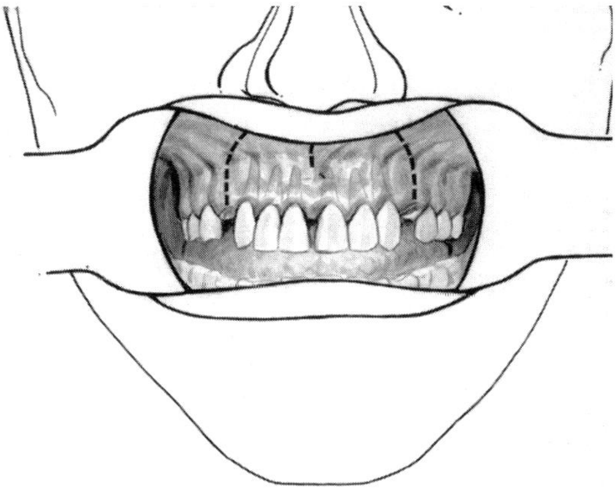

Figure 15 Maxillary segmental osteotomy. After extraction of the first premolar two vertical incisions are made on the vestibular gingival. A third small incision is made at the midline to access the nasal spine.

in a medial and slightly posterior direction to the midline. The same dissection is made on the opposite side, forming a subperiosteal tunnel 1-cm-wide crossing the palate transversally (Fig. 18). Bone resection is made by two vertical cuts including almost the full thickness of the bone with an oscillatory saw. The distance between the two vertical cuts represents the extent of the predicted posterior displacement of the maxillary segment. It is important during this maneuver to avoid injuring the root of the teeth to prevent postoperative morbidity. The mucosa is protected with a thin, malleable retractor (Fig. 19). Once the cut is above the dental roots, the osteotomy is directed horizontally to the nasal floor. At this time, a thin, malleable retractor is introduced into the tunnel made on the palatal mucosa, and with the use of the side-cutting burr, the osteotomy is completed into the palatine process (Fig. 20). The segment is finally freed with a thin osteotome, cutting the junction of the nasal spine with the septum. It is usually necessary to use a fine burr at this stage to eliminate minor irregularities of the bone to allow mobilization of the free segment into the previously planned position (Figs. 11 and 21A). The occlusal plate is placed at this time in order to place the free segment in the exact position corresponding to the preoperative plan. Contact between the segments is usually maintained with an orthodontic arch fixed to the plates, but it may be necessary sometimes to use one stainless steel wire suture on each side or to place a small microplate on each side. The mucosa is carefully sutured with thin, absorbable material and the occlusal plate is removed (Fig. 22). It is also important to have the required instruments, mainly saws, oscillatory and reciprocating.

MANDIBULAR SEGMENTAL OSTEOTOMIES

As with the maxilla the segmental osteotomy includes the incisors and canines, although it is possible to extend it posteriorly with a good margin of safety. An occlusal plate should be

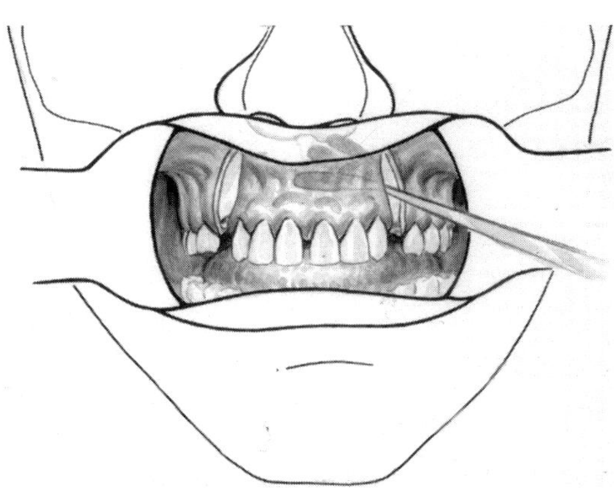

Figure 16 The mucoperiosteum is elevated, connecting the vertical incisions.

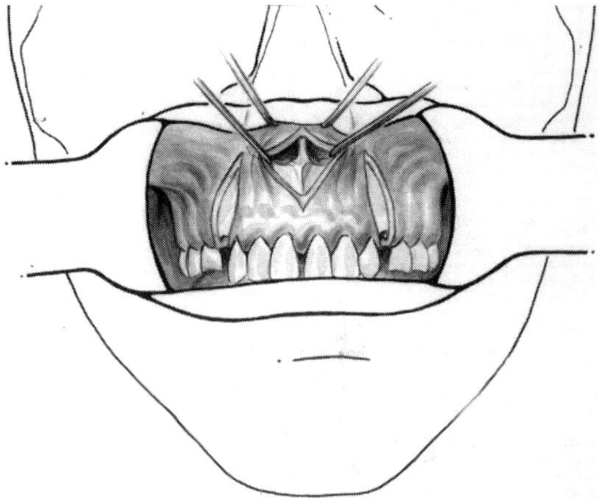

Figure 17 The periosteum is elevated from the nasal spine. The use of a small nasal speculum facilitates this maneuver. The vascular supply is maintained.

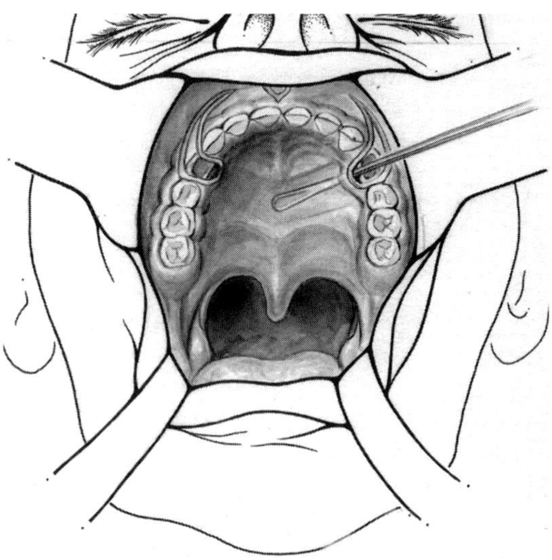

Figure 18 A tunnel is made on the mucoperiosteum of the palate entering through the gingiva of the extracted first premolar.

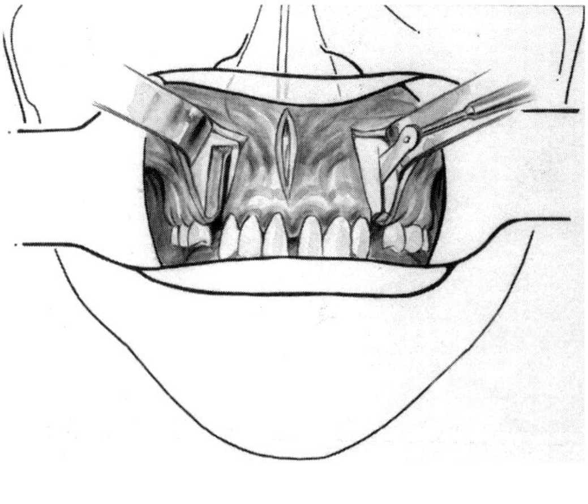

Figure 19 The preplanned bone resection is initiated with a reciprocating saw.

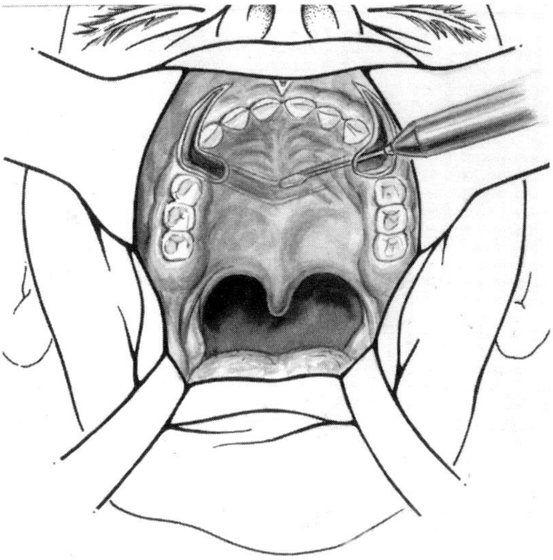

Figure 20 The osteotomy is completed with a side-cutting burr while the palatal mucoperiosteum is protected with a narrow, malleable retractor.

prepared in advance, and the two first premolars if present extracted before beginning the operation. The mucosa of the oral vestibulum is cut vertically from the midsection of the first premolar in a caudal direction to the sulcus of the buccal vestibulum (Fig. 14). Subperiosteal dissection of the anterior aspect of the mandible is made to join both incisions, avoiding trauma of the mucosa (Fig. 23). Subperiosteal dissection of the lingual aspect of the bone is done with a periosteal elevator designed in the shape of a golf club, allowing mucoperiosteal undermining without any incisions (Fig. 24). Bone resection is done, making two parallel vertical cuts on the segment between the canine and the second premolar (Fig. 25). The osteotomy is extended caudally beyond the dental roots. The posterior mucosa is protected during this stage with a thin, malleable retractor. A horizontal osteotomy is then made below the dental roots using a reciprocating saw while the mucosa is protected with a right angle nasal retractor (Fig. 26). The bone segment is then mobilized to the preplanned position using the occlusal plate, and an orthodontic bar is placed to achieve immobilization (Figs. 27 and 28).

For the simultaneous correction of maxillary and mandibular protrusion it is necessary to prepare two occlusal plates (Fig. 29A and B). The maxillary osteotomy is made first by placing the first splint to fix the maxillary segment in the proper position. The splint is then removed and the mandibular segmental osteotomy is performed using the second occlusal plate, to make sure that both segments are positioned in the previously determined position. Continuous irrigation with cold saline solution is important to control the temperature produced by the high-speed saws to prevent burning the tissues. We never use postoperative intermaxillary fixations. Patients leave the operating room with their mouths open, and they

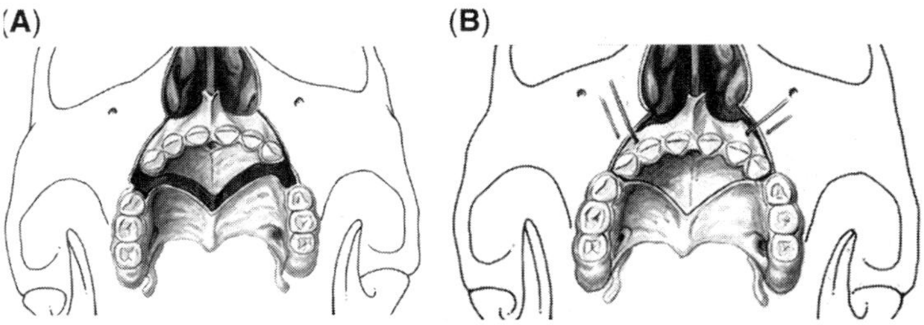

Figure 21 (**A**) Diagram showing the completed osteotomy. No incisions are made on the palatal mucosa. (**B**) The premaxillary segment is retropositioned and fixed with a wire suture on each side or with a microplate and monocortical screws.

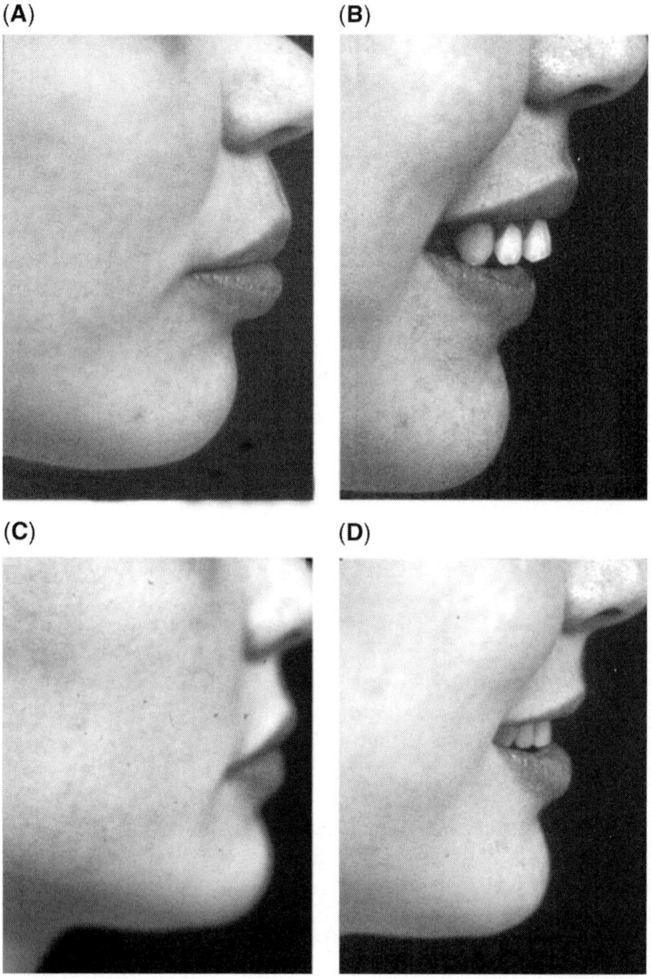

Figure 22 (**A** and **B**) Preoperative views of a patient with maxillary alveolar protrusion. Observe the abnormal position of the lower lip with the mouth closed. (**C** and **D**) Postoperative views after retropositioning the maxillary segment.

are discharged from the hospital the following day (Fig. 13). Corticosteroids are used the first few days, and antibiotics are prescribed for the first five postoperative days. A soft diet is recommended for six to eight weeks. With this technique the blood supply of the bone and of the mucosa is preserved, avoiding the necrosis previously reported (Fig. 30).

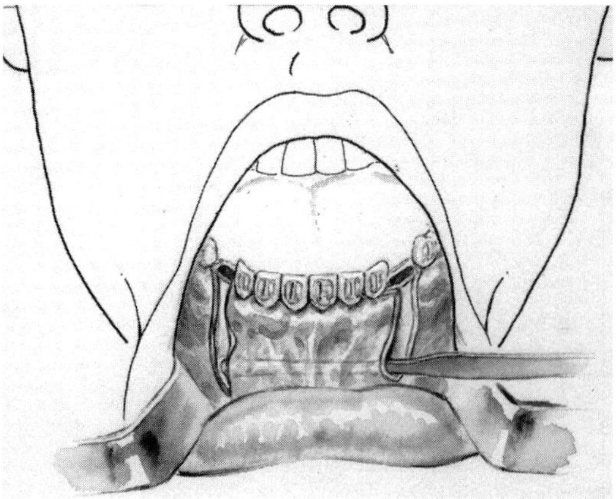

Figure 23 Segmental mandibular osteotomy. Two vertical incisions on vestibular mucosa. Subperiosteal dissection. Vascular supply is preserved.

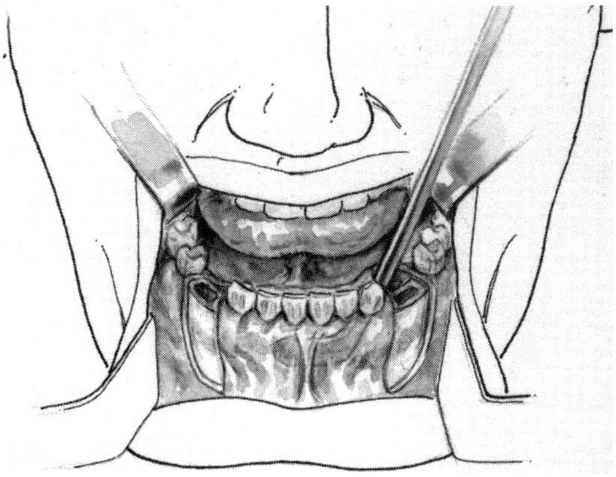

Figure 24 Segmental mandibular osteotomy. Subperiosteal dissection of the posterior aspect of the mandible is made with a golf club periosteal elevator. No incisions are made on the mucosa.

THE CHIN

The shape, the dimension, and the projection of the chin are important for facial aesthetics, and the surgical procedures of this area are a routine part of the aesthetic surgery of the facial skeleton.

Horizontal osteotomies of the chin are used to increase its projection or to decrease the vertical dimension of the mandibular symphisis. It is common to combine both concepts simultaneously. The patient desiring chin alterations should be examined on the full-face view, analyzing the anthropometric references of the medial and the lower third of the face—mainly the relationship between the subnasale, the stomion, and the menton. The exaggeration or the deficiency of the vertical dimension on the symphisis produces alterations of lip closure; the mouth should therefore be examined in the position of rest, during complete dental closure, and during the smile. It is also important to detect exhibition of the inferior incisors in the rest position. This usually results from the lack of tension and ptosis of the soft tissues of the face common in elderly persons (Fig. 31).

On the profile view, the assessment of the vertical dimensions is completed, analyzing the projection of the upper lip in relation to the lower lip and the menton. It should be remembered that the upper lip should project anteriorly in front of the lower lip. A vertical line perpendicular to the Frankfort plane beginning at the nasal root and extended in an inferior direction, touching tangentially the lower lip, should be at the level of the chin or discreetly in front of it. The sublabial sulcus is located between the mucocutaneous border of the lower lip and the prominence of the chin. When this sulcus is exaggerated as is the occlusal type 2 corresponding to retromandibulism, a mandibular advancement is required. Although the subject is slightly outside the aesthetic objectives of this work, it is worth mentioning that the new osseous distraction technique using intraoral devices allows the correction of

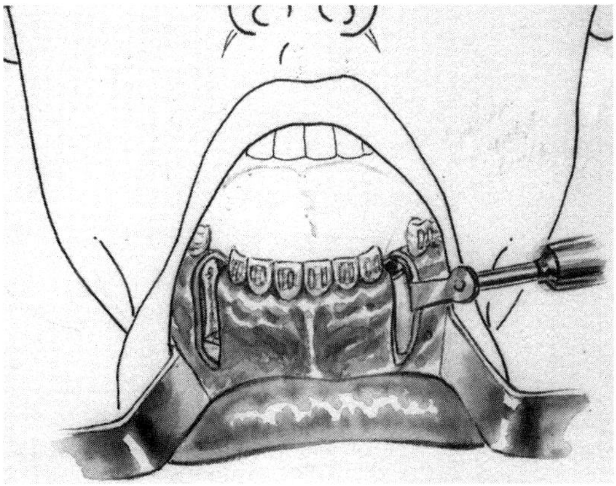

Figure 25 Segmental mandibular osteotomy. Bone resection is made with an oscillatory saw.

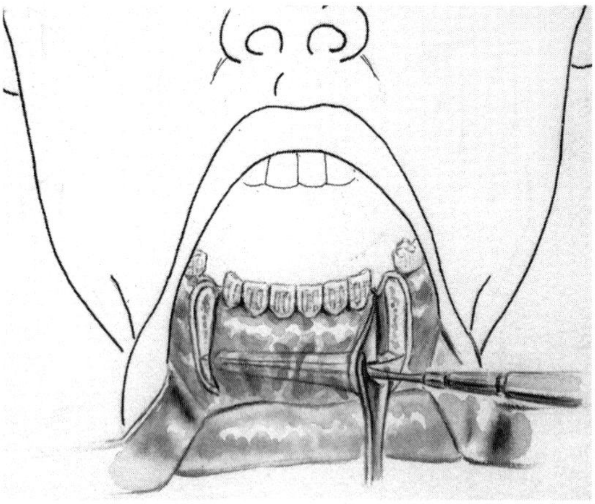

Figure 26 Segmental mandibular osteotomy. The mucoperiosteum is protected with a right angle retractor and a horizontal osteotomy is made.

retromandibulism in a manner much simpler than the old surgical techniques. The sublabial groove is also exaggerated when there is maxillary overprojection. The absence of the sublabial sulcus is aesthetically unpleasant, altering labial closure and the smile. It may be associated with mandibular prognathism or with overprojection of the mandibular dental arches. It may also be a result of microgenia, and the treatment varies in each case. Mandibular segmental osteotomies allow retroposition of the alveolar segment, decreasing the projection of the lower lip and improving its relation to the chin and the sublabial sulcus (Figs. 12, 31, and 32). In some cases of prognathism after mandibular retropositioning, it is necessary to advance the menton to produce the sublabial sulcus and to establish a harmonious lip–menton relationship. Over-projection of the menton may be partially corrected by shaving the bone at the level of the symphisis, although this procedure does not produce optimal results.

SLIDING GENIOPLASTY

The horizontal osteotomy of the mandibular symphisis is used to advance, to shorten, or to elongate the mandibular symphisis. We frequently combine this operation with other procedures such as a rhinoplasty, so we usually prefer general anesthesia (Fig. 31). The operative field is infiltrated with a 1:10,000 solution of adrenaline and a gull-wing incision 4–5 cm long is made slightly in front of the vestibular sulcus to include some of the submucous tissue at the edges to facilitate the suture and prevent adherence to the periosteum postoperatively (Fig. 32). A subperiosteal dissection is made in a caudal direction to the edge of the mandible and continued on each side, making a tunnel between the mandibular border and the emergence of the nerve (Figs. 33 and 34). This tunnel should extend well into the lateral aspect of the cmandibular body.

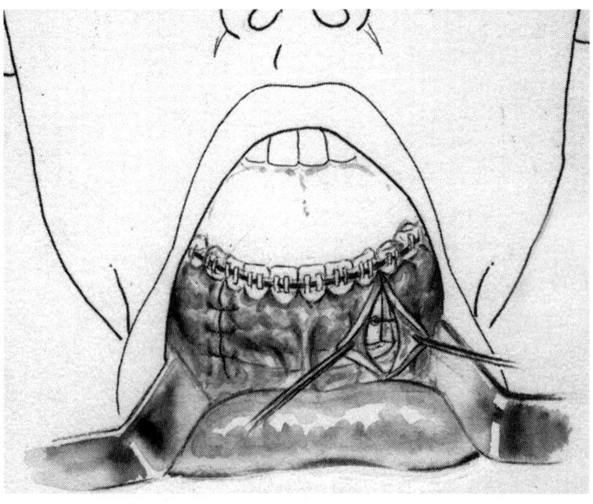

Figure 27 Segmental maxillary osteotomy. The free bone segment is mobilized to the preplanned position using an acrylic splint as a guide. Fixation is achieved by the orthodontic bar. Wire sutures or a microplate are used if necessary.

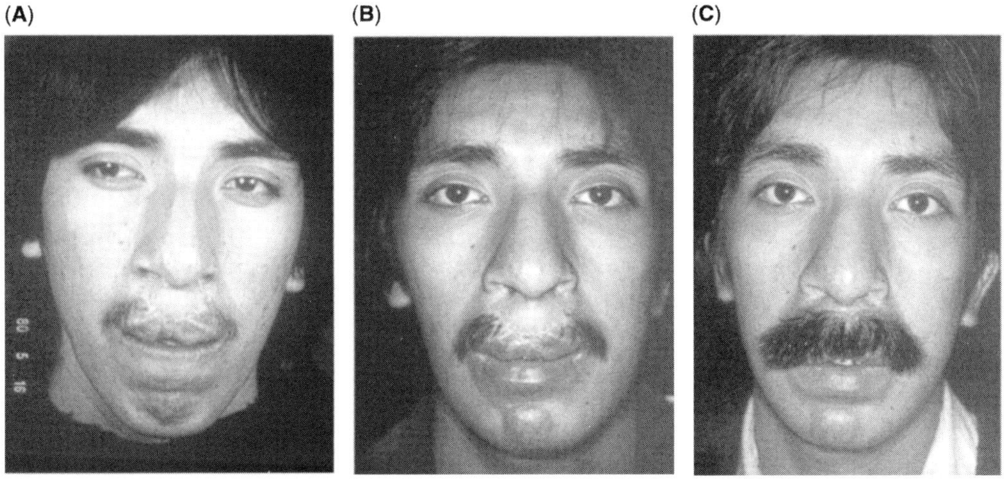

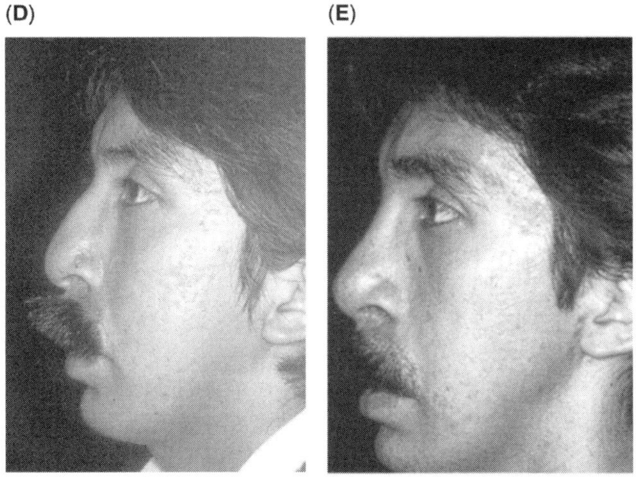

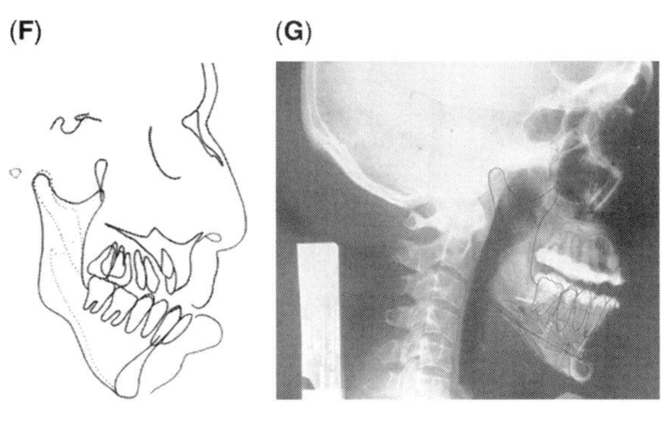

Figure 28 (**A**) Preoperative view of an adult male with severe sequelae of a bilateral cleft of the lip and palate. The lip is badly scarred and the nasal tip is underprojected. Maxillary hypoplasia is combined with mandibular alveolar protrusion. (**B**) Postoperative view after segmental mandibular osteotomy and sliding genioplasty. (**C**) Postoperative view after replacement of the upper lip skin with a scalp flap. (**D**) Postoperative view after osteotomies and scalp flap. (**E**) Final result after rhinoplasty. (**F**) Preoperative cephalometry. (**G**) X ray showing the final result.

In our experience it is important to extend the osteotomy in order to achieve a pleasant square chin and to maintain good contact between the bony segments, avoiding a palpable or visible step on the mandibular edge. Less extended osteotomies may achieve advancement or shortening of the bony segment but result in pointed chins that are not aesthetically pleasant. In order to decrease the vertical dimension, a horizontal resection is made; to augment the vertical dimension, a bone graft is interposed anteriorly between the two segments. Before starting the osteotomy, it is advisable to make a mark on the midline of the mandible, which is used as a reference to maintain symmetry at the time of the osteosynthesis (Fig. 34). This is also useful when there is an asymmetry of the inferior third of the face in order to determine with precision the extent of the lateral displacement after the osteotomy.

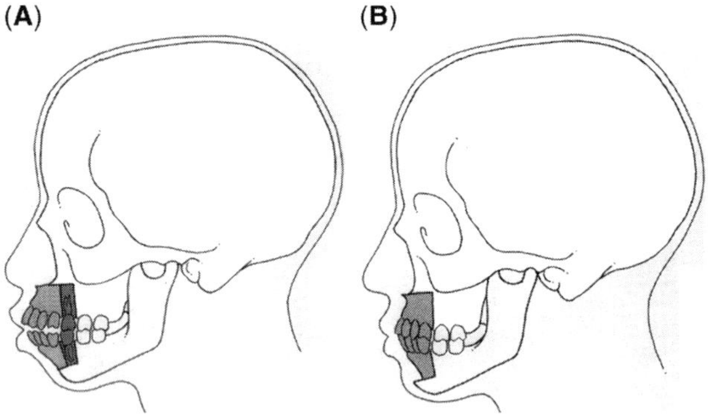

Figure 29 (**A**) Diagram showing the technique for simultaneous segmental maxillo-mandibular osteotomies. Dark areas are resected. (**B**) Bone segments are repositioned.

A right angle retractor is introduced into the subperiosteal tunnel to protect the nerve, and the osteotomy is performed with a reciprocating saw. The saw is maintained in a horizontal position following the previously determined direction, beginning at the lateral edge in a medial direction and finishing at the symphisis (Fig. 35). The maneuver is repeated on the contralateral side. Hemostasis is made by coagulation if there are some bleeding vessels or by applying wax on the bone. The segment is advanced to the desired position and the osteosynthesis made with stainless steel wire. We usually put one wire suture on each side at the level of the canine. A perforation is made on the anterior cortex of the fixed segment and another perforation on the posterior cortex of the free segment so the new position of the chin is maintained after fixation (Figs. 36–38). Titanium miniplates may be used to achieve fixation, especially when the bone graft is inserted to increase the vertical dimension, but in general, we prefer the wire osteosynthesis. The mucosa is sutured with absorbable material, and the chin is covered with a few strips of elastic tape. In the early postoperative period, it is convenient to remember that a dissecting hematoma of the floor of the mouth obstructing the airway may occur. This is an extremely rare complication that we have never seen in our experience, but it is worth observing the patient for a few hours.

With the right indication, the results of this operation are very satisfactory. It improves the projection of the chin and restores the sublabial sulcus. It also gives an excellent definition of the cervical angle because of the traction on the suprahyoid muscles that are inserted on the posterior aspect of the mobilized segment. This anterior projection of the skeleton stretches the soft tissues of the face and has a rejuvenating effect.

ELONGATING AND SHORTENING THE CHIN

To decrease the vertical dimension of the symphisis, the same osteotomy described above is performed. Once it is completed and the inferior segment is free, a second osteotomy parallel to the first is made on the superior edge, changing slightly the direction in such a way that the

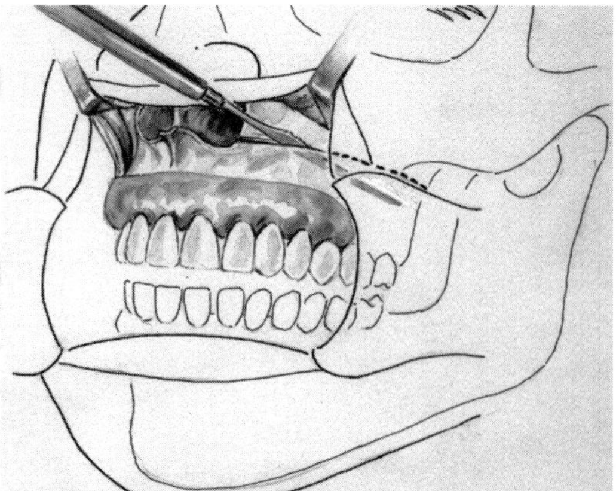

Figure 30 LeFort I osteotomy. The maxilla is cut horizontally with a fine reciprocating saw in a medial to lateral direction.

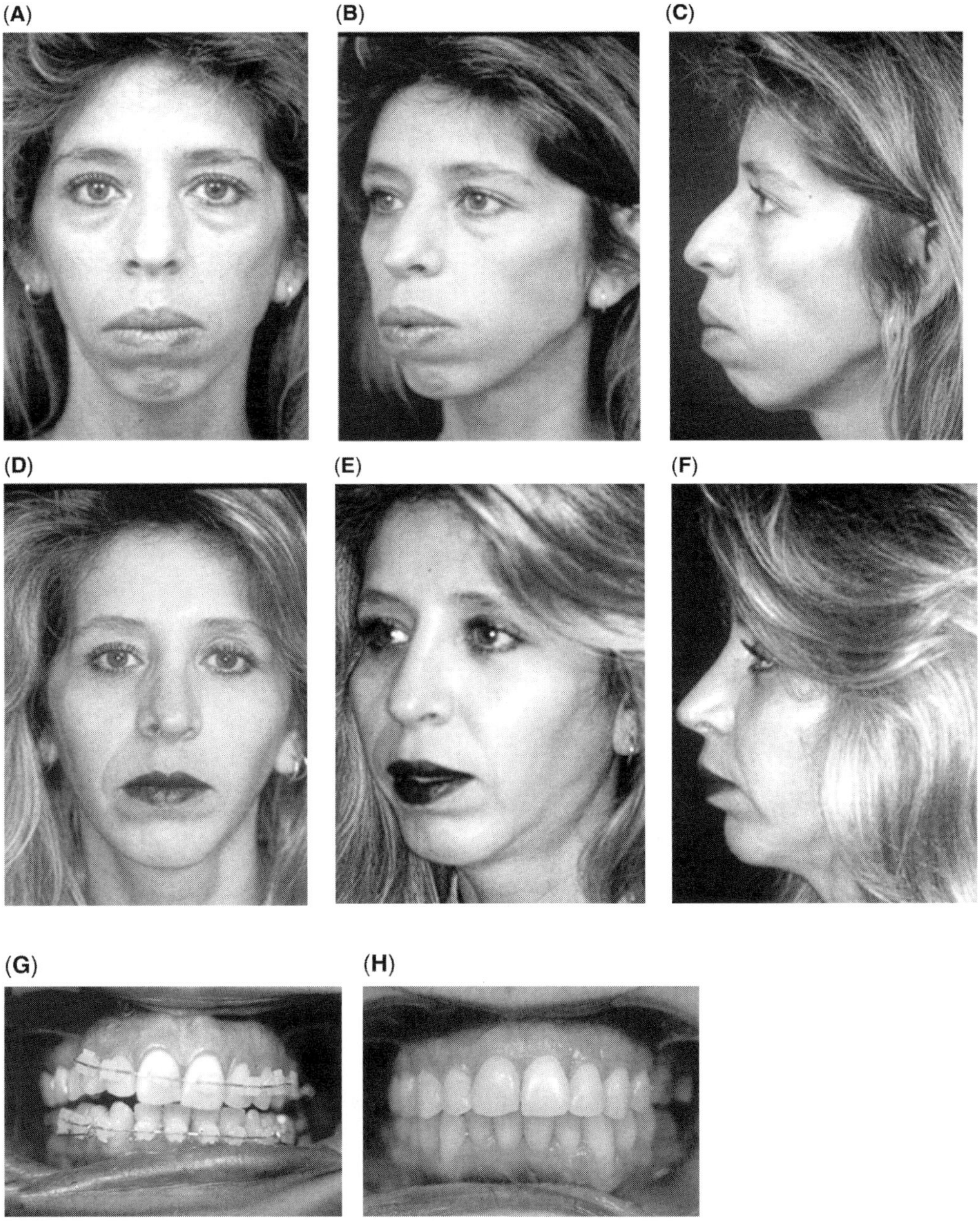

Figure 31 (**A–C**) Preoperative views of a female requesting nasal and chin correction. Observe the exaggerated facial convexity, biprocidence of the dental arches, absence of sublingual groove and severe microgenia. (**D–F**) Postoperative result after segmental maxillo-mandibular osteotomies, sliding genioplasty and rhinoplasty. (**G**) Preoperative orthodontic treatment. (**H**) Final occlusion.

lateral extreme of both osteotomies meet at the level of the free edge to achieve continuity and to prevent a step irregularity (Figs. 37 and 38). Fixation is done in the same way.

An important anatomical detail is the possible low localization of the intramandibular tract of the nerve. In preoperative X rays it is possible to determine the position of the canal to prevent injury of the nerve, and if necessary, a burr is used to open it and free the nerve before doing the superior osteotomy.

When it is necessary to increase the vertical dimension, the same horizontal osteotomy is made, interposing a bone graft anteriorly between the two segments. Fixation can be done

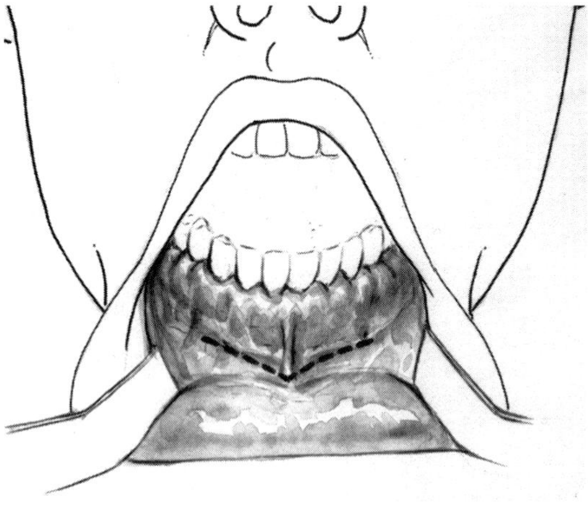

Figure 32 Sliding genioplasty. A gull-wing incision is made 5 mm in front of the vestibular sulcus.

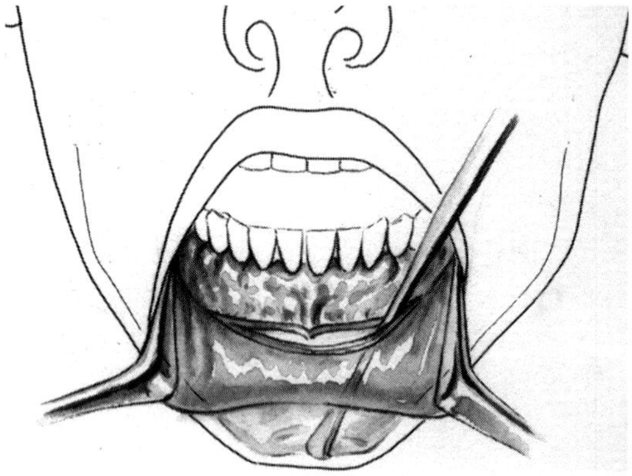

Figure 33 Sliding genioplasty. Subperiosteal dissection of the anterior aspect of the mandible.

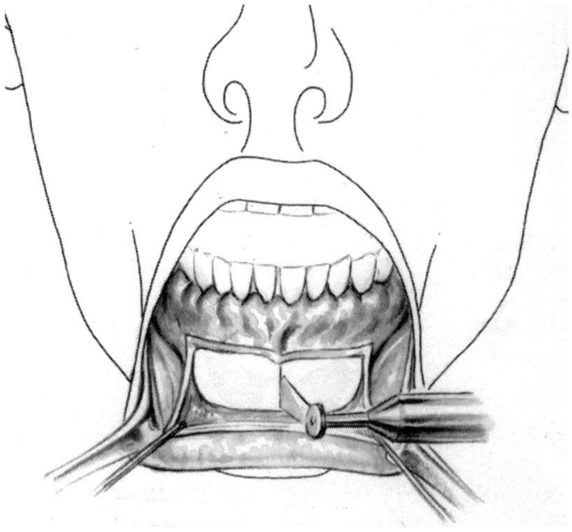

Figure 34 Sliding genioplasty. The subperiosteal dissection is extended laterally along the mandibular body forming a tunnel below the emergence of the nerve.

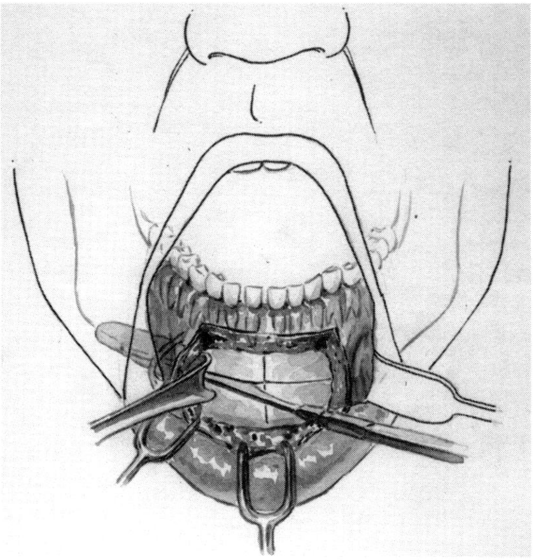

Figure 35 Sliding genioplasty. A vertical mark is made on the bone to insure symmetry. A reciprocating saw is used to perform the osteotomy while the nerve is protected with a right angle retractor.

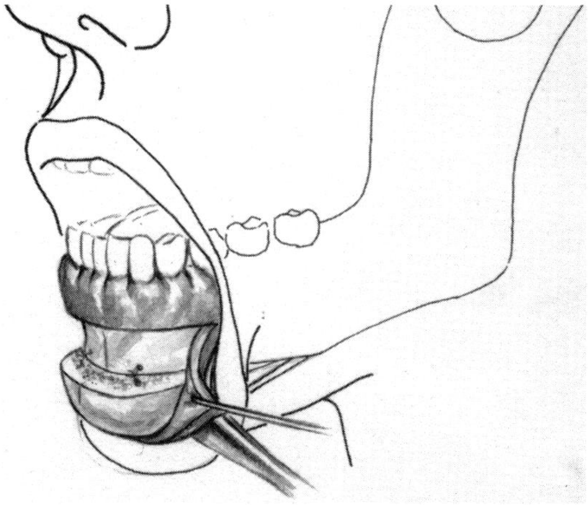

Figure 36 Sliding genioplasty. The free segment is mobilized anteriorly and fixed with two wire sutures.

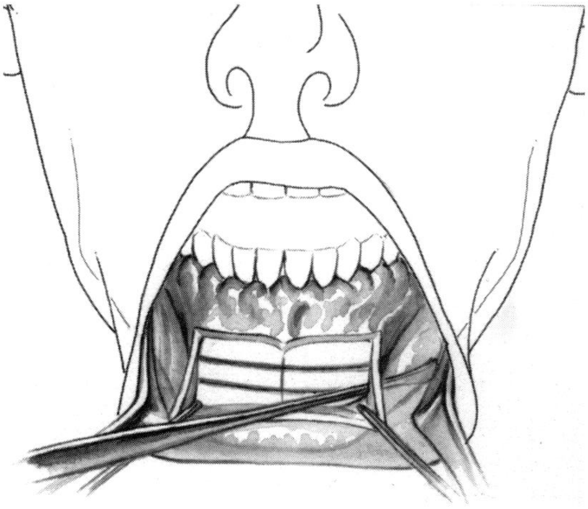

Figure 37 Sliding genioplasty. To shorten the chin two parallel osteotomies are made to achieve an edge resection.

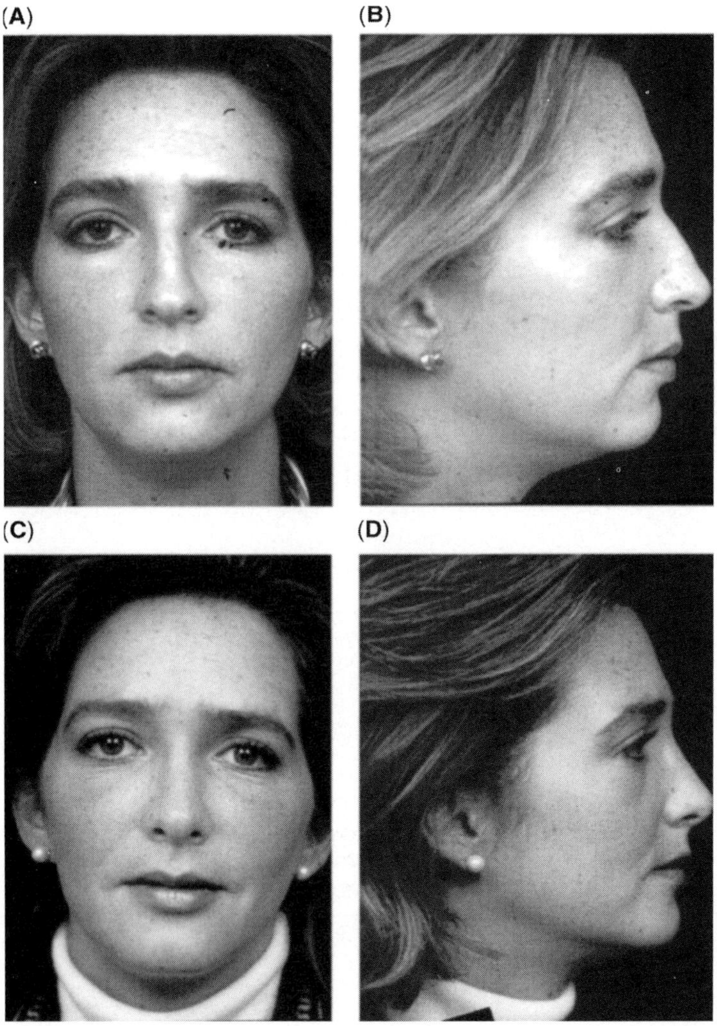

Figure 38 (**A** and **B**) Preoperative views of a patient requesting nasal correction and chin augmentation. (**C** and **D**) Postoperative result after a rhinoplasty and sliding genioplasty. Facial balance is improved combined with the rejuvenating effect of the genioplasty, which stretches the lower face tissues and enhances neck angle.

with stainless steel wire sutures, but the use of miniplates in the case of elongation allows better pressure between the two segments over the graft and its fixation.

OSTEOTOMIES ON THE MANDIBULAR BODY

Patients who require the correction of exaggerated mandibular width usually have normal dental occlusion, and the problem is purely aesthetic. On palpation, it is possible to detect the lateral projection of the mandibular angle and the insertion of a powerful masseter muscle. Manual palpation with a finger introduced into the buccal cavity confirms the impression of lateral displacement of the gonium and the thickness of the mandibular body. It is usual to find an increased thickness of the mandibular body along the oblique line. This malformation is usually bilateral and symmetrical although it may be present on only one side, resulting in facial asymmetry. This usually corresponds to congenital malformation of the type of hemifacial microsomia and congenital torticollis.

X-ray studies, especially postero-anterior(PA) cephalometry, are useful to confirm clinical impressions, allowing also the elimination of other pathological processes on the bone. The thickness of the bone of the mandibular body is usually increased. The mandibular angle is

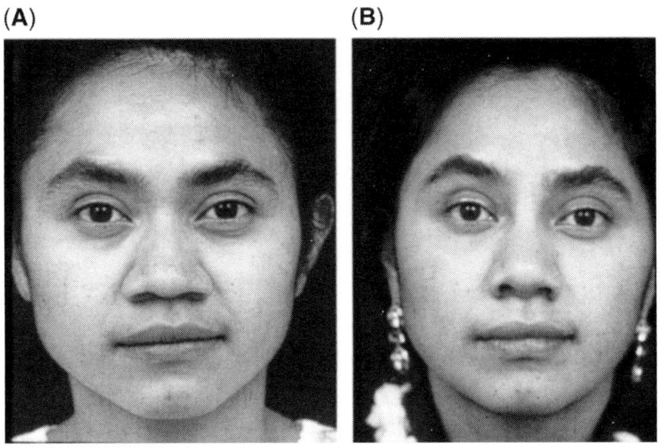

Figure 39 (**A**) Preoperative view of a patient with an exaggerated bigonial and hypertrophy of the masseters. She also has a low nasal dorsum and wide nasal base. (**B**) Result after remodeling of the mandible, chondrocostal graft to the nasal dorsum, and wedge resection of the nostril sills.

hypertrophic and also shows a curvature. It is important in the X-rays to localize the position of the duct of the dental nerve to avoid possible injury during surgery.

SURGICAL TECHNIQUE

Under general endotracheal anesthesia an incision is made on the mucosa of the mandibular vestibulum, exposing the lateral aspect of the mandibular body all the way to the gonial angle with a subperiosteal dissection. The dissection should be extended to the mandibular edge using the periosteal elevators especially designed for this purpose. The dissection should also extend to the posterior edge of the ramus. The insertion of the masseter muscle is entirely liberated. Protecting the soft tissues with an Obwegeser retractor, the hypertrophic section of the bone is modeled using a burr or a reciprocating saw. It is important to maintain continuous irrigation to prevent permanent injury to the bone and the soft tissues (Fig. 39).

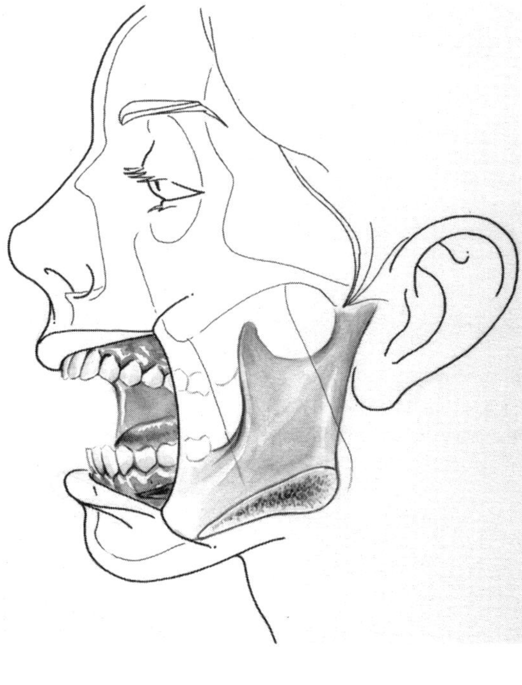

Figure 40 Through a vestibular incision, the mandibular periosteum is elevated to the posterior edge of the ramus with adequate protection of the soft tissues. The bone is remodeled with a burr or with a reciprocating saw.

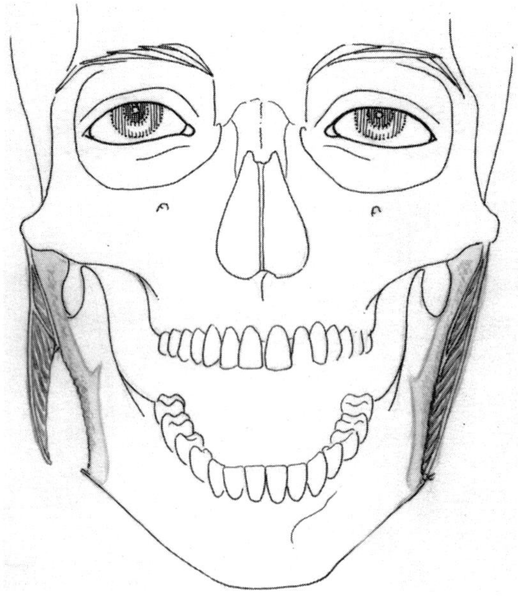

Figure 41 A wedge section of the masseter is resected.

Resection of the opposite side is done, taking care to maintain symmetry of the mandible. The final stage is a wedge resection of the medial aspect of the masseter muscle, preserving the integrity of the lateral aspect of the muscle and its facial cover (Fig. 40). A muscle resection may not be necessary, because the volume of the muscle will be decreased posteriorly as a result of its decreased mandibular insertion. The mucosa is closed with absorbable material, and an elastic bandage with moderate pressure is applied. If necessary, thin suction drains may be introduced percutaneously (Fig. 41).

REFERENCES

1. Ricketts RM. Divine proportion in facial aesthetics. Clin Plast Surg 1988; 81:500.
2. Whitaker LA, Bartlett SP. Aesthetic surgery of the facial skeleton. Perspect Plast Surg 1988; 2:23.
3. Whitaker LA, Pertschuk M. Facial Skeletal contouring for aesthetic purposes. Plast Reconstr Surg 1991; 87:268.
4. Barnett A, Whitaker LA. Facial form analysis of the lower middle face. Plast Reconst Surg 1986; 78:158.
5. Lefort René. Experimental study of fractures of the upper jaw. L'Echo Medical du North 1900; 4:470–473; Traducido por Tilson HB. DDS. The University of Texas, Dental Branch at Houston, 1972.
6. Dingman R. The history of the Le Fort I osteotomy. J Maxillofac Surg 1986; 14:119–122.
7. Obwegeser H. Surgical correction of the small or retrodisplaced maxillae. Plast Reconst Surg 1969; 43:352–365.
8. Ortiz Monasterio F. The long and narrow face. In: En Ousterhout DK, ed. Aesthetic Contouring of the Craniofacial Skeleton. Boston: Little Brown, 1991.
9. Tessier P. Osteotomies totales de la face. Syndrome de Crouzon, syndrome d'Apert, oxycephalies, scaphocephalies, turricephalies. Ann Chirurgie Plastique 1967; 12:269–286.
10. Köle K. Surgical operations on the alveolar ridge to correct occlusal abnormalities. J Oral Surg 1959; 12:515.
11. Köle H. Results, experience and problems in the operative treatment of anomalies with severe overbite. J Oral Surg 1965; 19:427.
12. Wassmund M. Lehrbuch der praktischen Chirurgie des Mundes und der Kiefer. Barth Vol. 1. Leipzig: H. Meusser, 1935.
13. Wunderer S. Profile correction of the midfacial area with the help of a pediculated maxillary fragment method. Transactions of the Fifth International Congress of Plastic and Reconstructive Surgery, Rome, 1967.
14. Straith RD, Lawson JN. Surgical orthodontia: a new horizon for plastic surgery. Plast Reconstr Surg 1967; 39:366.

15 Body Image as Seen by the Anatomists, the Artists, and the Surgeons

Fernando Ortiz-Monasterio
School of Medicine, Universidad Nacional Autónoma de México, Mexico City, Mexico

INTRODUCTION

I don't intend to write about beauty, much less attempt to define it. My purpose is to present a general perspective of the concept of body image as seen by the anatomists and by the artists and, to some extent, by the surgeons. Implicit in this overview is the fact that all of them, anatomists and artists, represented in their work the ideal of beauty at their particular time and culture.

The notion of the perfect body is not only the territory of modern plastic surgery; it appears in the history of art from the most ancient times. This concept was developed by the Greeks associating anatomy and art. The anatomical terms used to describe the different parts of the human body appear early in Greek literature. Homer's detailed descriptions of injuries in the battle of Troy are closer to a medical record than to a poetic expression. In fact, many of the terms we currently use in anatomy were employed by Homer.

The Greeks had a passion for beauty and explored the rules for the harmonious proportions applicable to all artistic manifestations. The mathematical studies of Pythagoras and Euclid established the basis for the Golden Rule of proportions applicable to all things in nature (1). This rule was consistently used by Vitruvio and Marco (2) and by Palladio (3) in their architectural designs. This concept has been used by all the classic artists like Donatello, della Robbia, Verocchio, da Vinci, Raphael, Buonarrotti, and many others in modern times (4). Le Corbusier, the famous French architect, with a group of artists and anthropologists erected a stella in Marseilles in the late 1930s inscribed with the measurements of what was considered the ideal proportions of the human body (5).

Greek anatomical knowledge, based on keen observation of the human figure, was originally copied by the Romans, and lost during the Middle Ages. Anatomy was taught in the European universities in the 15th century following the text of Mondino, published in 1423. He may have dissected a few cadavers, but his book is full of errors following the Galenic concepts accepted as dogmas for more than 1000 years. The scarce anatomical illustrations in Mondino's work demonstrate a poor concept of the human body.

Modern anatomy was born in Padua in the 16th century during the explosion of ideas of the Renaissance. America was discovered; Galileo proved that the earth orbits around the sun; Galenic dogmas were questioned; Vesalius conducted cadaver dissections and published his Fabrica in 1543 with the marvelous illustrations of von Kalkar (6). For the first time the human body was represented as a well-proportioned athletic figure similar to the classic Greek statues. The "Ecorché," the skinless muscle man, represents a connection between the reality of the living model and the imagined reality of a postmortem object of autopsy (Fig. 1). This trend was followed by his disciple Eustachio (7), although his work was published much later (Fig. 2) and by the brilliant anatomist Casserius (8) also working in Padua (Fig. 3). Feminine anatomy was illustrated in detail; his dissected madonnas were well-proportioned, almost athletic young women.

The "Fabrica Anatomica" of Petraglia included illustrations of nondissected females in splendorous femininity (Figs. 4 and 5) (9). Mascagni, in the 18th century, published a series of outstanding anatomical illustrations in two versions, one of them in color, emphasizing the well-developed muscles of the masculine body (10).

In his work "Anatomy for Artists" published in 1723 (Fig. 6), Genga (11) selected Roman copies of classical sculptures of the late Hellenistic period: the powerful relaxed Hercules fatigued after a battle, the young man in a position of attack (Fig. 7), and the thoroughly trained athlete were the Greek ideal of harmony of the body and soul. Genga represented Aphrodite

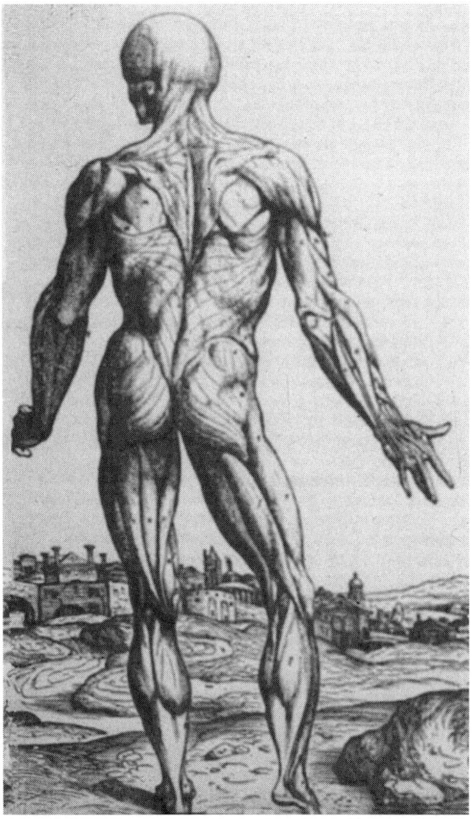

Figure 1 Anatomical plate from Vesalius, "Humani Corporis Fabrica." The marvelous woodcarvings by von Kalkar represent the "Ecorché," the skinless man, a connection between the reality of the living model and the imaginate reality of an autopsy.

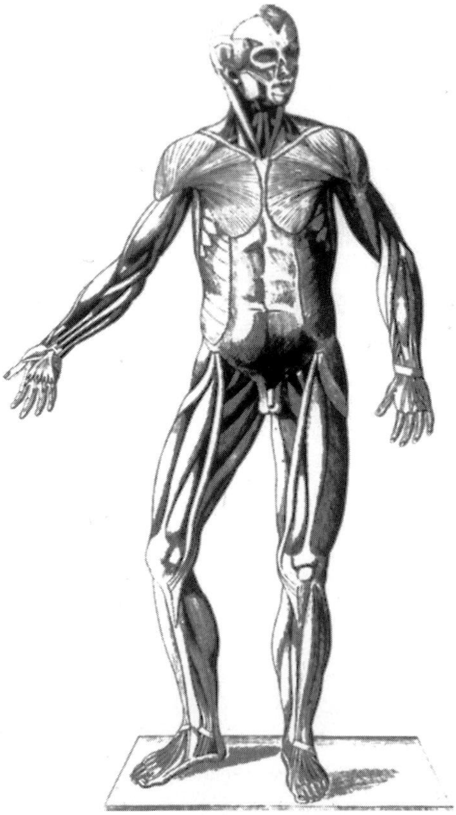

Figure 2 A less realistic but more precise copper etching in the "Anatomy" by Barthomaeo Eustachi Bartolomeo.

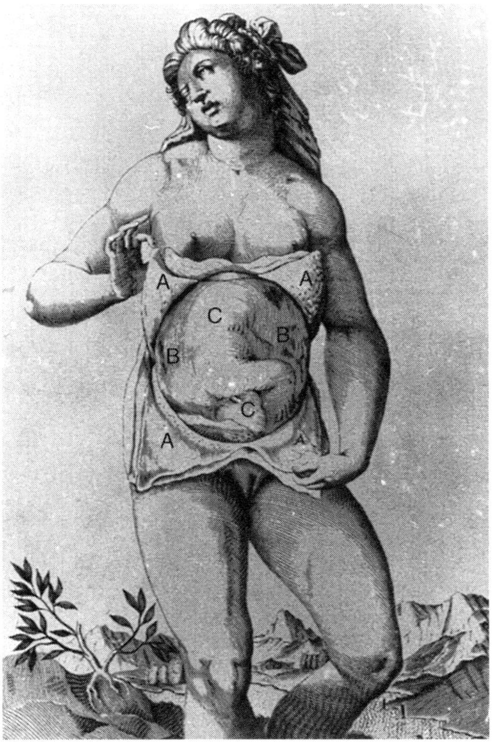

Figure 3 In contrast with the 16th-century anatomists, Casserius used sensual models to depict precise information on fetal development.

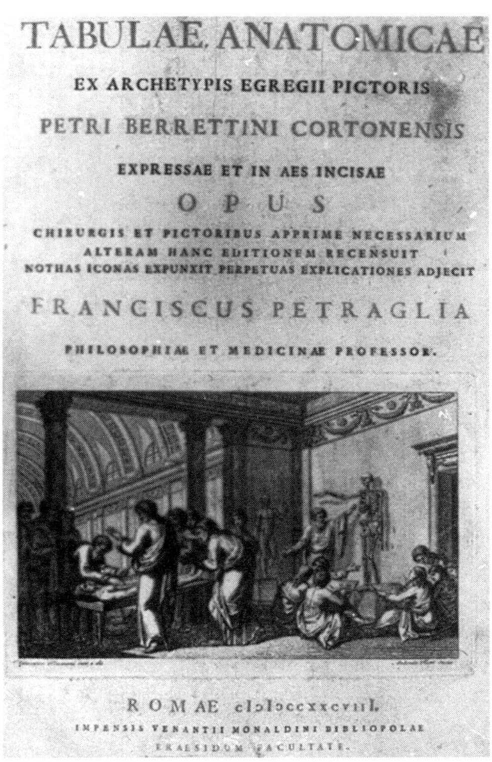

TABULAE ANATOMICAE
EX ARCHETYPIS EGREGII PICTORIS
PETRI BERRETTINI CORTONENSIS
EXPRESSAE ET IN AES INCISAE
OPUS
CHIRURGIS ET PICTORIBUS APPRIME NECESSARIUM
ALTERAM HANC EDITIONEM RECENSUIT
NOTHAS ICONAS EXPUNXIT PERPETUAS EXPLICATIONES ADJECIT
FRANCISCUS PETRAGLIA
PHILOSOPHIAE ET MEDICINAE PROFESSOR.
ROMAE cIↄIↄccxxcviii.
IMPENSIS VENANTII MONALDINI BIBLIOPOLAE
PRAESIDUM FACULTATE.

Figure 4 Title page of the "Anatomy" by Franciscus Petraglia.

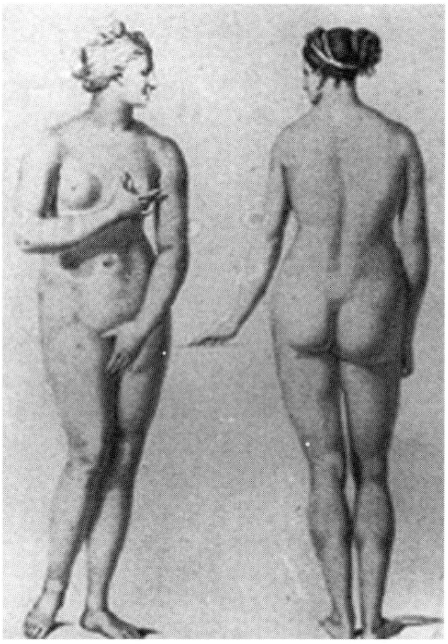

Figure 5 Women in Petraglia's Anatomy are represented in splendorous femininity.

(Fig. 8) as a serene being, not troubled by the gaze of the spectators, alone in her human divinity. She has just undressed to take a bath. She appears as a mature woman with voluptuous feminine curves but with small breasts.

Artists have been also involved in anatomy. Leonardo studied human proportions and produced marvelous illustrations. His own face was probably used as a model in the "Divina Proportione" of Pacioli (Fig. 9) (12).

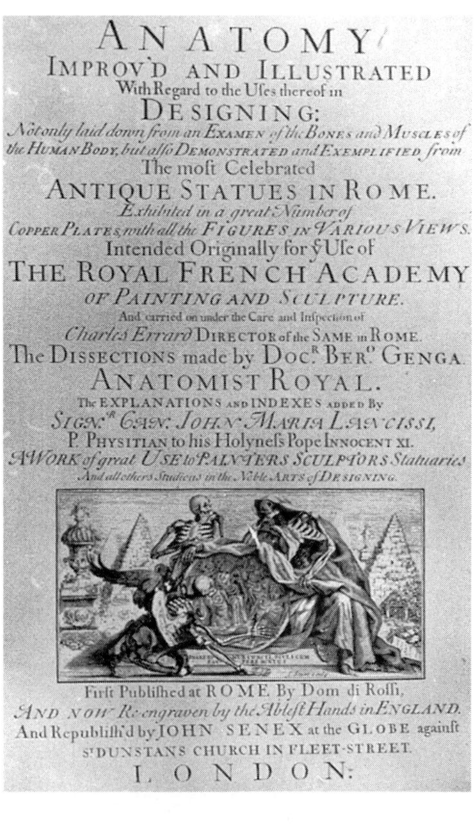

ANATOMY
IMPROV'D AND ILLUSTRATED
With Regard to the Uſes thereof in
DESIGNING:
Not only laid down from an EXAMEN *of the* BONES *and* MUSCLES *of the* HUMAN BODY, *but alſo* DEMONSTRATED *and* EXEMPLIFIED *from*
The moſt Celebrated
ANTIQUE STATUES IN ROME.
Exhibited in a great Number of
COPPER PLATES, with all the FIGURES IN VARIOUS VIEWS.
Intended Originally for ye Uſe of
THE ROYAL FRENCH ACADEMY
OF PAINTING AND SCULPTURE.
And carried on under the Care and Inſpection of
Charles Errard DIRECTOR of the SAME in ROME.
The DISSECTIONS made by DOC^R^ BER^O^ GENGA
ANATOMIST ROYAL.
The EXPLANATIONS AND INDEXES ADDED By
SIGN:^R^ CAN: JOHN MARIA LANCISSI,
P. PHYSITIAN to his Holyneſs Pope INNOCENT XI.
A WORK of great USE to PAINTERS SCULPTORS Statuaries
And all others Studious in the Noble ARTS of DESIGNING.

First Publiſhed at ROME By Dom di Roſſi,
AND NOW Re-engraven by the Ableſt Hands in ENGLAND.
And Republiſh'd by JOHN SENEX at the GLOBE againſt
S^T^ DUNSTANS CHURCH IN FLEET-STREET.
LONDON:

Figure 6 Genga in the 18th century published a beautiful "Anatomy for Artists."

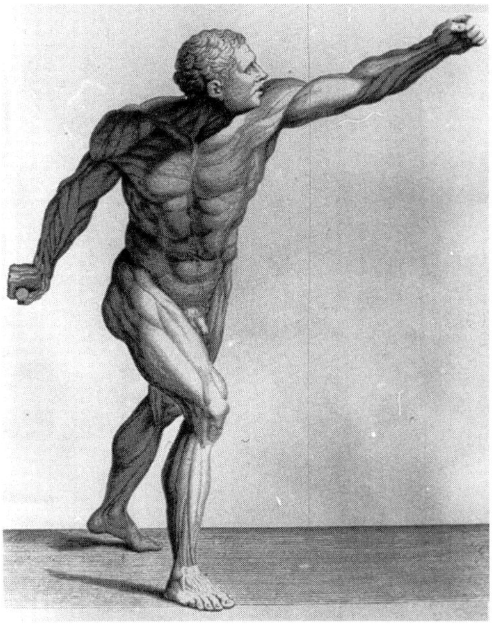

Figure 7 Roman copies of the classic Hellenistic period were chosen by Genga to represent the masculine body as a strong, well-trained athlete.

Albert Dürer, the most important and original theoretician of the history of art, published very detailed physical, anthropological data on the human body, both masculine and feminine, at rest and in motion, as well as the overweight and underweight variants (13). Reading Dürer's methodical text requires patience and determination. Reading Leonardo's notes written in the exquisitely educated Tuscan language is a pleasure (Figs. 10 and 11).

The human figure has been represented by artists since time immemorial, from the lipodystrophic Venus of Lespugue suggesting fertility to the stylized females of the cicladic art of 2000 B.C. and the early Greek tanagras (Figs. 12 and 13).

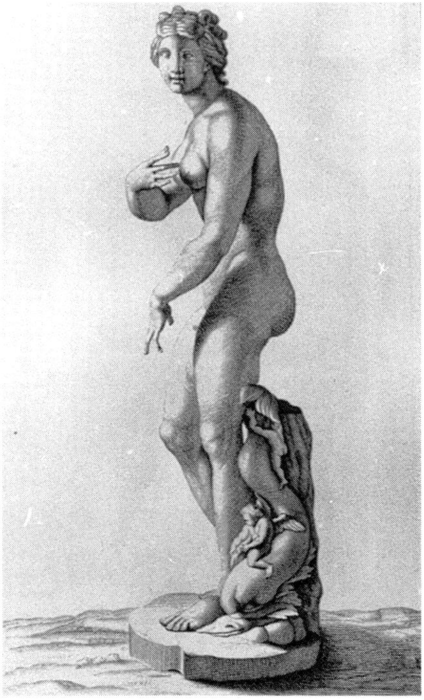

Figure 8 For the female body Genga presented Aphrodite as a serene being, alone in her human divinity.

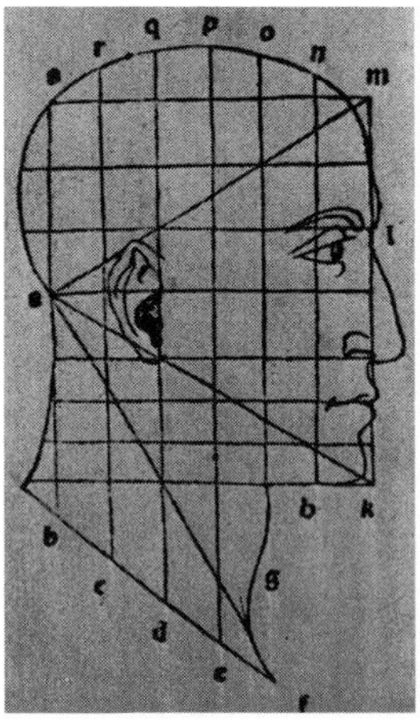

Figure 9 Leonardo may have been the model represented in the "Divina Proportione" by Pacioli.

The female body was an extensive representative of Mesoamerica. The deliciously erotic maidens from the pre-classic period of Mexico, molded around 500 B.C. with their wide hips, not only represented fertility but also an aesthetic ideal (Fig. 14).

Lean, idealized Adam and Eve were represented in the marvelous painting of Dürer, whereas a rather overmuscled androgynous female was sculptured by Michelangelo for the funeral monument of the Medici family in Florence.

The "Ladies in a Turkish Bath" by Ingres and "The Three Graces" by Rubens represented the aesthetic ideal for their time. The reclining feminine figure, dressed or nude, has been a favorite subject for the painters throughout the ages. Artists tend to select beautiful models or to improve them. It is pertinent to mention some representative works, because they represent the ideal feminine body image at different epochs.

The "Venus de Urbino" by Titian in the 16th century (Fig. 15), "Danae Waiting for Her Lover" by Rembrandt in the 17th, the lovely, voluptuous "Maja Desnuda" by Goya in 18th (Fig. 16), and the magnificent "Olympia" by Manet in the 19th are all excellent examples of feminine beauty in their particular time and culture.

The trend continues in the 20th century: the mysterious inexpressive ladies with big eyes of Delvaux; the sweet, obese Colombian women by Botero, which may represent a trend to a more varied aesthetic concept of body image (14). According to Botero, volume is a promise of

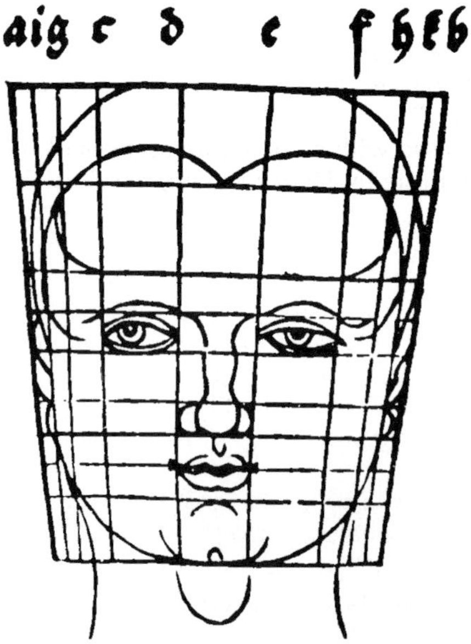

Figure 10 Detailed physical anthropological studies of the human face were published by Albert Dürer in the 16th century.

(**A**)

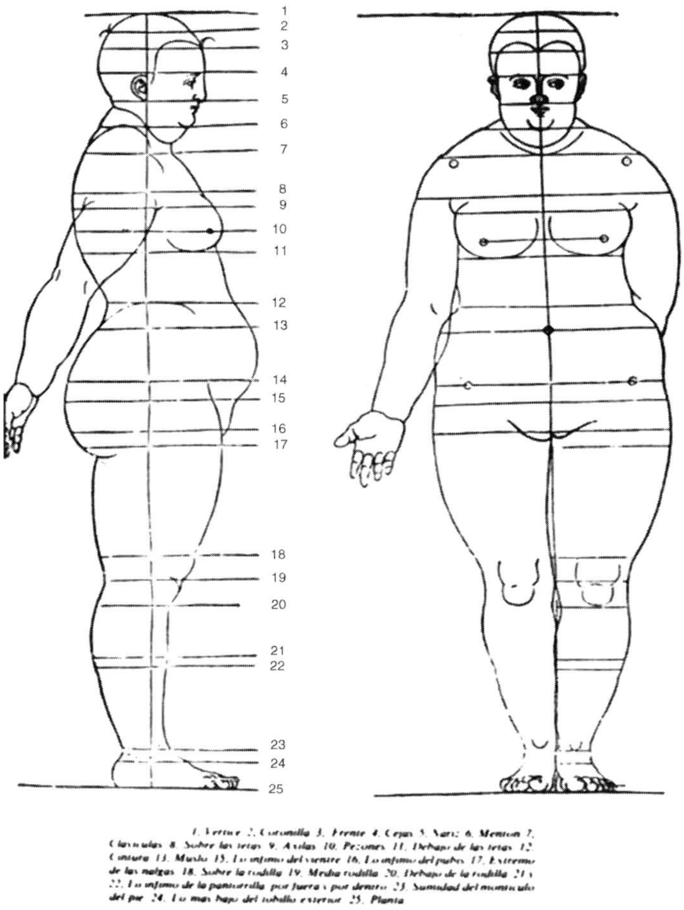

Figure 11 The superb studies by Dürer on the human figure, at rest and in motion, lean and overweight. (*Continued on next page.*)

sensuality, of happiness; weight gives stability, and more extended skin gives more aperture to sensations. Evidently obese persons, like thin people, also live delicious love affairs, mystical obsessions, and imaginative paradises. As expressed by Shakespeare in the tragedy of Julius Caesar: "I want fat people around me, with tight skin, who sleep well; Cassius has a lean and hungry air; he thinks too much, is jealous and dangerous."

This is also emphasized in the reclining lady of Picasso with some reminiscences of his analytic cubism period and the almost abstract reclining nude by Henry Moore, possibly the most important sculptor of the 20th century (Fig. 17).

The masculine body has also been extensively represented in art. From the mythic Greek sculptor Daidalos in the 7th century B.C. to the works of Phydias and Praxiteles, man in his god-human figure is represented as a strong, well-trained, and intelligent athlete.

The Renaissance recovered the concept of the ideal body image, closer to the classical Greek as sculptured by Michelangelo in the powerful, relaxed David after slaying Goliath. The expression of a strong body was emphasized in the manneristic paintings of Domenico Teotocopoulos, called "El Greco" in Spain, using disproportionate relations between the small heads and long bodies.

In the late 20th century the trend to show the not-so-beautiful human body is present in the work of Freud, nephew of the famous psychoanalyst, or in the lean men of Giacometti. At the beginning of the third millennium the ideal masculine body image remains close to the classical Greek sculptures of the late period corresponding to the young, well-trained athlete similar to his counterpart in the original Olympic Games.

(**B**)

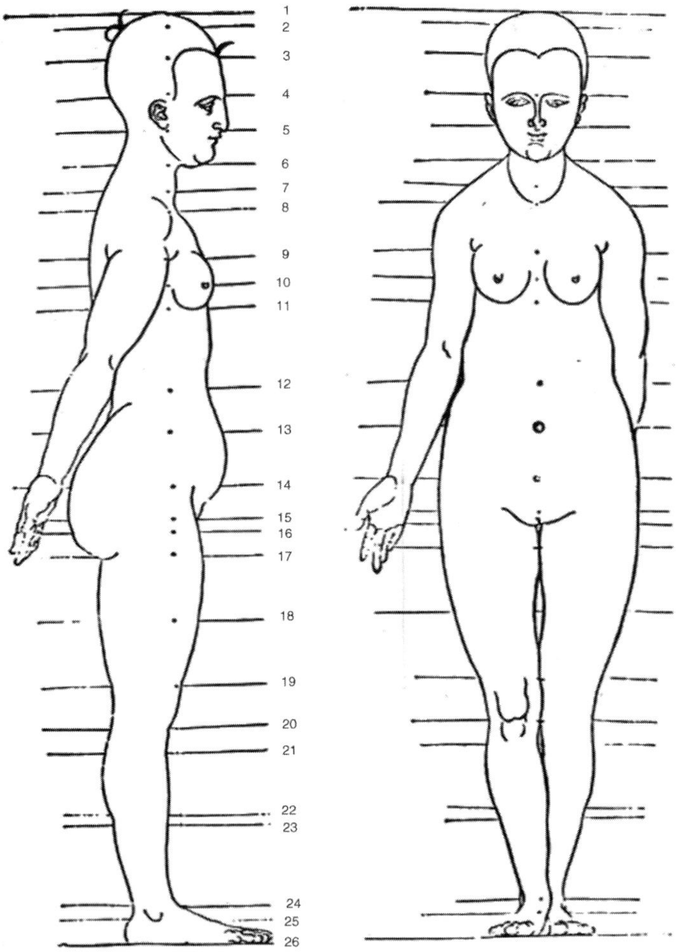

1. Vértice. 2. Coronilla. 3. Frente. 4. Cejas. 5. Nariz. 6. Mentón. 7. Sumidad de los hombros. 8. Clavículas. 9. Axilas. 10. Pezones. 11. Debajo de las tetas. 12. Cintura. 13. Ombligo. 14. Sumidad del muslo. 15. Abertura. 16. Lo más bajo del pubis. 17. Extremidad de las nalgas. 18. Surco del muslo. 19. Sobre la rodilla. 20. Media rodilla. 21. Bajo la rodilla. 22 y 23. Lo ínfimo de la pantorrilla por fuera, por dentro. 24. Monte del pie. 25. Lo más alto del tobillo externo. 26. Planta.

Figure 11 (*Continued from previous page*)

The face, being possibly the most important element, at least the most visible of the body and the main subject of our surgical endeavors, deserves special consideration (Fig. 18). Physiognomists in the past have given great emphasis to the relation between facial features and temperament (15). Hippocrates described five well-defined facial types. Giovanni Battista della Porta related facial features and temperament to animal resemblance, and in modern times Lavatier devised a complex system to assess the temperament of a person by the facial features (Fig. 19). Following this system, Gallet (16) analyzed three interesting examples: Louis XIII, Voltaire, and Mirabeau with the Lavatier system.

God-like resemblance was represented in art in many cultures, like in the beautiful Olmec mask of a ruler carved 3000 years ago, deliberately emphasizing the features of the jaguar, their totemic god (Fig. 20).

The marked slanting of the eyes, present in the pre-Columbian population, was enhanced in the beautiful ladies from Veracruz who also had their teeth filed to achieve a more seductive smile. Fruit and floral fantasies were used by Archimboldo to depict the human face, and Picasso purposefully distorted the noses "to shock the viewer and force him to, finally, see a nose."

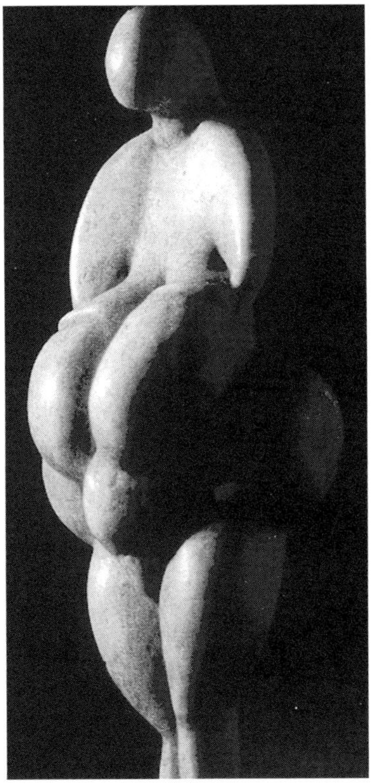

Figure 12 The "Venus of Lespugue." Glacial age.

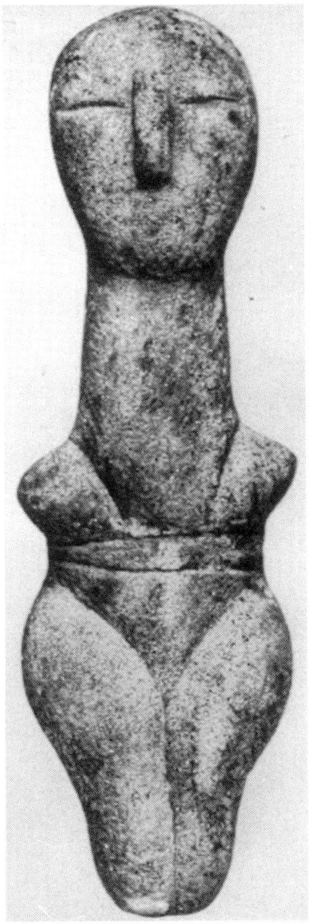

Figure 13 Feminine figure. Cicladic art, around 2000 B.C.

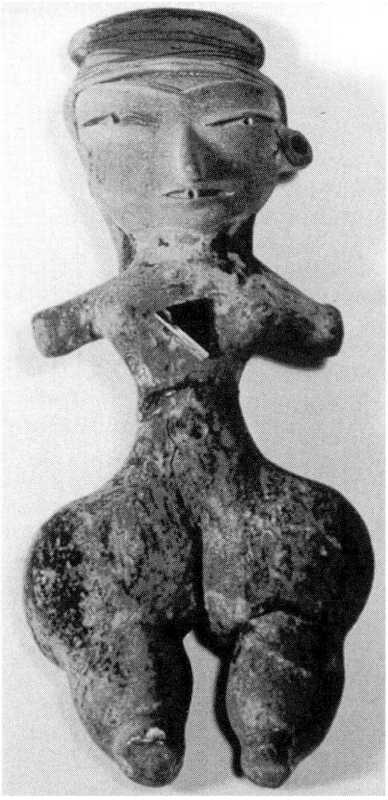

Figure 14 Feminine figure suggesting fertility and maybe also an aesthetic standard. Tlatilco, México. Pre-classic period.

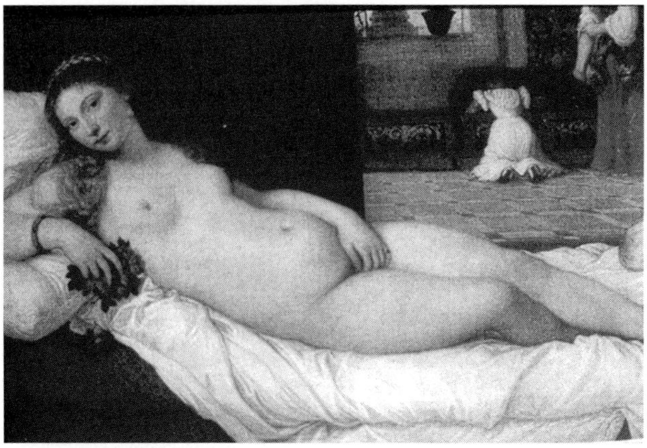

Figure 15 The "Venus of Urbino" by Titian, 16th century.

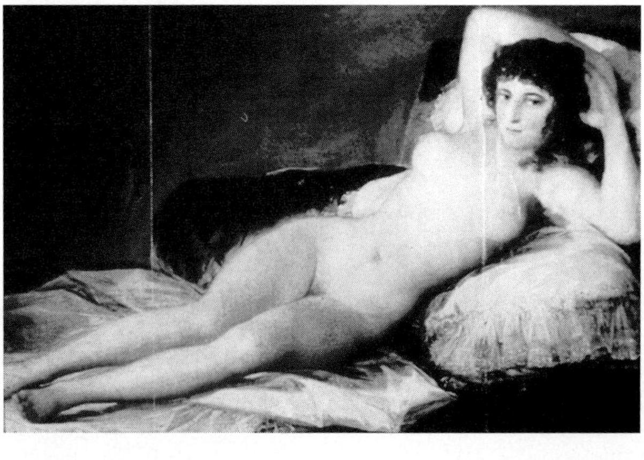

Figure 16 "The Maja Desnuda" painted by Francisco de Goya in the 16th century.

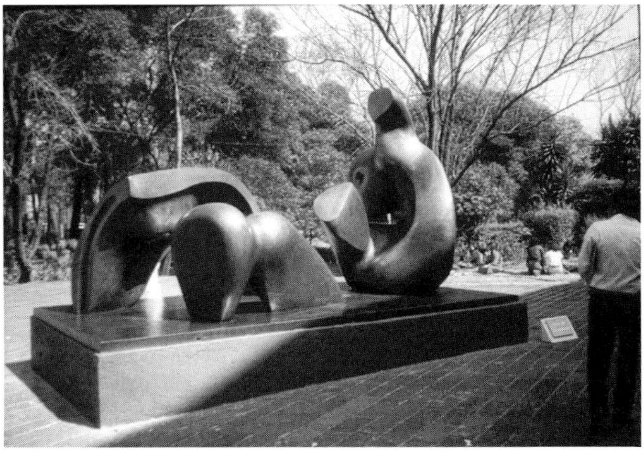

Figure 17 Reclining nude by Henry Moore.

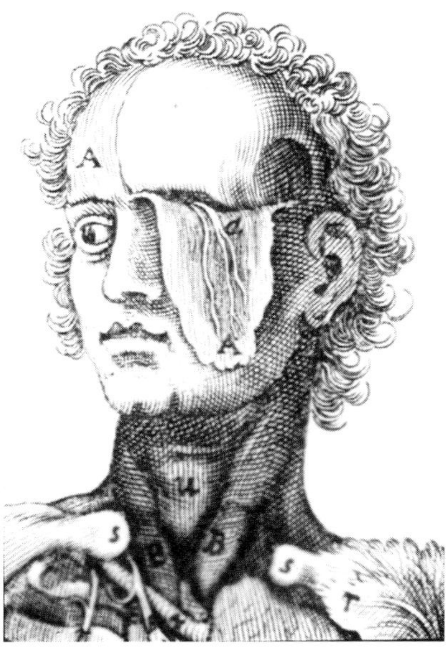

Figure 18 The human face in the Tabulae Anatomicae by Pietro da Cortona.

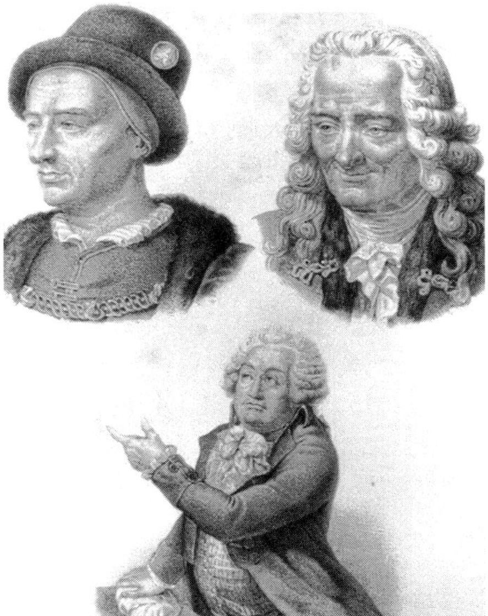

Figure 19 Gallet analyzed the temperament of Louis XIII, Voltaire, and Mirabeau with the Lavatier system.

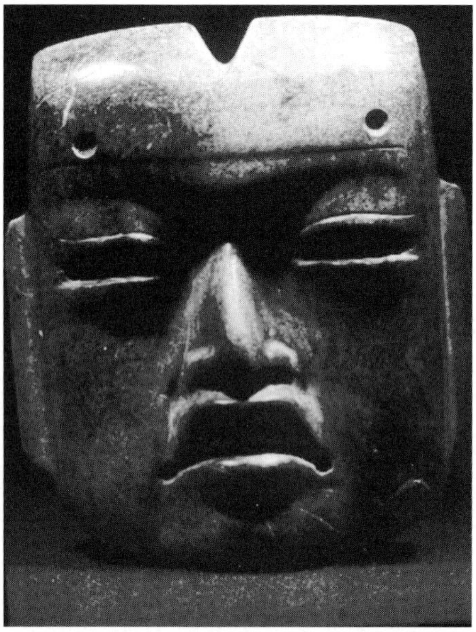

Figure 20 Jadeite mask of a ruler emphasizing the attributes of a jaguar. México, Olmec culture, around 1000 B.C.

I have mentioned the variations of the body image as perceived by the anatomists and by the artists.

For the surgeon, it is evident that the basic shape of the human body is related to the shape of the skeletal support. Returning to the mathematical concepts of Euclid, Leonardo, Fibonacci, Palladio, and Le Corbusier, we can see how the Golden Rule of proportions applies to the beautiful face. In the "Mute Lady" by Raphael, we perceive a perfect skeletal support, the ratio between the upper, middle, and lower thirds of the face is Golden as well as the relation between the height and width of the face (Fig. 21). When the face is in motion, especially during smiling, which is the ultimate test of beauty, a harmonious skeleton will produce a perfect smile as frequently shown in modern models.

The skin is the marvelous cover of the anatomical complex of skeleton and muscles. It is also the field where the art of wound healing of plastic surgery originated. The skin has

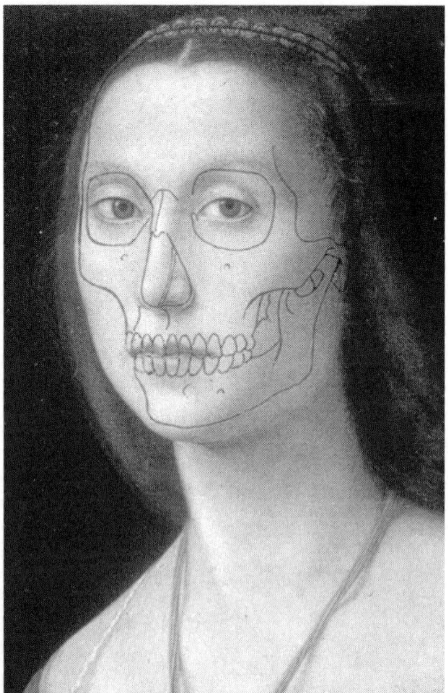

Figure 21 The "Mute Lady" by Raphael. The tracing of her facial skeleton shows perfect Golden Proportions.

adnexae, such as hair, that contribute to its aesthetic value. It also has pigment that filters the sunrays and that may be enhanced by cosmetics for ritual reasons or to achieve the perfection of white skin in the Japanese geishas. Our sun-worshiping culture with all its attractions is in contrast with the perfectly preserved, well-lubricated skin of the elegant women painted by Zurbaran and by Madrazo, in the Prado Museum in Madrid, and the immaculate texture of the faces and hands of the Countess of Newcastle and of the Viscountess of Redford in the portraits by William Larkin in the Tate Gallery in London.

Aesthetic appreciation of the skin is a visual, tactile, and olfactory experience. There are pheromones, perfumes, and body odors greatly admired in other times among the favorites of the kings of France: Agnes Sorel, Diane de Poitiers, and especially Gabrielle d'Estree whose irresistible attraction to Henry IV is documented in a letter he wrote to her: "Please, my lady, do not take a bath; I will arrive in three weeks."

The skin is not only an elastic and resistant tissue, it is the barrier of individuality, an armor and mechanism of contact, a site of beauty, and the playground for the perpetuation of our species. Skin is the soft cover, passionately attractive to surgeons, painters, photographers, lovers, and poets.

Domingo Gundisalvo in the 12th century defined the artist as the one who works over materials with tools (17). In the words of Galen men have hands to knit their dresses and their nets controlling territorial and marine animals, to write the laws, to build altars and ships and instruments, and to leave written records for posterity.

Body image is the territory of the work of the plastic surgeon. We work with our hands and talk about the art of surgery, but a more humble approach seems indicated. We are craftsmen with pretensions of artistic understanding.

REFERENCES

1. Ricketts RM. Divine proportion in facial aesthetics. Clin Plast Surg 1998; 81:500.
2. Vitruvio P, Marco L. Los diez libros de la arquitectura. Madrid: Alianza Editorial, 1995.
3. Palladio A. I quatro libri dell'architettura, en Murano, M. Venetian Villas, Magnus, Udine, 1986.
4. Da Vinci L. In: Ludwig H, ed. Trattato della Pittura. Codex Vaticanus (Urbinas), 1883.
5. Le Corbusier: 1910–1960. Zurich: Editions Girsberger, 1960.
6. Vesalius A. In: De Humanis Corpoiris FabricaVenice1543.
7. Eustaquio B. Tabulae AnatomicaeRoma1714.
8. Casserii J. Daniel Bucretius, ed. Tabulae Anatomicae. Venice, 1626.
9. Petraglia F. Tabulae Anatomicae. Impresis Venantii Menaldini, Bibliopole, Roma.
10. Mascagni P. Anatomia del Corpo Umano. In Nuovo Giornale dei Litterati. Pisa: Nistri, 1823.
11. Genga B. Anatomy improved for artists. 1672. Reingraved in London, 1723, by Senex, John.
12. Paccioli L. De divina proportione. 1509. In: Wintenberg, ed., 1889.
13. Durero A. Los cuatro libros de la simetría de las partes del cuerpo humano. Universidad Nacional Autónoma de México, 1987.
14. Lascault G. "Botero". Madrid: Lerner & Lerner, 1993.
15. Da Cortona P. Tabulae Anatomicae. Roma: Bibliographae, 1741.
16. Gallet D. Cuerpo del Hombre. Imprenta de Antonio Berdeguer. Barcelona, 1844.
17. Gundisalvo. In: Akal SA, ed. Tatarkiewicz Historia de la Estética. Madrid, España: Ediciones, 1987.

16 Aesthetic Osteotomies of the Malar Region

Fernando Molina

Department of Plastic, Aesthetic, and Reconstructive Surgery, Hospital General "Dr. Manuel Gea Gonzalez," Mexico City, Mexico

INTRODUCTION

In the middle third of the face, the malar region constitutes an area of extreme variability in projection and form. The malar midface can be divided in three subregions, blending imperceptibly with each other: inner (paranasal), middle (malar), and outer (zygomatic arch) (1–3).

The malar eminences are visible highlight points and are positioned anterior and medial in the bizygomatic distance, which is the widest portion of the face (3).

Several surgeons, artists, and experts in physical anthropometrics (4–7) have brought attention to the malar area and its significance in providing the aesthetically pleasing oval shape of the face. Actually, this oval shape represents the more harmonic, pleasing, equilibrated, and cherished face in our civilization. Therefore, the malar area holds an important key to the youthful look of the face. Surgeons should, therefore, seek three-dimensional treatment for each problem.

Aesthetically the malar area is very important; it provides not only a high point for the cheeks but also the anterior projection and transverse dimension of the face through the zygoma (8).

The correction of malar deficiencies, however, not only deals with the effects of gravity but also may involve developmental problems and occlusal abnormalities. The treatment of these patients must, therefore, be individualized according to the skeletal and soft-tissue requirements gleaned from a careful examination of each patient.

The use of osteotomies to address the morphology of the face was pioneered by Tessier (9,10). The evolution of osteotomies to correct occlusal abnormalities in combination with midface hypoplasia for purely aesthetic aims is actually part of the therapeutic armamentarium of a surgeon with craniomaxillofacial training. The knowledge gained in the past has allowed surgeons today to modify only specific areas of the facial skeletal to produce a more pleasing appearance without disturbing the natural architecture of the essential areas such as the orbits, the maxilla, and the mandible to obtain a better relationship between the different thirds of the face; according to the "Golden Rule" from the divine proportions in facial aesthetics (11).

Maxillary and malar osteotomies with interpositional bone grafting (12,13) has been used to broaden the horizontal projection of the middle third of the face; however, this technique has failed to obtain a better anterior projection of the malar-zygoma complex. A more complete osteotomy of the malar complex that allows not only an increase in transverse dimension but also an advancement to address the antero–posterior projection was initially utilized by Tessier (10) and then after widely used by Wolfe and Vitenas (14) to correct malar hypoplasia of a different etiology. We have performed some modifications to the original technique and it has been adapted to our group of patients, most of them with non-Caucasian characteristics, who are the ethnic group that we treat more frequently.

SURGICAL TECHNIQUE

We perform a combined surgical access, first through a coronal incision and subperiosteal dissection until we reach the zygomatic arch. Then through a second incision at the superior vestibular sulcus, we complete the subperiosteal dissection of the maxilla and malar zygomatic bones. These dissections permit a complete visualization of the malar structure, its relationship with the orbit, and its contents and the infraorbitary nerve foramen (Fig. 1).

The osteotomy design includes the malar bone going from inferior orbital rim to the lateral portion at the foramen of the infraorbital nerve, then it continues over to the superior aspect of the maxillary buttress. From this point it continues to the middle third of the

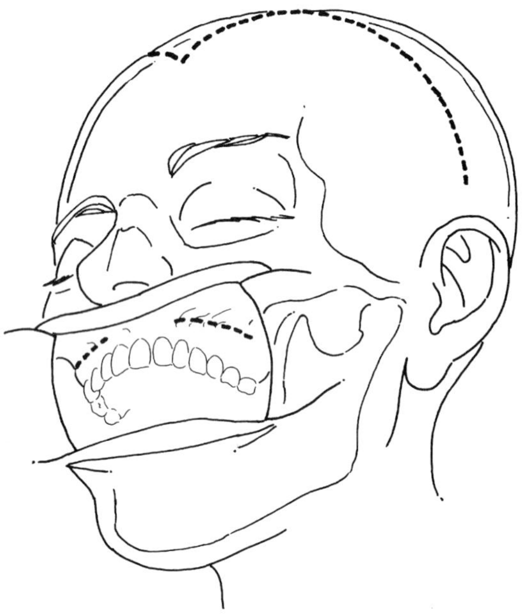

Figure 1 Drawing showing a combined surgical access: the coronal incision and a superior vestibular access. Both incisions allow subperiosteal dissection in the maxilla, zygomatic, and malar regions.

zygomatic arch. Cephalically the osteotomy includes a 5- to 6-mm width of the orbital floor and lateral wall, ending in the midportion of the lateral rim (Fig. 2). Through an intraoral route we begin the osteotomy with a reciprocating saw; the blade is positioned obliquely in front of the most caudal portion of the osteotomy and with a direction toward the orbit. The bone cut includes the entire width of the malar bone until the orbital rim and zygomatic arch (Fig. 3). Then, using a curved chisel the osteotomy is completed at the level of the orbital floor and the lateral wall, taking care to leave a bony union at the level of the midportion of the lateral orbital rim (Fig. 4), that produces the effect of a pivot.

The pedicle of this osteotomy is the periosteal layer of the orbital floor. The aim of preserving vascularity is always mandatory to conserve the continuity of the periosteum at

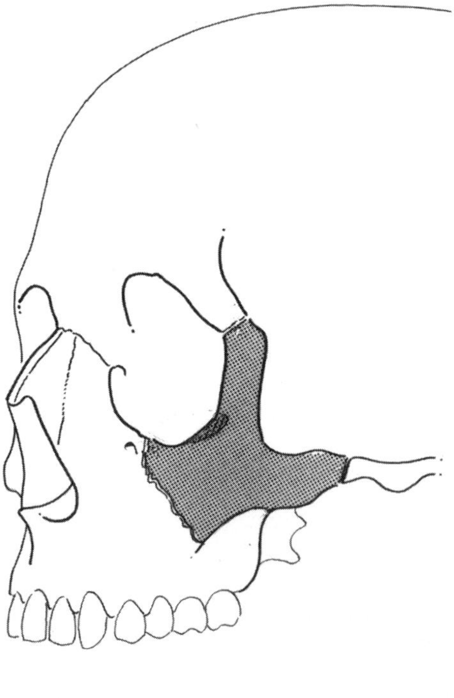

Figure 2 The drawing shows the osteotomy of the malar bone, which includes the orbital floor and the lateral wall, ending in the midportion of the lateral rim.

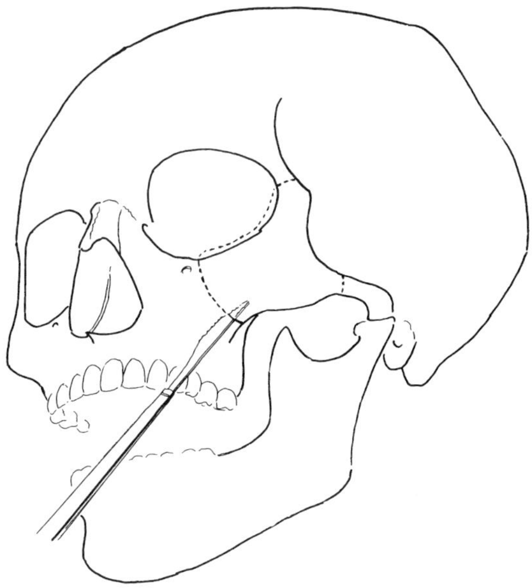

Figure 3 Using a reciprocating saw, we initiate the bone cut in the inferior border of the malar bone.

this level. Ideally the osteotomy must be completed with a "green stick" fracture at the midportion of the lateral wall of the orbit. This maneuver is achieved by introducing a 7-mm chisel in the transverse section of the malar bone. The malar bone is then pivoted superiorly with the access of rotation being the infraorbital rim (Fig. 5).

Cranial bone grafts from the parietal region can then be placed beneath the osteotomy, between the maxilla and the osteotomized malar bone (Fig. 6). The graft can be extended 4–8 mm below the inferior border of the osteotomy. When a larger bone graft is used, the malar bone projection in antero–posterior projection as well as in the bizygomatic transverse dimension will be greater.

After verification of the proper position of the grafts a gentle and constant pressure is applied with the hand over the skin and muscles on the malar area. This maneuver will produce the inverse mechanism of the fracture and will fix the bone grafts in place avoiding the use of rigid fixation material. Simultaneously, it allows the surgeon to verify intraoperatively that the malar augmentation is symmetric.

Then an absorbable suture is used to close the vestibular incision. In the selected cases for simultaneous facial rejuvenation, we immediately proceed to perform the subperiosteal

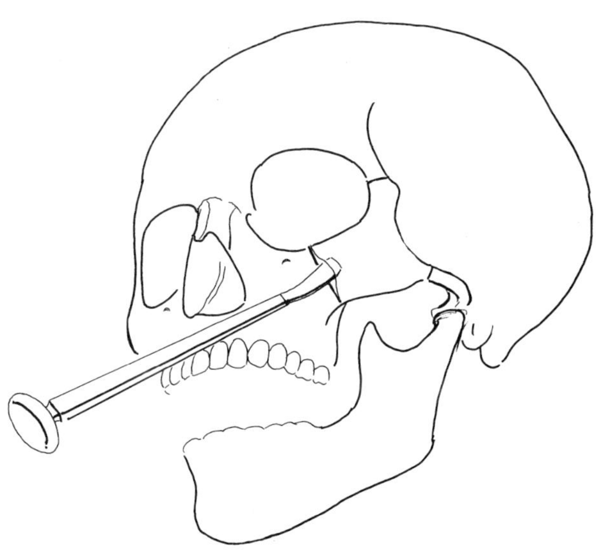

Figure 4 With a curved chisel, the osteotomy is completed at the level of the orbital floor and the lateral wall.

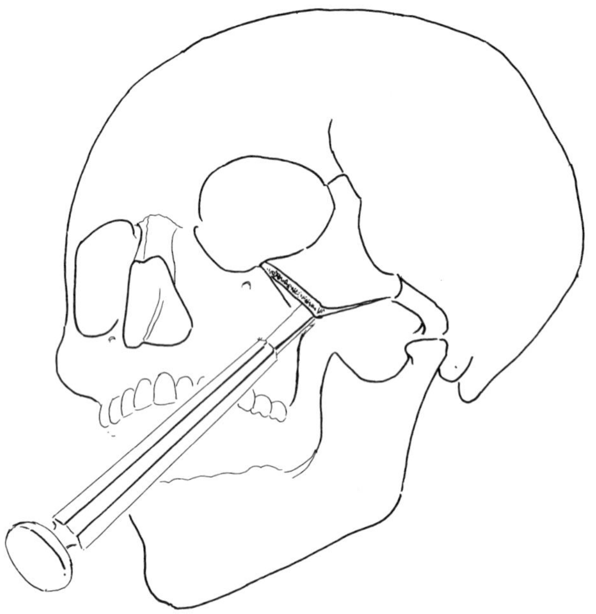

Figure 5 With a straight chisel of 7 mm we use a maneuver to complete the osteotomy with a "green stick" fracture.

suspension of the midface soft tissues followed with closure of the coronal incision with nonabsorbable sutures.

The results obtained with the malar augmentation osteotomy produce changes in facial contour with a natural appearance. The achieved volume gradually increases because the inferior half of the lateral orbital rim reaches the highest point of projection at the level of the zygomatic arch (Fig. 7A and B). In the cases where subperiosteal lifting is associated with a simultaneous correction of a lateral canthus dystopia, together with volume enhancement of the malar region, a pleasant rejuvenation change simultaneously results around the orbits, cheeks, and nasolabial folds. The sagging of the tissues of the middle and upper face are corrected (Fig. 8A and B).

This technique is also very useful for treating congenital malar deficiencies present with major facial clefts. The malar augmentation procedure can be combined with other reconstructive techniques producing very satisfactory aesthetic and functional results (Fig. 9A and B). The resulting face is more attractive and in better proportion.

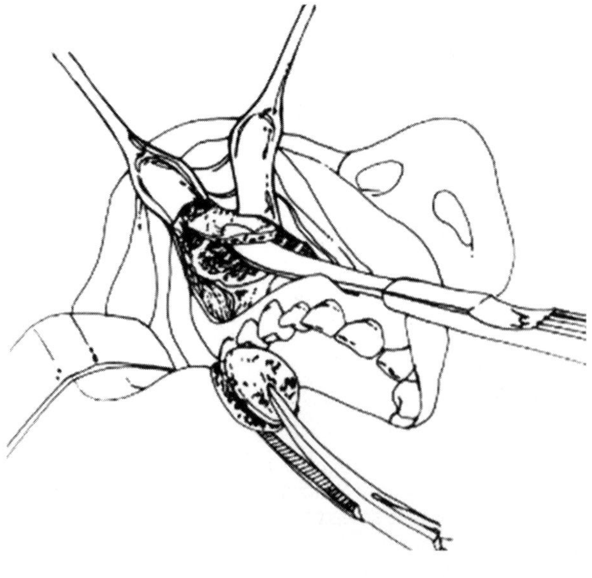

Figure 6 Beneath the osteotomy, cranial bone grafts are placed in the parietal region.

(A) (B)

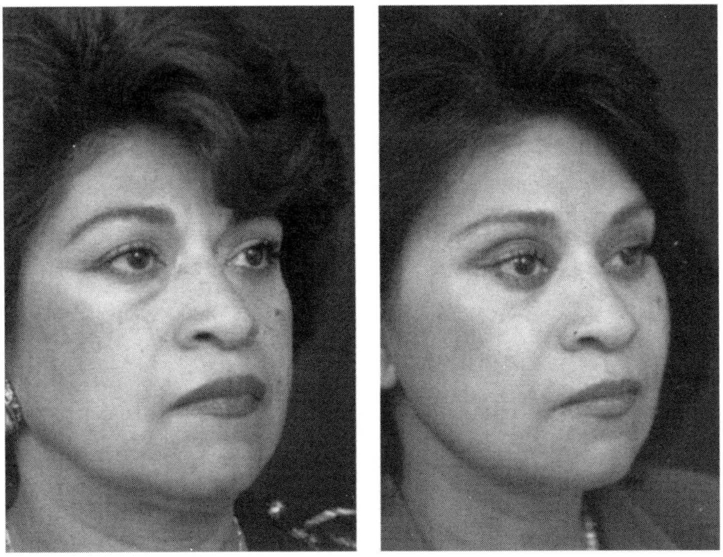

Figure 7 (**A**) Preoperative view of a 52-year-old female patient, with malar hypoplasia, sagging, and sadness of periorbital tissues and midface. (**B**) Postoperative view after malar augmentation osteotomy and subperiosteal face-lift. Notice the changes in the facial contour. The appearance of the soft tissues has a natural relationship with the underlying bone structure.

In some particular cases, perhaps related to ethnicity, the patients can present with an exaggerated projection of the malar-zygomatic region. This condition is more frequently observed in Asians. In these countries it represents a common cause of consultation for the plastic surgeons. Different techniques have been proposed to diminish the projection of the malar bone and to obtain a smooth natural contour of the face (15–18). To improve the aes-

(A) (B)

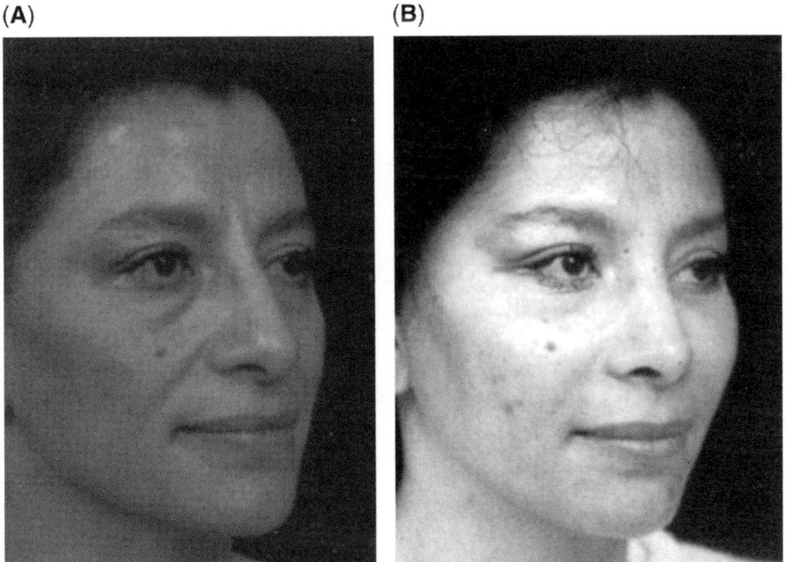

Figure 8 (**A**) Preoperative view of a 48-year-old female, with severe soft-tissues ptosis of the midface and periorbital sadness. (**B**) Postoperative view after subperiosteal lifting and osteotomy of bone augmentation. A remarkable difference is obtained in the malar and zygoma areas, also the sad look has disappeared. Notice the enhancement in the facial contour.

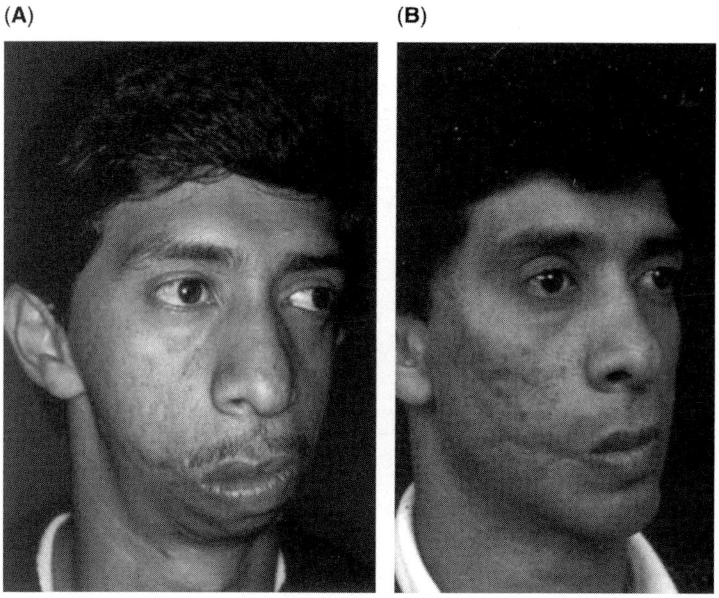

Figure 9 (**A**) Male patient, 20 years old, showing sequelae of facial clefts presenting a microgenia and severe malar deficiency. (**B**) Osteotomies of malar bone augmentation, combined with a chin osteotomy and gonion reconstruction, produces a better aesthetic appearance.

thetic results, frequently these techniques are associated with chin and mandibular angle osteotomies.

In our experience there are two main indications to modify the malar-zygoma contour: (*i*) when it is necessary to reduce the transverse bizygomatic distance, or (*ii*) when it is only necessary to reduce the antero–posterior projection.

In the first group of patients, the surgical technique and the osteotomy design is very similar to the one utilized for augmentation. In performing malar reduction, once the dissection is completed, we outline the portion of malar bone to be removed, and 5–8 mm of the caudal border of the bone are resected in most cases (Fig. 10). Using a reciprocating saw we

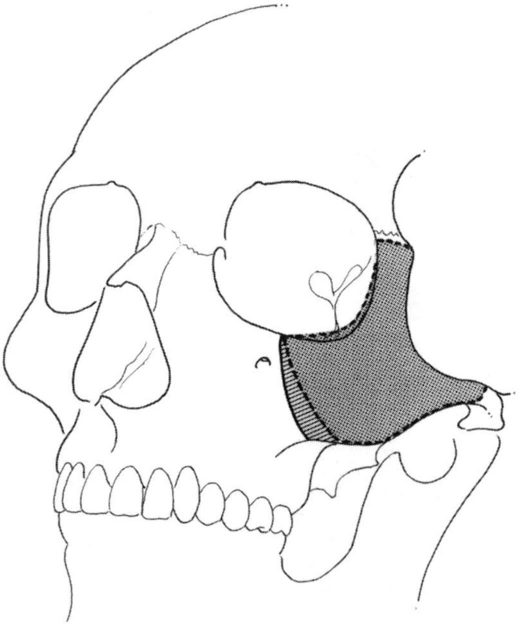

Figure 10 The dotted line shows the osteotomy reduction of the malar bone. The inferior bone fragment will be removed.

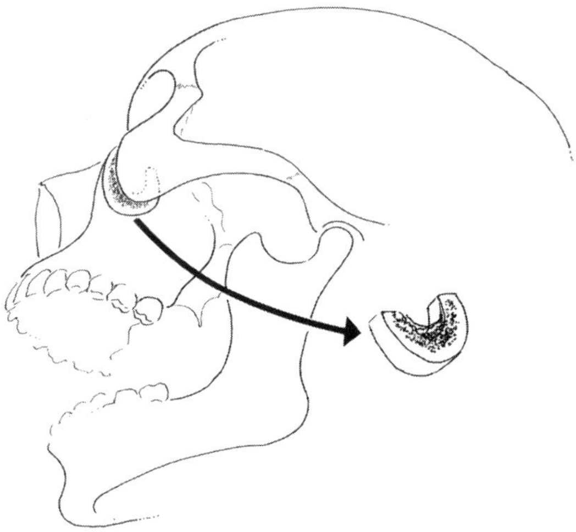

Figure 11 The removed fragment involves the external cortical layer and its union with the maxila and the cancellous bone.

perform the cut of this bone fragment until it is removed as a "cake slice," including the external cortical layer and the cancellous bone but not including the orbital floor (Fig. 11). Once this maneuver has been completed, a curved chisel is used to osteotomize the zygomatic arch and the lateral orbital wall. Again a "green stick" fracture is created using hand pressure over the malar region until obtained bone contact is attained and in continuity between the maxilla and the malar portions. In cases where there is instability of the bone fragments, we recommend fixing the osteotomy with a wire or miniplates.

A reduction malar osteotomy performed with a subperiosteal lifting produces pleasing aesthetic results. It reduces the transverse bizygomatic dimension allowing a better relationship between the midface and the rest of the facial structures. Soft-tissue changes around the orbits correct the sagging and sadness in the patients' appearances (Fig. 12A–D). Reduction of the malar region associated with sliding genioplasty and rhinoplasty often produces a more attractive face than natural heredity and offers the patients a more refined appearance.

(A)

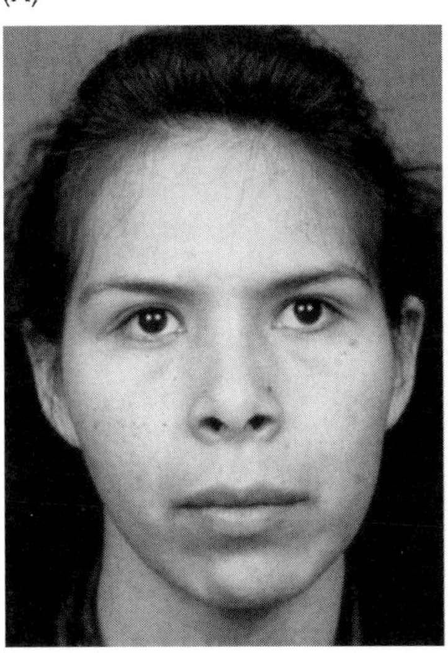

(B)

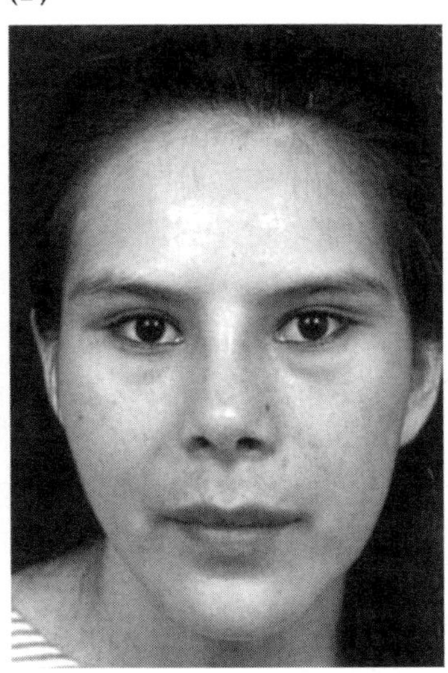

Figure 12 (*Continued on next page*) (**A**) Preoperative frontal photograph of a 28-year-old female patient with the bizygomatic distance augmented. (**B**) Postoperative view after malar reduction osteotomy; 9 mm of bone malar was removed obtaining a new bizygomatic dimension. The relationship of the vertical and transverse dimension of the face is now well proportioned and in harmony. (**C**) Three-quarter view. The augmented dimension of the bone structure (zygomatic malar area) produces a hard-looking appearance in the face of this young patient. (**D**) Reduction of the malar region associated with sliding osteotomy produces a better distribution of soft tissues. A rhinoplasty was also performed in this patient.

(C) (D)

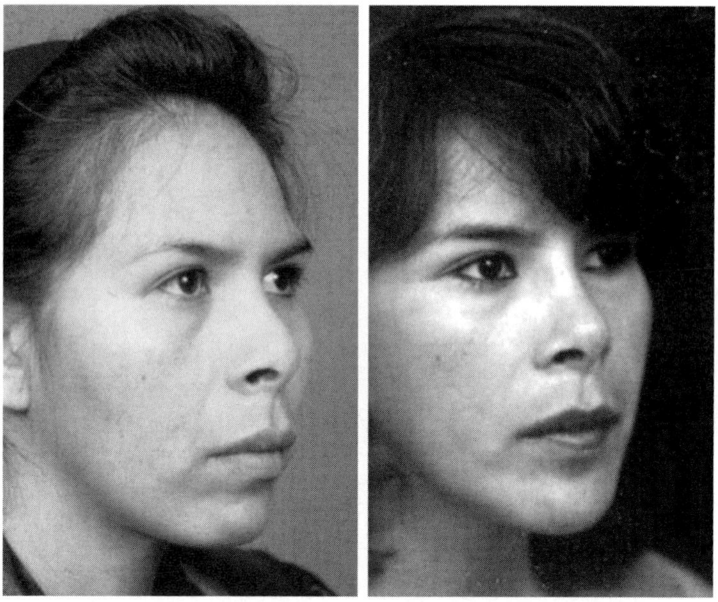

Figure 12 (*Continued from previous page*)

(A)

(B)

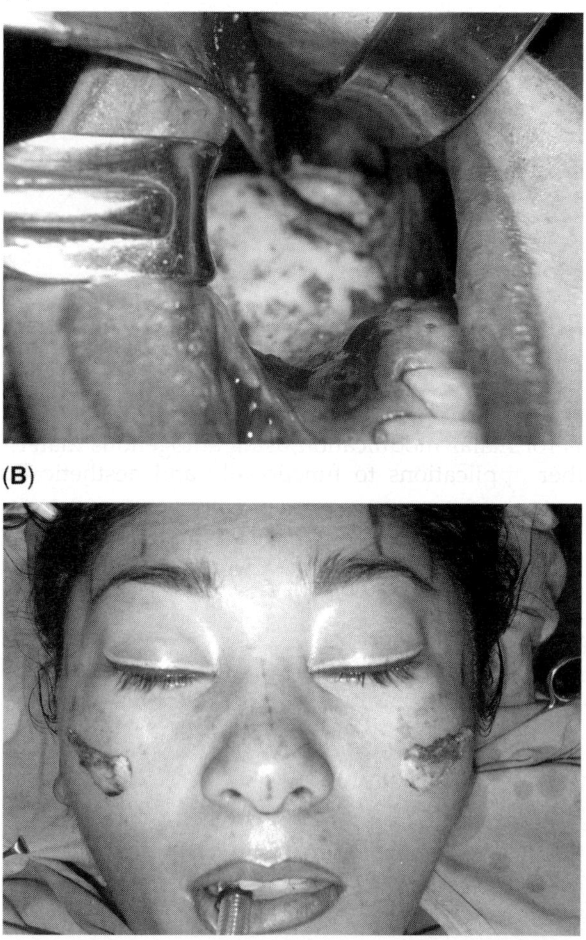

Figure 13 (**A**) Intraoperative photograph showing malar bone fragment to be removed through the vestibular incision. (**B**) Intra-operative photograph showing two malar bone fragments resected.

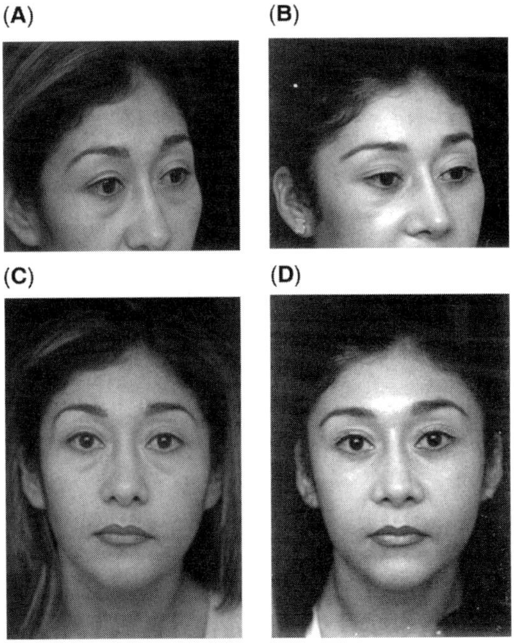

Figure 14 (**A**) Preoperative photograph of a 42-year-old female patient. It shows an exaggerated anterior projection of the malar bone. (**B**) Postoperative photograph with the bone structure corrected at the zygomatic area. Fat resection in the inferior eyelid was also done. (**C**) Preoperative frontal picture of the patient. (**D**) Postoperative frontal view showing the final correction obtained.

When we only want to diminish the antero–posterior projection of the malar region without disturbing the transverse dimension of the face, we use only an intraoral approach to the malar region. Through this access, a wide subperiosteal dissection is performed until the inferior orbital rim and the first portion of the zygomatic arch is exposed. Then we outline the portion of bone to be resected and with a reciprocating saw a precise osteotomy is performed from caudal to cephalic, without intrusion on the maxillary sinus (Fig. 13A and B). Posteriorly a burr is used to remodel the borders of the osteotomy and create a smooth surface on the malar bone. When 5–7 mm of bone is removed the face becomes more delicate in appearance. The acute projection of the malar zygomatic structure changes into a softer contour with a pleasing oval shape to the face (Fig. 14A–D).

A surgeon who uses this group of osteotomies has to produce desirable changes in facial shape without the need for being concerned about late problems. With these techniques, we are using modifications of the patients' own tissues to avoid secondary problems, which sometimes occurs when using foreign materials. At the present time, these techniques are safe and predictable.

Precise anatomic knowledge together with surgical expertise in the craniomaxillofacial field provides this wide variety of methods for malar modification using autogenous materials, which will certainly evolve into further applications to functionally and aesthetically improve our patients.

REFERENCES

1. Cash TF, Horton CE. Aesthetic surgery: effects of rhinoplasty on social perception of patients by others. Plast Reconstr Surg 1983; 72:543–548.
2. Edgerton MT, Jacobson WE, Meyer E. Surgical-psychiatric study of patients seeking plast (cosmetic) surgery: ninety-eight consecutive patients with minimal deformity. Br J Plast Surg 1960; 13:136–145.
3. Edgerton MT, Langman MW, Pruzinsky T. Patients seeking symmetrical recontouring for "perceived" deformities in the width of the face and skull. Aesth Plast Surg 1994; 6:172.
4. Obwegeser HL. Surgical correction of small or retrodisplaced maxillae. Plast Reconstr Surg 1969; 43:351.
5. Phillips JH, Rahn BA. Fixation effects on membranous and endochondral onlay bone graft resorption. Plast Reconstr Surg 1988; 82:872.
6. Powell NB, Riley RW, Laub DR. A new approach to evaluation and surgery of the malar complex. Ann Plast Surg 1988; 20:3.

7. Prendergast M, Schoenrock LD. Malar augmentation patient classification and placement. Arch Otolaryngol Head Neck Surg 1989; 115:964.
8. Whitaker LA. Aesthetic augmentation of the malar midface structures. Plast Reconstr Surg 1987; 80:337.
9. Tessier P. Transactions of the Fourth International Congress of Plastic Surgery in Rome, 1967. Amsterdam: Excerpta Medica, 1968.
10. Tessier P. Autogenous bone graft taken from the calvarium for facial and cranial applications. Clin Plast Surg 1982; 9:531.
11. Ricketts RM. Divine proportion in facial aesthetics. Clin Plast Surg 1982; 9:401.
12. Epkel BN, Wolford LM. Middle-third facial osteotomies: their use in correction of acquired and developmental dentofacial and craniofacial deformities. J Oral Surg 1975; 33:491.
13. Powell NB, Riley RW, Laub DR. A new approach to evaluation and surgery of the malar complex. Ann Plast Surg 1988; 20:3.
14. Wolfe SA, Vitenas P Jr. Malar Augmentation using autogenous materials. Clin Plast Surgery 1991; 18:39.
15. Onizuka T, Watanabe K, Takasu K, et al. Reduction malarplasty. Aesthetic Plast Surg 1983; 7:121.
16. Sumiya N, Kondo S, Ito Y, et al. A new method for reduction malarplasty for facial contouring. Jpn J Plast Reconstr Surg 1993; 36:305.
17. Whitaker LA. Temporal and malar-zygomatic reduction and augmentation. Clin Plat Surg 1991; 18:55.
18. Yang DB, Park HS, Parf CG. Technical refinements of infracture for the zygomatic body and arch reduction. Aesthetic Plast Surg 1998; 22:381.

Index